Endoscopy in the Diagnosis and Management of Acute and Chronic Pancreatitis

Editor

MARTIN L. FREEMAN

GASTROINTESTINAL ENDOSCOPY CLINICS OF NORTH AMERICA

www.giendo.theclinics.com

Consulting Editor
CHARLES J. LIGHTDALE

October 2013 • Volume 23 • Number 4

ELSEVIER

1600 John F. Kennedy Boulevard • Suite 1800 • Philadelphia, Pennsylvania, 19103-2899

http://www.theclinics.com

GASTROINTESTINAL ENDOSCOPY CLINICS OF NORTH AMERICA Volume 23, Number 4
October 2013 ISSN 1052-5157, ISBN-13: 978-0-323-22718-6

Editor: Kerry Holland
Developmental Editor: Donald Mumford

Photocopying
Single photocopies of single articles may be made for personal use as allowed by national copyright laws. Permission of the Publisher and payment of a fee is required for all other photocopying, including multiple or systematic copying, copying for advertising or promotional purposes, resale, and all forms of document delivery. Special rates are available for educational institutions that wish to make photocopies for non-profit educational classroom use. For information on how to seek permission visit www.elsevier.com/permissions or call: (+44) 1865 843830 (UK)/(+1) 215 239 3804 (USA).

Derivative Works
Subscribers may reproduce tables of contents or prepare lists of articles including abstracts for internal circulation within their institutions. Permission of the Publisher is required for resale or distribution outside the institution. Permission of the Publisher is required for all other derivative works, including compilations and translations (please consult www.elsevier.com/permissions).

Electronic Storage or Usage
Permission of the Publisher is required to store or use electronically any material contained in this periodical, including any article or part of an article (please consult www.elsevier.com/permissions). Except as outlined above, no part of this publication may be reproduced, stored in a retrieval system or transmitted in any form or by any means, electronic, mechanical, photocopying, recording or otherwise, without prior written permission of the Publisher.

Notice
No responsibility is assumed by the Publisher for any injury and/or damage to persons or property as a matter of products liability, negligence or otherwise, or from any use or operation of any methods, products, instructions or ideas contained in the material herein. Because of rapid advances in the medical sciences, in particular, independent verification of diagnoses and drug dosages should be made.

Although all advertising material is expected to conform to ethical (medical) standards, inclusion in this publication does not constitute a guarantee or endorsement of the quality or value of such product or of the claims made of it by its manufacturer.

Gastrointestinal Endoscopy Clinics of North America (ISSN 1052-5157) is published quarterly by Elsevier Inc., 360 Park Avenue South, New York, NY 10010-1710. Months of issue are January, April, July, and October. Business and Editorial Offices: 1600 John F. Kennedy Blvd., Suite 1800, Philadelphia, PA, 19103-2899. Periodicals postage paid at New York, NY and additional mailing offices. Subscription prices are $319.00 per year for US individuals, $441.00 per year for US institutions, $169.00 per year for US students and residents, $351.00 per year for Canadian individuals, $538.00 per year for Canadian institutions, $445.00 per year for international individuals, $538.00 per year for international institutions, and $235.00 per year for Canadian and foreign students/residents. To receive student/resident rate, orders must be accompanied by name of affiliated institution, date of term, and the *signature* of program/residency coordinator on institution letterhead. Orders will be billed at individual rate until proof of status is received. Foreign air speed delivery is included in all *Clinics* subscription prices. All prices are subject to change without notice. **POSTMASTER:** Send address change to *Gastrointestinal Endoscopy Clinics of North America*, Elsevier Health Sciences Division, Subscription Customer Service, 3251 Riverport Lane, Maryland Heights, MO 63043. **Customer Service: 1-800-654-2452 (US). From outside the United States, call 1-314-447-8871. Fax: 1-314-447-8029. E-mail: JournalsCustomerService-usa@elsevier.com (for print support) or JournalsOnlineSupport-usa@elsevier.com (for online support).**

Reprints. For copies of 100 or more, of articles in this publication, please contact the Commercial Reprints Department, Elsevier Inc., 360 Park Avenue South, New York, NY 10010-1710. Tel. 212-633-3874; Fax: 212-633-3820; E-mail: reprints@elsevier.com.

Gastrointestinal Endoscopy Clinics of North America is covered in *Excerpta Medica, MEDLINE/PubMed (Index Medicus), and MEDLINE/MEDLARS.*

Printed and bound by CPI Group (UK) Ltd, Croydon, CR0 4YY

Transferred to digital print 2012

Contributors

CONSULTING EDITOR

CHARLES J. LIGHTDALE, MD
Professor of Clinical Medicine, Director of Clinical Research, Division of Digestive and Liver Diseases, Department of Medicine, New York-Presbyterian Hospital/Columbia University Medical Center, New York, New York

EDITOR

MARTIN L. FREEMAN, MD
Professor of Medicine, Director, Division of Gastroenterology, Hepatology and Nutrition; Director, Advanced Endoscopy and Pancreaticobiliary Endoscopy Fellowship, University of Minnesota, Minneapolis, Minnesota

AUTHORS

DEEPAK K. BHASIN, MD, DM, FASGE, AGAF
Professor, Department of Gastroenterology, Post Graduate Institute of Medical Education and Research (PGIMER), Chandigarh, India

IVO BOŠKOSKI, MD, PhD
Digestive Endoscopy Unit, Gemelli University Hospital, Università Cattolica del Sacro Cuore, Rome, Italy

VINCENZO BOVE, MD
Digestive Endoscopy Unit, Gemelli University Hospital, Università Cattolica del Sacro Cuore, Rome, Italy

GUIDO COSTAMAGNA, MD, FACG
Digestive Endoscopy Unit, Gemelli University Hospital, Università Cattolica del Sacro Cuore, Rome, Italy

JEAN-MARC DUMONCEAU, MD, PhD
Division of Gastroenterology and Hepatology, Geneva University Hospitals, Geneva, Switzerland

B. JOSEPH ELMUNZER, MD
Assistant Professor, Internal Medicine, Division of Gastroenterology, University of Michigan Medical Center, Ann Arbor, Michigan

PIETRO FAMILIARI, MD, PhD
Digestive Endoscopy Unit, Gemelli University Hospital, Università Cattolica del Sacro Cuore, Rome, Italy

JESSICA M. FISHER, MD
Division of Gastroenterology, Department of Medicine, University of Washington, Seattle, Washington

TIMOTHY B. GARDNER, MD
Director Pancreatic Disorders, Section of Gastroenterology, Department of Medicine, Dartmouth-Hitchcock Medical Center, Lebanon, New Hampshire

MICHEL KAHALEH, MD, AGAF, FACG, FASGE
Professor of Clinical Medicine, Chief, Endoscopy, Medical Director Pancreas Program, Division of Gastroenterology and Hepatology, Department of Medicine, Weill Cornell Medical College, New York, New York

MYUNG-HWAN KIM, MD, PhD
Department of Internal Medicine, Asan Medical Center, University of Ulsan College of Medicine, Songpa-Gu, Seoul, South Korea

NISA M. KUBILIUN, MD
Clinical Lecturer, Internal Medicine, Division of Gastroenterology, University of Michigan Medical Center, Ann Arbor, Michigan

VINCENT C. KUO, MD
Gastroenterology Fellow, Methodist Dallas Medical Center, Dallas, Texas

SUNG-HOON MOON, MD
Department of Internal Medicine, Hallym University Sacred Heart Hospital, Hallym University College of Medicine, Anyang, South Korea

SURINDER S. RANA, MD, DM, FASGE
Assistant Professor, Department of Gastroenterology, Post Graduate Institute of Medical Education and Research (PGIMER), Chandigarh, India

JASON R. ROBERTS, MD
Division of Gastroenterology, Hepatology, and Nutrition, University of Louisivlle School of Medicine, Louisville, Kentucky

JOSEPH ROMAGNUOLO, MD, MSc, FASGE
Division of Gastroenterology and Hepatology, Medical University of South Carolina, Charleston, South Carolina

REEM Z. SHARAIHA, MD, MSc
Assistant Professor of Clinical Medicine, Division of Gastroenterology and Hepatology, Department of Medicine, Weill Cornell Medical College, New York, New York

TYLER STEVENS, MD
Assistant Professor, Department of Gastroenterology and Hepatology, Cleveland Clinic, Cleveland, Ohio

PAUL R. TARNASKY, MD
Program Director, Gastroenterology Fellowship, Digestive Health Associates of Texas, Methodist Dallas Medical Center, Dallas, Texas

SHYAM VARADARAJULU, MD
Medical Director, Center for Interventional Endoscopy, Florida Hospital, Orlando, Florida

JESSICA WIDMER, DO
Clinical Instructor of Medicine, Division of Gastroenterology and Hepatology, Department of Medicine, Weill Cornell Medical College, New York, New York

Contents

> Endoscopic ultrasonography (EUS) can be a useful tool for detecting the underlying causes of acute pancreatitis and establishing the severity of fibrosis in chronic pancreatitis. Ancillary techniques include fine needle aspiration and core biopsy, bile collection for crystal analysis, pancreatic function testing, and celiac plexus block. This review focuses on the role of EUS in the diagnosis of acute and chronic pancreatitis.

 Videos of the needle-knife precut sphincterotomy and standard sphincterotomy techniques accompany this article

> Acute pancreatitis represents numerous unique challenges to the practicing digestive disease specialist. Clinical presentations of acute pancreatitis vary from trivial pain to severe acute illness with a significant risk of death. Urgent endoscopic treatment of acute pancreatitis is considered when there is causal evidence of biliary pancreatitis. This article focuses on the diagnosis and endoscopic treatment of acute biliary pancreatitis.

> Post–endoscopic retrograde cholangiopancreatography (ERCP) pancreatitis is a common and potentially devastating complication of ERCP. Advances in risk stratification, patient selection, procedure technique, and prophylactic interventions have substantially improved the endoscopists' ability to prevent this complication. This article presents the evidence-based approaches to preventing post-ERCP pancreatitis and suggests timely research questions in this important area.

> Endoscopic therapy has become an essential component in the management of post-pancreatitis complications, such as infected and/or symptomatic pancreatic pseudocysts and walled-off necrosis. However, although

there have been 2 recent randomized, controlled trials performed, a general lack of comparative effectiveness data regarding the timing, indications, and outcomes of these procedures has been a barrier to the development of practice standards for therapeutic endoscopists managing these issues. This article reviews the available data and expert consensus regarding indications for endoscopic intervention, timing of procedures, endoscopic technique, periprocedural considerations, and complications.

Endoscopy plays an important role in both the diagnosis and the initial management of recurrent acute pancreatitis, as well as the investigation of refractory disease, but it has known limitations and risks. Sound selective use of these therapies, complemented with other lines of investigation such as genetic testing, can dramatically improve frequency of attacks and associated quality of life. Whether endoscopic therapy can reduce progression to chronic pancreatitis, or reduce the risk of malignancy, is debatable, and remains to be proven.

Endoscopic therapy is recommended as the first-line therapy for painful chronic pancreatitis with an obstacle on the main pancreatic duct (MPD). The clinical response should be evaluated at 6 to 8 weeks. Calcified stones that obstruct the MPD are first treated by extracorporeal shockwave lithotripsy; dominant MPD strictures are optimally treated with a single, large, plastic stent that should be exchanged within 1 year even in asymptomatic patients. Pancreatic pseudocysts for which therapy is indicated and are within endoscopic reach should be treated by endoscopy.

Chronic pancreatitis (CP)-related common bile duct (CBD) strictures are more difficult to treat endoscopically compared with benign biliary strictures because of their nature, particularly in patients with calcific CP. Before any attempt at treatment, malignancy must be excluded. Single plastic stents can be used for immediate symptom relief and as "bridge to surgery and/or bridge to decision," but are not suitable for definitive treatment of CP-related CBD strictures because of long-term poor results. Temporary simultaneous placement of multiple plastic stents has a high technical success rate and provides good long-term results.

Over the last 2 decades there has been continuing development in endoscopic ultrasonography (EUS). EUS-guided pancreatic drainage is an evolving procedure that can be offered to patients who are high-risk surgical candidates and in whom the pancreatic duct cannot be accessed by endoscopic retrograde pancreatography. Although EUS-guided pancreatic drainage is a minimally invasive alternative option to surgery and interventional radiology, owing to its complexity and potential for fulminant complications, it is recommended that these procedures be performed by highly skilled endoscopists. Additional data are needed to define risks and long-term outcomes more accurately via a dedicated prospective registry.

Pancreatitis, whether acute or chronic, can lead to a plethora of complications, such as fluid collections, pseudocysts, fistulas, and necrosis, all of which are secondary to leakage of secretions from the pancreatic ductal system. Partial and side branch duct disruptions can be managed successfully by transpapillary pancreatic duct stent placement, whereas patients with disconnected pancreatic duct syndrome require more complex endoscopic interventions or multidisciplinary care for optimal treatment outcomes. This review discusses the current status of endoscopic management of pancreatic duct leaks and emerging concepts for the treatment of disconnected pancreatic duct syndrome.

This review addresses the role of endoscopy in the diagnosis and treatment of autoimmune pancreatitis (AIP) and provides a diagnostic process for patients with suspected AIP. When should AIP be suspected? When can it be diagnosed without endoscopic examination? Which endoscopic approaches are appropriate in suspected AIP, and when? What are the roles of diagnostic endoscopic retrograde pancreatography, endoscopic biopsies, and IgG4 immunostaining? What is the proper use of the steroid trial in the diagnosis of AIP in patients with indeterminate computed tomography imaging? Should biliary stenting be performed in patients with AIP with obstructive jaundice?

Pancreatic stenting for patients with obstructive pain secondary to a malignant pancreatic duct stricture is safe and effective, and should be considered a therapeutic option. Although pancreatic stenting does not seem to be effective for patients with chronic pain, it may be beneficial in those with obstructive type pains, pancreatic duct disruption, or smoldering pancreatitis. Fully covered metal stents may be an option, but data on their use are limited. Further studies, including prospective randomized studies comparing plastic and metal stents in these indications, are needed to further validate and confirm these results.

GASTROINTESTINAL ENDOSCOPY CLINICS OF NORTH AMERICA

NOW AVAILABLE FOR YOUR iPhone and iPad

Foreword
Advances in Pancreatic Endoscopy

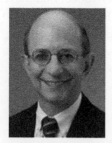

Charles J. Lightdale, MD
Consulting Editor

"Risky Business" is a title that springs to mind when considering an issue of the *Gastrointestinal Endoscopy Clinics of North America* on the subject of "Endoscopy in Pancreatic Diseases." The pancreas is such a complex and "touchy" organ, that for years, gastrointestinal endoscopists have tended to avoid the risks of diagnosing and treating pancreatic diseases. Times have changed! Interventional endoscopists have learned to approach the pancreas with a strategy of "treat it with respect" rather than "avoid the pancreas at all costs." Using improved instruments and new understanding of pancreatic pathophysiology, these endoscopists have harnessed endoscopic retrograde cholangiopancreatography and endoscopic ultrasonography to improve diagnosis and treatment of many pancreatic diseases: acute and chronic, inflammatory, and neoplastic. Patients with pancreatic diseases have gained tremendous benefit from their efforts. Of course, the management of pancreatic diseases takes a multispecialty effort, and for endoscopists, the classic Kenny Rogers anthem: "know when to hold 'em, know when to fold 'em," is particularly apt.

I feel so fortunate that the great gastrointestinal endoscopist from Minnesota, Martin Freeman, agreed to be guest editor for this issue of *Gastrointestinal Endoscopy Clinics of North America* on pancreatic diseases. Dr Freeman has an extraordinary grasp of this evolving field and has gathered an outstanding group of experts to provide a comprehensive coverage of pancreatic diseases and the possibilities and limitations of endoscopic interventions. I understand that sweetbreads are not for every taste, but for gastroenterologists in general, and for radiologists and surgeons,

Gastrointest Endoscopy Clin N Am 23 (2013) ix–x
http://dx.doi.org/10.1016/j.giec.2013.06.012
1052-5157/13/$ – see front matter © 2013 Elsevier Inc. All rights reserved.

giendo.theclinics.com

and especially for pancreatologists and interventional endoscopists, this issue is made to order.

Charles J. Lightdale, MD
Department of Medicine
Columbia University Medical Center
161 Fort Washington Avenue, Room 812
New York, NY 10032, USA

E-mail address:
CJL18@columbia.edu

Preface
Effective Endoscopic Management of Pancreatic Diseases

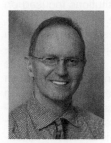

Martin L. Freeman, MD
Editor

I had the honor of being invited by Dr Lightdale to edit the current issue of *Gastrointestinal Endoscopy Clinics of North America* on the role of endoscopy in pancreatic diseases. This is a very timely topic as endoscopists are becoming increasingly involved in both diagnosis and therapy of acute pancreatitis, chronic pancreatitis, pancreatic neoplasms, and autoimmune pancreatitis to name a few entities. Endoscopic ultrasound has evolved from a purely diagnostic procedure to include fine-needle aspiration as an essential tool for the diagnosis of neoplastic diseases and autoimmune pancreatitis. Most importantly now, EUS is a vital component of endoscopic therapy, particularly for access into and debridement of walled off necrosis, and for ductal access into the pancreas when other techniques fail. EUS has thus allowed gastrointestinal endoscopists to perform the first true "NOTES" procedures to achieve widespread applicability and efficacy. For ERCP, therapy has expanded dramatically into the pancreas itself, for applications such as treatment of chronic pancreatitis, acute recurrent pancreatitis, pancreatic duct leaks, and treatment of biliary strictures associated with pancreatic disease. Central to all these techniques is safety. Prevention of post-ERCP pancreatitis has evolved dramatically in the last decade so that both effective endoscopic methods, such as pancreatic stent placement, and pharmacologic prevention, such as use of rectal nonsteroidal anti-inflammatory agents, are now not only shown to be effective in reducing risk of postprocedure pancreatitis but also are increasingly becoming the "standard of care." These measures have allowed greatly improved safety of procedures once viewed as universally prohibitively dangerous. We have evolved substantially beyond the old axiom of "don't mess with the pancreas."

Although great strides have been made in the diagnosis and management of pancreatic diseases, several important cautionary notes should be stressed. First,

Gastrointest Endoscopy Clin N Am 23 (2013) xi–xiii
http://dx.doi.org/10.1016/j.giec.2013.06.009
1052-5157/13/$ – see front matter © 2013 Elsevier Inc. All rights reserved.

effective endoscopic management of pancreatic diseases requires substantial under-standing of the disease processes in the pancreas, which is highly variable among endoscopists focused primarily on therapeutic endoscopy rather than the discipline of pancreatology. It is becoming increasingly clear that acute recurrent and chronic pancreatitis are the result of multifactorial predisposing factors, including genetics, environment, dietary, and toxic exposures as well as structural. Endoscopists tend to focus primarily on structural causes or consequences of disease. Thus education regarding diseases and management of the pancreas is highly desirable for practi-tioners and is ideally accomplished within organizations and institutions focused on pancreatic diseases rather than solely on therapeutic endoscopy.

Second, effective management of pancreatic disease requires a team approach with active cooperation among multiple specialties including specialized surgery, crit-ical care, oncology, and diagnostic and interventional radiology. Probably no single entity exemplifies this more than management of necrotizing pancreatitis, for which morbidity and mortality is potentially very high, but endoscopic intervention is evolving as the procedure of choice in many circumstances, such as infected walled off necro-sis. Before, during, and after pancreatic endoscopic interventions such as endoscopic necrosectomy, close cooperation with all of the above specialties is absolutely essen-tial for good outcomes. Furthermore, the efficacy of endoscopic therapy of the pancreas is highly variable. The decision to pursue endoscopic therapy in the pancreas should be a multidisciplinary one, considering alternatives to endoscopic therapy. Once a decision to pursue endoscopic therapy has been made, it is essential to have a clear goal, an endpoint such that procedures such as ERCP with pancreatic stenting are not repeated excessively. Many pancreatic centers have seen patients with chronic pancreatitis who have undergone in excess of 50 ERCPs without sub-stantial long-term improvement. There must be a plan for alternative treatment such as surgical or other management if and when endoscopic therapy fails to achieve the hoped goal. Particularly challenging is relief of chronic intractable pain associated with acute recurrent and chronic pancreatitis, which represent a continuum of dis-eases. Increasingly, new alternatives such as total pancreatectomy with islet auto-transplantation are becoming feasible. If patients are appropriate for these alternative treatments, endoscopists should always question the value of embarking on long and expensive courses of endoscopic therapy. It is likely that reimbursement for such practices will eventually end.

Finally, the difficult question of who should be performing these advanced pancre-atic endoscopic procedures? The demand for extreme technical expertise and perfor-mance of a high volume of these specialized procedures is probably greater than for any other area of gastrointestinal endoscopy. The potential for complications, some-times severe or fatal, is enormous. There is probably no procedure in gastrointestinal endoscopy that carries a higher risk-to-benefit ratio. In fact, in some entities such as recurrent acute pancreatitis, due to a lack of randomized controlled trials, there are lingering questions as to whether there is any substantial benefit from commonly per-formed interventions such as minor papillotomy for pancreas divisum. As a result, it is recommended that the procedures discussed in this issue be performed only by highly specialized endoscopists at advanced medical centers, and with a deep understand-ing of the underlying disease processes they are addressing, and ideally with ongoing collection of data.

In this issue, I have had the privilege of including contributions from many of the world's leaders in specific topics and procedures covering most of the spectrum of endoscopy in the diagnosis and treatment of pancreatic diseases. I am hopeful that readers will find this issue informative and instructive, with insights, analyses, tips, and tricks that will potentially improve their patients' outcomes. I am very grateful to Dr Charles Lightdale for the opportunity to bring this issue to light.

Martin L. Freeman, MD
Division of Gastroenterology, Hepatology and Nutrition
University of Minnesota
MMC 36, 406 Harvard Street SE
Minneapolis, MN 55455

E-mail address:
freem020@umn.edu

Role of Endoscopic Ultrasonography in the Diagnosis of Acute and Chronic Pancreatitis

Tyler Stevens, MD

KEYWORDS

- Pancreatitis • EUS • Gallstones • Pancreas divisum • Cause • Diagnosis
- Pancreatic function test • Elastography

KEY POINTS

- Endoscopic ultrasonography (EUS) is a valuable screening test for biliary and structural causes in patients with idiopathic acute pancreatitis.
- EUS is a sensitive test for detecting parenchymal and ductal changes found in minimal change chronic pancreatitis (CP).
- The true accuracy of EUS for diagnosing CP is not well defined and its reliability is limited by lack of specificity and interobserver variability.

INTRODUCTION

Pancreatitis represents a continuum from the first inflammatory episode progressing to parenchymal fibrosis and functional insufficiency. Patients referred to gastroenterology offices present at some point along this spectrum. They may lack obvious risk factors such as gallstones or heavy alcohol consumption. The primary clinical goals are to detect and reverse underlying causes, establish the severity of fibrosis and functional loss, improve abdominal pain, and optimize nutrition.

Endoscopic ultrasonography (EUS) can be a useful tool in achieving these goals. It serves as an efficient and safe screen for structural causes of pancreatitis, as well as a relatively sensitive test for chronic pancreatitis (CP). Ancillary techniques include fine-needle aspiration and core biopsy, bile collection for crystal analysis, pancreatic function testing (PFT), and celiac plexus block. This review focuses on the role of EUS in the diagnosis of acute and CP.

Financial Disclosures: The author has no financial conflicts of interest pertaining to this article.
Department of Gastroenterology and Hepatology, Cleveland Clinic, 9500 Euclid Avenue, A31, Cleveland, OH 44195, USA
E-mail address: stevent@ccf.org

Gastrointest Endoscopy Clin N Am 23 (2013) 735–747
http://dx.doi.org/10.1016/j.giec.2013.06.001
1052-5157/13/$ – see front matter © 2013 Elsevier Inc. All rights reserved.

ACUTE PANCREATITIS
Diagnosis and Prognosis of Acute Pancreatitis

EUS is not necessary for the diagnosis of acute pancreatitis (AP), which is usually accomplished by serum enzyme levels, characteristic abdominal pain, or conventional imaging such as computed tomography (CT). The most common EUS feature of AP is hypoechogenicity of the pancreas, indicating edema.[1] Less common findings include pancreatic enlargement and peripancreatic fluid. EUS may also reveal a normal-appearing pancreas in mild cases.

A few studies have explored the role of EUS in predicting the severity of AP. Although imaging with CT and magnetic resonance imaging (MRI) is of greater practical value in this setting, EUS has benefits of no radiation or contrast. One study found that a geographic hyperechoic area within the pancreas was an adverse clinical predictor of severity.[2] Another showed that the presence of peripancreatic edema, parenchymal heterogeneity, dilation of the common bile duct (CBD), and ascites was associated with severe AP in a univariable analysis.[3] These findings require validation before widespread application in the early phase of AP. EUS has a significant role in the management of acute pancreatic pseudocysts and walled-off necrosis, discussed in depth in another section.

Determining Causes of AP

In most cases, the cause of AP is obvious and successfully eliminated, preventing future attacks. For example, if there is radiographic evidence of gallstones, a cholecystectomy usually resolves the issue. Even in these clear-cut cases, it may still be reasonable to check a triglyceride level, screen the medication list, and make sure cancer has been ruled out with appropriate imaging. Beyond these basic considerations, further costly or invasive testing to look for coexisting etiologic factors is not required.

In about 20% of cases of AP, an obvious cause is not found, even after a careful history, ultrasonography, and routine laboratory studies. Although some advocate expectant management after a single episode of unexplained AP, most concur that further evaluation is necessary in those with recurrent idiopathic bouts. This evaluation may include blood tests for metabolic, autoimmune, and genetic causes, and additional structural testing to look for biliary and ductal obstructive disease.

In the past, endoscopic retrograde cholangiopancreatography (ERCP) was the structural test of choice for evaluation of idiopathic recurrent AP (IRAP). Now, EUS and magnetic resonance cholangiopancreatography (MRCP) are advocated as safer options. There are limited studies comparing EUS and MRCP for etiologic diagnosis of AP. In 1 study,[4] EUS and MRCP were performed prospectively in 49 patients with idiopathic AP. The overall yield was significantly higher for EUS compared with MRCP (51% vs 20%, $P = .001$), mostly because of biliary causes found with EUS and missed with MRCP. Another similar study[5] showed a higher yield overall and for biliary causes in patients with idiopathic AP compared with MRCP and ERCP. Based on these and other studies, EUS may be a preferred test in the evaluation of IRAP, and has a yield considered adequate to justify its cost and minimal risk.[6] Some of the causes of AP detectable with EUS are discussed in the following sections.

Biliary Pancreatitis

Transabdominal ultrasonography (TAUS) is routinely and correctly performed to look for a biliary source for AP. However, AP may result from very small stones missed with TAUS. It may even be inferred that tiny stones smaller than 2 mm (microlithiasis) would be most likely to traverse the cystic duct and impact at the ampullary orifice. EUS provides complete imaging of the gallbladder body, neck, and fundus like TAUS, and superior imaging of the CBD. The finding of echogenic layering sludge in the gallbladder or CBD is strongly suggestive of coexisting microlithiasis and should prompt consideration of cholecystectomy (**Fig. 1**).

Several studies have suggested that EUS has incremental value in uncovering a biliary source even after TAUS, CT, or MRCP are negative. In a study of 35 patients with biliary-type pain and negative TAUS,[7] 33 (95%) were found to have sludge or microlithiasis in the gallbladder or CBD on EUS. In 246 patients with idiopathic AP and negative TAUS, EUS revealed sludge or stones in the gallbladder or CBD in 46 (19%) with gallbladder in situ.[8] In 223 patients with suspected mild biliary AP (alanine transaminase level >120 U/L), a definite biliary cause was not found on TAUS, CT, or MRCP in 37 (17%). Thirty-three of these patients underwent an EUS, and stones or sludge in the gallbladder or CBD were found in more than a third.[9]

The yield of the EUS in AP is higher in those with intact gallbladders compared with those who have undergone a cholecystectomy.[4,8,10] However, EUS may still identify a biliary source even in a postcholecystectomy patient. EUS carries 94% sensitivity and 95% specificity for detecting CBD stones (**Fig. 2**).[11] Although MRCP also provides excellent imaging of the biliary tree, EUS is more sensitive for small CBD stones and is better for visualizing the gallbladder.[12]

EUS is often reserved for IRAP, but it may reveal a biliary cause even in those with a single unexplained attack. In 134 patients with their first attack and intact gallbladders, 27 (21%) were found to have GB or bile duct stones/sludge.[8] Based on these and other data, a recent technical review suggested that EUS should be considered for patients after their first unexplained bout.[6]

Cholecystokinin (CCK)-stimulated collection of bile for crystal analysis may be performed during EUS in those with intact gallbladders. CCK is administered intravenously at a dose of 0.02 µg per kilogram, producing gallbladder contraction and expression of bile into the duodenal lumen within a few minutes. Five or 10 mL of bile is suctioned through the scope into a fluid trap and placed on ice. The specimen is centrifuged and examined under a polarized microscope for detection of cholesterol and bilirubinate crystals. The addition of bile collection increases sensitivity for microlithiasis, and may be routinely performed if EUS imaging does not reveal gallbladder

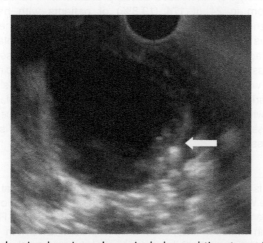

Fig. 1. Gallbladder showing layering echogenic sludge and tiny stones (*arrow*).

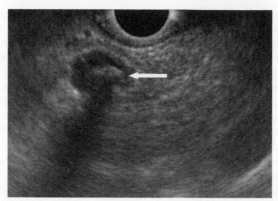

Fig. 2. Head of pancreas showing a shadowing stone in the distal CBD (*arrow*).

sludge. In 80 patients with single or recurrent AP (RAP) who had no obvious sludge or stones on EUS, bile analysis revealed crystals in 38 (48%).[8] CCK can cause uterine contractions, so women of childbearing age should have a negative pregnancy test immediately before the endoscopy. Crystal analysis has limited reproducibility and clinical implications and as a result is not widely performed.

Occasionally, patients are referred for ERCP while in the throes of biliary AP to detect and extract retained stones. Cautious endoscopists may think twice about this procedure, because most stones pass spontaneously and ERCP may worsen existing AP. ERCP is warranted when signs of cholangitis are present or liver function tests are increasing, but if clinical suspicion for a retained stone is low, a preliminary EUS may help in decision making. If a stone is present, ERCP with extraction can be performed in the same endoscopic session. If no stone is found, the patient can be spared the added risk. This stepwise strategy has been shown to be beneficial, avoiding ERCP in most patients.[13]

Pancreatic Neoplasms

A pancreatic tumor that obstructs the main pancreatic duct (PD) may produce recurrent pancreatitis, likely from increased ductal pressure. In 1 series,[14] AP was a presenting in symptom in 24 of 174 (13.8%) of patients with pancreatic cancer. Pancreatic neuroendocrine tumors may also cause AP.[15] Cancer is of particular concern in patients older than 40 years who develop an unexplained attack, and cross-sectional imaging is recommended if no other obvious cause is found.[16] However, standard cross-sectional imaging tests may miss a pancreatic mass if it is a small lesion, contrast is withheld, or significant inflammation and necrosis masks its presence. EUS is superior for the detection of small pancreatic neoplasms smaller than 2 cm compared with dual-phase CT scan and contrast-enhanced MRI (**Fig. 3**).[17] EUS also allows tissue sampling through fine-needle aspiration of suspicious hypoechoic areas or masses.

Pancreas Divisum

Pancreas divisum is a congenital malunion of the dorsal and ventral PDs and is found in up to 10% of the Western population. It may be a primary cause or a risk modifier in conjunction with genetic or environmental factors in the genesis of RAP.[18] MRCP with or without secretin injection has essentially replaced ERCP in the diagnosis of pancreas divisum. However, EUS may also be helpful in detecting pancreas divisum

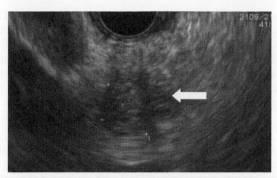

Fig. 3. This 53-year-old patient presented with an unexplained bout of AP. The CT was negative except for slight PD prominence. EUS revealed this small mass in the head of the pancreas smaller than 1.5 cm (*arrow*).

and evaluating its significance. One study showed superior sensitivity of EUS compared with MRCP (86.7% vs 60%, P<.001) in 45 patients with pancreas divisum confirmed by ERCP.[19]

Several technical criteria have been proposed for radial and linear endosonography, such as the absence of a stack sign (presence of CBD, PD, and portal vein in 1 image), presence of a crossing duct sign (crossed appearance of CBD and PD), or a separate insertion of PDs and bile ducts into the duodenal wall. Existing studies of these criteria are difficult to interpret because of their small sample sizes. The most logical approach may be to trace the PD from its union with the bile duct at the major papilla proximally into the dorsal pancreas. If the PD can be traced, pancreas divisum has been ruled out by definition. One study[20] evaluated this criterion or the visualization of the duct crossing a distinct demarcation of the ventral and dorsal pancreas (dorsal-ventral anlage) in 162 patients using ERCP as the reference standard. The reported sensitivity was 95% (n = 19 with divisum) and specificity was 97%. However, these test performance estimates were calculated only in the 78% of patients in whom adequate endosonographic ductal visualization was obtained. Almost a quarter of the patients were not included because their ductal anatomy could not be adequately assessed, even in expert hands. Based on these results, EUS may be considered useful to rule out divisum if the above maneuver (tracing PD from ampulla to body) can be accomplished. But because many patients have ductal anatomy that cannot be traced adequately with EUS, it may not be as useful to rule in pancreas divisum.

Most patients with pancreas divisum do not experience symptoms. After diagnosing pancreas divisum in a patient with AP, a secondary diagnostic dilemma is to determine its clinical significance. Endoscopic and EUS findings such as a santorinicele and dorsal duct dilation may help clarify if impaired drainage is causing AP, to justify ERCP with minor papillotomy.

Other Structural Causes

Additional structural causes that can be diagnosed with EUS include annular pancreas, choledochocele with anomalous insertion of the PD, and PD strictures.

Also, the endoscopic examination can offer clues. Duodenal or ampullary disease can obstruct pancreatic outflow and produce recurrent bouts of AP. EUS should begin with a careful upper endoscopic examination using a standard upper endoscope. A side-viewing endoscopy can usually be avoided if adequate ampullary views are obtained with the oblique-viewing echoendoscope. Examples of disease that may cause AP diagnosed with endoscopy include upper gastrointestinal Crohn disease,[21] penetrating peptic ulcer,[22] ampullary polyps,[23] ampullary carcinoma,[24] intraluminal windsock diverticulae, and extraluminal periampullary diverticulae.[25] Another significant endoscopic finding is a gaping major papilla with extrusion of mucin, which indicates main-duct intraductal papillary mucinous neoplasm, which may produce AP through mucin plugging. Endoscopy also permits periampullary biopsies, which may assist in the diagnosis of autoimmune pancreatitis.[26]

Sphincter of Oddi Dysfunction

Sphincter of Oddi dysfunction (SOD) and ampullary stenosis may cause RAP, which is a particular consideration after cholecystectomy. ERCP of any kind in patients with suspected sphincter of Oddi manometry (SOM) with or without sphincterotomy comes with a substantial risk of pancreatitis, and efficacy of sphincterotomy is uncertain. Although EUS can neither reliably diagnose nor treat SOD, it does offer a safe and accurate visualization and measurement of the CBD and PD. Proximal enlargement of these ducts may suggest underlying outflow obstruction to support the SOD diagnosis, as in the Milwaukee criteria.[27] EUS with side-viewing endoscopy may help diagnose restenosis after a previous sphincterotomy.

Some investigators have included secretin injection at the time of EUS, with timed measurement of ductal diameters to determine if there is delayed emptying of the duct.[5,28,29] One study[28] included ductal measurements every 1 minute after secretin in multiple patients with various conditions producing PD outflow delay. There were 20 patients with suspected SOD who underwent a previous ERCP with SOM as gold standard. In 13 patients with normal SOM, the secretin EUS was normal in 12 (92% specificity). In 7 who had abnormal SOM, the secretin EUS was abnormal in 4 (57% sensitivity). This test is time consuming, requires meticulous performance to ascertain ductal drainage delays, and has not been externally validated to justify its widespread use. There are multiple factors other than the sphincter of Oddi that may affect the results. For example, patients with CP may have less fluid production in response to secretin and a more fibrotic duct wall, and thus less ductal enlargement after secretin.

CP

CP is a painful disorder that usually occurs after recurrent inflammatory episodes and is defined histologically based on chronic inflammation and fibrosis. Most patients undergo CT scan in the initial evaluation of abdominal pain. CP is easily diagnosed if the CT scan shows calcifications, main-duct dilation, and atrophy, the cardinal structural features of severe or calcific CP. The diagnosis of mild CP is more challenging, because these major structural changes may be lacking. Also, a minimal change variant has been recognized, often seen in patients lacking typical environmental risk factors like smoking and alcohol.[30] In these groups, more sensitive second-line tests such as EUS are needed to detect subtle structural and functional abnormalities.

There is now a long experience with EUS for the diagnosis of CP, but there remains widespread controversy regarding its accuracy and reliability. EUS images of the pancreas are scored based on the presence of parenchymal and ductal features. The most common scoring system includes 5 ductal and 4 parenchymal criteria (**Fig. 4, Table 1**).[31] The features are counted in an equally weighted fashion and compared with a diagnostic threshold. The cut point used to diagnose CP varies in the literature and in practice. A lower cut point (eg, ≥3 criteria) maximizes sensitivity, whereas a higher cut point (≥6 criteria) maximizes specificity.

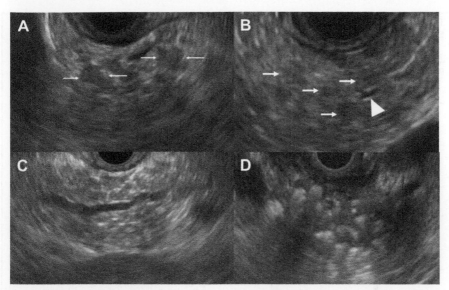

Fig. 4. Examples of EUS CP criteria. (*A*) Honeycombed lobularity in the head of the pancreas. The arrows delineate hypoechoic lobules separated by hyperechoic strands. (*B*) Diffuse lobularity (*arrows*) and strands in body of the pancreas. The duct wall is echogenic (*triangle*). (*C*) Irregular duct with hyperechoic wall in body of the pancreas. The parenchyma contains hyperechoic foci and strands. (*D*) Heavily calcified head of the pancreas in patient with advanced CP.

Histologic Comparison

The accuracy of EUS is not clear, because of the lack of histologic comparison in a wide spectrum of disease severity. Most early studies used a nonhistologic reference standard such as ERCP or hormone-stimulated PFT, and reported sensitivities and specificities greater than 80%.[32,33] More recently, histologic comparison studies have reported sensitivities ranging from 71% to 91%, and specificities from 86% to 100%.[34–36] A more recent study published in abstract form suggests only that EUS may be less accurate then previously believed.[37] Investigators compared preoperative EUS scoring with histology in 50 patients undergoing total pancreatectomy with autologous islet cell transplantation, with histology obtained from wedge biopsies of the harvested pancreas. The discrimination of EUS scoring was poor in this study (receiver operating characteristic area under the curve 0.59) as were the negative and positive predictive values. A limitation of these histologic comparisons is that they consisted primarily of patients undergoing surgical resection. They are heavily weighted with severe disease, which may falsely increase sensitivity and limit extrapolation of the test performance estimates in typical patients with abdominal pain. Because of the impracticality of obtaining pancreatic biopsies in consecutive patients with abdominal pain, the real sensitivity and specificity of EUS criteria may never be clearly defined.

Reliability Issues

Aside from indefinite test performance, there are several other noted controversies surrounding EUS CP criteria. First, conditions besides CP may create a similar sonographic appearance. CP criteria may be observed in patients who are elderly[38,39] and those who regularly consume alcohol or smoke but lack symptoms of pancreatitis.[40] Patients with high body mass index or high triglyceride levels and chronic alcohol

Table 1
EUS standard and Rosemont criteria for CP

	Standard	Rosemont
Parenchyma	Hyperechoic foci	Hyperechoic foci without shadowing (minor). Echogenic structures ≥2 mm long and wide with no shadowing
		Hyperechoic foci with shadowing (major A). Echogenic structures ≥2 mm long and wide that shadow
	Hyperechoic strands	Stranding (minor). Hyperechoic lines of ≥3 mm in length in ≥2 different directions with respect to the imaged plane
	Cysts	Cysts (minor). Anechoic, rounded/elliptical structures with or without septations
	Parenchymal lobularity	Lobularity with honeycombing (major B). Well-circumscribed, ≥5 mm structures with enhancing rim and relatively echo-poor center, with ≥3 contiguous lobules
		Lobularity without honeycombing (minor). Well-circumscribed, ≥5 mm structures with enhancing rim and relatively echo-poor center, with noncontiguous lobules
Duct	MPD dilation	MPD dilation (minor). ≥3.5 mm in body or >1.5 mm in tail
	Irregular MPD margins	Irregular MPD contour (minor). Uneven or irregular outline and ecstatic course
	Hyperechoic MPD margins	Hyperechoic MPD margin (minor). Echogenic, distinct structure >50% of entire MPD in the body and tail
	Shadowing calcifications	MPD calculi (major A). Echogenic structures within MPD with acoustic shadowing
	Visible side branches	Dilated side branches (minor). ≥3 tubular anechoic structures each measuring ≥1 mm wide, budding from the MPD

Abbreviation: MPD, main pancreatic duct.
Adapted from Catalano MF, Sahai A, Levy M, et al. EUS-based criteria for the diagnosis of chronic pancreatitis: the Rosemont classification. Gastrointest Endosc 2009;69:1251–61.

drinkers may also have hyperechoic changes in the pancreas because of fatty infiltration.[41] These extraneous factors decrease specificity and should be taken into account when interpreting EUS images. A second issue is high interobserver variability. In a study of multiple readers interpreting the same still-frame images, [42] the κ score (agreement beyond chance) for global diagnosis of CP was only moderate (κ = 0.45), and less for most individual criteria. A more recent study of back-to-back examinations performed by 2 endosonographers in patients without suspected pancreatic disease also revealed modest agreement for most individual criteria.[43] As a result of these issues, EUS remains a controversial test for diagnosis of minimal change CP.

Rosemont Classification

An expert consensus conference was convened in 2009 in the village of Rosemont near Chicago, Illinois to address these controversies and improve EUS scoring. The result was a more elaborate and quantitative scoring system.[44] The Rosemont classification expands on previous criteria, classifying them as major and minor (see **Table 1**). Instead of a diagnostic cut point, it integrates these features into a 4-level diagnostic stratification, with categories for normal, indeterminate, suggestive, and most consistent. Potential strengths of the Rosemont classification are the use of weighted criteria, and the incorporation of a probability-based rating rather than an arbitrary cut point. Also, the definitions for each criterion were made more stringent through the use of quantitative thresholds. For example, to diagnose echogenic stranding, the endosonographer must visualize at least 3 echogenic strands greater than 2 mm visible within at least 2 planes. It was hoped that these more rigorous definitions would decrease interobserver variability. However, 3 studies[45–47] have failed to reveal significant improvement in κ scores compared with conventional scoring. Although the Rosemont classification refines past criteria and may help standardize EUS scoring for clinical and research purposes, it needs further validation.

Ancillary Imaging Techniques

Adjunctive imaging technologies have recently been tested in CP to determine if they enhance standard subjective B mode image interpretation. Such approaches may produce more quantitative results, and potentially decrease interobserver variability. Digital imaging analysis (DIA) involves computerized algorithmic interpretation of the number and distribution of white and black pixels within a region of interest to assess the degree of fibrotic (hyperechoic) change. In 1 study, the echogenicity assessed using DIA was significantly higher in patients with CP compared with controls, and correlated with worsening disease severity.[48]

Elastography measures the hardness of tissue, and would naturally seem useful for diagnosing a fibrotic condition like CP. This technique requires specialized hardware and software available in conjunction with Pentax scopes (Pentax, Inc, Tokyo, Japan) and Hitachi processors (Hitachi, Inc, Chiyoda, Tokyo, Japan). Colorized images are generated based on the degree of strain that occurs with compression of tissue by the scope. These images can be interpreted subjectively or through neural network analysis to distinguish different pancreatic diseases.[49] Initial cross-sectional studies have focused on differentiating inflammatory from neoplastic masses. For example, 1 study[50] revealed that a honeycombing pattern was characteristic of CP and was not found in pancreatic cancer or in control patients. Elastography has not been adequately studied in patients with minimal change CP to determine its incremental value over standard B mode imaging. Also, the operator dependency of elastography performance has not been well defined. Another obstacle has been the lack of compatibility of elastography technology with all types of EUS systems to allow widespread adaptation.

Endoscopic Secretin Pancreatic Function Test

The diagnosis of minimal change CP is sometimes a data-gathering exercise rather than a dichotomous test result. A reasonable clinical diagnosis is made based on the preponderance of the evidence, including the presence of risk factors, preceding AP or lipase fluctuations, and EUS changes. Another piece of evidence that may support CP is exocrine insufficiency, which may be present in a mild form even at the onset of pancreatic fibrosis. The gold standard for detecting mild exocrine insufficiency is direct PFT using hormonal secretagogues such as secretin and CCK.

An endoscopic secretin PFT can be combined with EUS (EUS-ePFT), which allows a simultaneous structural and functional assessment of the pancreas.[51] The usual protocol involves intravenous administration of synthetic secretin in a dose of 0.2 μg/kg, followed by collection of duodenal aspirates after 15, 30, and 45 minutes.

The fluid can be analyzed for bicarbonate concentration on a hospital autoanalyzer. A peak bicarbonate concentration (the highest concentration from the 3 samples) less than 80 mM is suggestive of exocrine insufficiency.

At our center, we typically administer secretin when EUS shows minimal abnormalities (<4 standard criteria or indeterminate Rosemont class). In this setting, an abnormal ePFT result may lend further credence to the equivocal structural findings seen with EUS. One could argue whether it is beneficial to add 1 imperfect test to another, because neither secretin PFT nor EUS is 100% sensitive or specific and the true performance characteristics of either test are not known. However, performing both methods may help optimize sensitivity for CP. We compared preoperative EUS and secretin ePFT with histology in 25 patients undergoing pancreatic resection or biopsy (36). Both EUS and ePFT had sensitivity of ~85%, but combining the tests produced 100% sensitivity for pancreatic fibrosis.

EUS Versus MRCP

MRCP is a less-invasive structural test used by many centers in the diagnosis of CP. The use of heavily T2-weighted imaging produces an ERCP-like pancreatogram, which allows a determination of the Cambridge classification of main-duct and side-branch abnormalities.[52] Visualization of these ductal changes is enhanced with secretin injection.[53] The use of secretin also allows an estimation of exocrine function by quantification of duodenal filling.[54] Other MRI parameters that have been reported to aid in CP diagnosis include diminished T1 signal in the parenchyma, delayed post-contrast enhancement, and diffusion-weighted imaging after secretin.[55] Despite cross-sectional studies comparing various MRI parameters in healthy individuals and established CP, their accuracy (alone or in combination) has not been well validated. Furthermore, the ideal MRCP CP protocol has not been standardized.

EUS and MRCP may be considered competing structural tests for diagnosing minimal change CP. EUS has been compared with MRCP in a 1 prospective study, in which 99 patients evaluated for CP underwent both tests.[56] The results were compared with a composite gold standard of ERCP findings, histologic fibrosis, or calcifications on follow-up. EUS showed higher sensitivity (93% vs 65%) and similar specificity (93% vs 90%) when compared with MRCP. Despite this study, it would be disingenuous to conclude that EUS is superior based on the concerns regarding its accuracy and reliability. It is possible that based on their individual strengths, these tests may offer complementary benefit in the workup of pancreatitis.

SUMMARY

EUS is a useful second-line evaluation for patients with RAP. In 1 endoscopic session, several important causes can be elucidated that may contribute to recurrent attacks. EUS is especially helpful in detecting a biliary source, even when other tests are unrevealing.

It is clear that EUS is not a panacea in the diagnosis of CP, and controversy abounds in this area. However, clinicians at many centers rely on EUS because it provides a safe and close-up view and can detect subtle findings, helping to build the case for CP as a source of debilitating pain. EUS CP criteria must be interpreted with caution in view of their known shortcomings, and put in context with other relevant clinical information.

REFERENCES

1. Kotwal V, Ralukdar R, Levy M, et al. Role of endoscopic ultrasound during hospitalization for acute pancreatitis. World J Gastroenterol 2010;16:4888–91.

2. Cho JH, Jeon TJ, Choi JS, et al. EUS finding of geographic hyperechoic area is in early predictor for severe acute pancreatitis. Pancreatology 2012;12:495–501.
3. Sotoudehmanesh R, Hooshyar A, Kalahdoozan S, et al. Prognostic value of endoscopic ultrasound in acute pancreatitis. Pancreatology 2010;10:702–6.
4. Ortega AR, Gomez-Rodriguez R, Romero M. Prospective comparison of endoscopic ultrasonography and magnetic resonance cholangiopancreatography in the etiological diagnosis of idiopathic acute pancreatitis. Pancreas 2011;40:289–94.
5. Mariani A, Arcidiacono PG, Curioni S, et al. Diagnostic yield of ERCP and secretin-enhanced MRCP and EUS in patients with acute recurrent pancreatitis of unknown aetiology. Dig Liver Dis 2009;41:753–8.
6. Wilcox CM, Varadarajulu S, Eloubeidi M. Role of endoscopic evaluation in idiopathic pancreatitis: a systematic review. Gastrointest Endosc 2006;63:1037–45.
7. Mirbagheri SA, Mohmadnejad M, Nasiri J, et al. Prospective evaluation of endoscopic ultrasonography in the diagnosis of biliary microlithiasis in patients with normal transabdominal ultrasonography. J Gastrointest Surg 2005;9:961–4.
8. Yusoff IF, Raymond G, Sahai AV. A prospective comparison of the yield of EUS in primary vs. recurrent idiopathic acute pancreatitis. Gastrointest Endosc 2004;60:673–8.
9. Zhan X, Guo X, Chen Y, et al. EUS in exploring the etiology of mild acute biliary pancreatitis with the negative finding of biliary origin by conventional radiologic methods. J Gastroenterol Hepatol 2011;26:1500–3.
10. Tandon M, Topazian M. Endoscopic ultrasound in idiopathic acute pancreatitis. Am J Gastroenterol 2001;109:196–200.
11. Tse F, Liu L, Barkun AN, et al. EUS: a meta-analysis of test performance in suspected choledocholithiasis. Gastrointest Endosc 2008;67:235–44.
12. Maple JT, Ben-Menachem T, Anderson MA, et al. The role of endoscopy in the evaluation of suspected choledocholithiasis. Gastrointest Endosc 2010;71:1–9.
13. De Lisi S, Leandro G, Buscarini E. Endoscopic ultrasonography versus endoscopic retrograde cholangiopancreatography in acute biliary pancreatitis: a systematic review. Eur J Gastroenterol Hepatol 2011;23:367–74.
14. Kohler H, Lankisch PG. Acute pancreatitis and hyperamylasaemia in pancreatic carcinoma. Pancreas 1987;2:177–9.
15. Bravo MT, Justo LM, Lasala JP, et al. Acute pancreatitis secondary to neuroendocrine pancreatic tumors. Report of 3 cases and literature review. Pancreas 2012;41:485–9.
16. Forsmark CE, Baillie J. AGA institute technical review on acute pancreatitis. Gastroenterology 2007;132:2002–44.
17. Dewitt J, Devereaux B, Chriswell M, et al. Comparison of endoscopic ultrasonography and multi-detector computed tomography for detecting and staging pancreatic cancer. Ann Intern Med 2004;141:753–63.
18. DiMagno MJ, DiMagno EP. Pancreas divisum does not cause pancreatitis, but associates with CFTR mutations. Am J Gastroenterol 2012;107:318.
19. Kushnir VM, Vani SB, Fowler K, et al. Sensitivity of endoscopic ultrasound, multi-detector computed tomography, and magnetic resonance cholangiopancreatography in the diagnosis of pancreas divisum: a tertiary care experience. Pancreas 2013;42(3):436–41.
20. Lai R, Freeman ML, Cass OW, et al. Accurate diagnosis of pancreas divisum by linear array endoscopic ultrasonography. Endoscopy 2004;46:705–9.
21. Eisner TD, Boldman IS, McKinley MJ. Crohns disease and pancreatitis. Am J Gastroenterol 1993;88:583–6.

22. Singh T, Mendelson R. Case report: confined penetration of a duodenal ulcer causing pancreatitis. J Med Imaging Radiat Oncol 2010;54:47–9.
23. Guzzardo G, Kleinman MS, Krackov JH, et al. Recurrent acute pancreatitis caused by ampullary villous adenoma. J Clin Gastroenterol 1990;12:200–2.
24. Petrou A, Bramis K, Williams T, et al. Acute recurrent pancreatitis: a possible clinical manifestation of ampullary cancer. JOP 2011;12:593–7.
25. Uomo G, Manes G, Rogozzino A, et al. Periampullary extraluminal duodenal diverticula and acute pancreatitis: an underestimated association. Am J Gastroenterol 1996;91:1186–8.
26. Moon SH, Kim MH, Park DH, et al. IgG4 immunostaining of duodenal papillary biopsy specimens may be useful for supported diagnosis of autoimmune pancreatitis. Gastrointest Endosc 2010;71:960–6.
27. Peterson BT. Sphincter of Oddi dysfunction, part 2: evidence-based review of the presentations, with "objective" pancreatic findings (types I and II) and of presumptive type III. Gastrointest Endosc 2004;59(6):670–87.
28. Catalano MF, Lahoti S, Alcocar E, et al. Dynamic imaging of the pancreas using real-time endoscopic ultrasonography with secretin stimulation. Gastrointest Endosc 1998;48:580–7.
29. Garder TB, Purich ED, Gordon SR. Pancreatic duct compliance after secretin stimulation. A novel endoscopic ultrasound diagnostic tool for chronic pancreatitis. Pancreas 2012;41:290–4.
30. Walsh TN, Rode J, Theis BA, et al. Minimal change chronic pancreatitis. Gut 1992;33:1566–71.
31. Sahai AV, Zimmerman M, Aabakken L, et al. Prospective assessment of the ability of endoscopic ultrasound to diagnose, exclude, or establish the severity of chronic pancreatitis found by endoscopic retrograde cholangiopancreatography. Gastrointest Endosc 1998;48:18–25.
32. Catalano MF, Lahoti S, Geenen JE, et al. Prospective evaluation of endoscopic ultrasonography, endoscopic retrograde pancreatography, and secretin test in the diagnosis of chronic pancreatitis. Gastrointest Endosc 1998;48:11–7.
33. Wiersema MJ, Hawes RH, Lehman GA, et al. Prospective evaluation of endoscopic ultrasonography and endoscopic retrograde cholangiopancreatography in patients with chronic abdominal pain of suspected pancreatic origin. Endoscopy 1993;25:555–64.
34. Chong AK, Romagnuolo J, Hoffman BJ, et al. Diagnosis of chronic pancreatitis with endoscopic ultrasound: a comparison with histopathology. Gastrointest Endosc 2007;65:808–14.
35. Varadarajulu S, Eltoum I, Tamhane A, et al. Histopathologic correlates of noncalcific chronic pancreatitis by EUS: a prospective tissue characterization study. Gastrointest Endosc 2007;66:501–9.
36. Albashir S, Bronner M, Parsi M, et al. Endoscopic ultrasound, secretin endoscopic pancreatic function test, and histology: correlation in chronic pancreatitis. Am J Gastroenterol 2010;105:2498–503.
37. Vega-Peralta J, Manivel C, Attam R, et al. Accuracy of EUS for diagnosis of minimal change chronic pancreatitis (MCCP): correlation with Histopathology in 50 patients undergoing total pancreatectomy (TP) with Islet Autotransplantion (IAT) [abstract]. 42nd Annual Meeting of the American Pancreatic Association. Volume Pancreas. Chicago: Lippincott Williams & Wilkins; November 3, 2011.
38. Bhutani MS, Arantes VN, Verma D, et al. Histopathologic correlation of endoscopic ultrasound findings of chronic pancreatitis in human autopsies. Pancreas 2009;38:820–4.

39. Rajan E, Clain JE, Levy MJ, et al. Age-related changes in the pancreas identified by EUS: a prospective evaluation. Gastrointest Endosc 2005;61:401–6.
40. Yusoff IF, Sahai AV. A prospective, quantitative assessment of the effect of ethanol and other variables on the endosonographic appearance of the pancreas. Clin Gastroenterol Hepatol 2004;2:405–9.
41. Al-Haddad M, Khashab M, Zyromski N, et al. Risk factors for hyperechogenic pancreas on endoscopic ultrasound. Pancreas 2009;38:672–5.
42. Wallace MB, Hawes RH, Durkalski V, et al. The reliability of EUS for the diagnosis of chronic pancreatitis: interobserver agreement among experienced endosonographers. Gastrointest Endosc 2001;53:294–9.
43. Gardner TB, Gordon SR. Interobserver agreement for pancreatic endoscopic ultrasonography determined by same day back-to-back examinations. J Clin Gastroenterol 2011;45:542–5.
44. Catalano MF, Sahai A, Levy M, et al. EUS-based criteria for the diagnosis of chronic pancreatitis: the Rosemont classification. Gastrointest Endosc 2009; 69:1251–61.
45. Stevens T, Adler DG, Al-Haddad MA, et al. Multicenter study of interobserver agreement of standard endoscopic ultrasound scoring and Rosemont classification for diagnosis of chronic pancreatitis. Gastrointest Endosc 2010;71:519–26.
46. Del Pozo D, Poves E, Tabernero S, et al. Conventional versus Rosemont endoscopic ultrasound criteria for chronic pancreatitis: interobserver agreement in same day back-to-back procedures. Pancreatology 2012;12:284–7.
47. Klamin B, Hoffman B, Hawes R, et al. Conventional versus Rosemont endoscopic ultrasound criteria for chronic pancreatitis: comparing interobserver reliability and intertest agreement. Can J Gastroenterol 2011;25:261–4.
48. Irisawa A, Mishra G, Hernandez LV, et al. Quantitative analysis of endosonographic parenchymal echogenicity in patients with chronic pancreatitis. J Gastroenterol Hepatol 2004;19:1199–205.
49. Saftoiu A, Vilmann P, Gorunescu F, et al. Neural network analysis of dynamic sequences of EUS elastography used for the differential diagnosis of chronic pancreatitis and pancreatic cancer. Gastrointest Endosc 2008;65:971–8.
50. Janssen J, Schlorer E, Greiner L. EUS elastography of the pancreas: feasibility and pattern description of the normal pancreas, chronic pancreatitis, and focal pancreatic lesions. Gastrointest Endosc 2008;65:971–8.
51. Stevens T, Dumot JA, Parsi MA, et al. Combined endoscopic ultrasound and secretin endoscopic pancreatic function test in the evaluation of chronic pancreatitis. Dig Dis Sci 2010;55:2681–7.
52. Axon AT, Classen M, Cotton P, et al. Pancreatography in chronic pancreatitis. International definitions. Gut 1984;25:1107–12.
53. Matos C, Metens T, Deviere J, et al. Pancreatic duct: morphologic and functional evaluation with dynamic MR pancreatography after secretin stimulation. Radiology 1997;203:435–41.
54. Sanyal R, Stevens T, Novak E, et al. Secretin enhanced MRCP: review of technique and application with proposal for quantification of exocrine function. AJR Am J Roentgenol 2012;198:124–32.
55. Balci C. MRI assessment of chronic pancreatitis. Diagn Interv Radiol 2011;17: 249–54.
56. Pungpapong S, Wallace MB, Woodward TA, et al. Accuracy of endoscopic ultrasonography and magnetic resonance cholangiopancreatography for the diagnosis of chronic pancreatitis. A prospective comparison study. J Clin Gastroenterol 2007;41:88–93.

Endoscopic Management of Acute Biliary Pancreatitis

Vincent C. Kuo, MD[a], Paul R. Tarnasky, MD[b],*

KEYWORDS

- Biliary pancreatitis • ERCP • Sphincterotomy • Timing of ERCP
- Pancreatic duct stenting

KEY POINTS

- Acute pancreatitis is considered an endoscopic emergency when a biliary cause is likely and there is suspected cholangitis or ongoing biliary obstruction.
- Elective endoscopic retrograde cholangiopancreatography (ERCP) should be considered when there is jaundice or proven choledocholithiasis by noninvasive imaging or intraoperative cholangiography.
- There remains some debate regarding the role of early ERCP in the setting of acute biliary pancreatitis without evidence of biliary obstruction.
- Further studies should better establish the indicators for ampullary obstruction and predictors for severe attacks.
- Additional prospective endoscopic trials are needed to clarify the optimal timing of biliary intervention, the potential benefit of biliary sphincterotomy in all cases independent of biliary obstruction, and the usefulness of pancreatic stenting.

Videos of the needle-knife precut sphincterotomy and standard sphincterotomy techniques accompany this article at http:// www.giendo.theclinics.com/

OBJECTIVES

- Understand the pathophysiology of acute biliary pancreatitis
- Recognize important factors in the clinical evaluation of a patient with acute biliary pancreatitis
- Know the available literature on the role of early endoscopic retrograde cholangiopancreatography (ERCP) versus conservative management for acute biliary pancreatitis

---

[a] Gastroenterology Fellowship, Methodist Dallas Medical Center, 1441 North Beckley Avenue, Dallas, TX 75203, USA; [b] Gastroenterology Fellowship, Digestive Health Associates of Texas, Methodist Dallas Medical Center, 221 West Colorado Boulevard, Pavilion II, Suite #630, Dallas, TX 75208, USA
* Corresponding author.
E-mail address: paul.tarnasky@dhat.com

Gastrointest Endoscopy Clin N Am 23 (2013) 749–768
http://dx.doi.org/10.1016/j.giec.2013.06.002
1052-5157/13/$ – see front matter © 2013 Elsevier Inc. All rights reserved.

- Understand the types of endoscopic therapy available for ERCP in acute biliary pancreatitis

INTRODUCTION

Acute pancreatitis represents numerous unique challenges to the practicing digestive disease specialist. Clinical presentations of acute pancreatitis vary from trivial pain to severe acute illness with a significant risk of death. Management goals are 4-fold:

1. Identify patients with a mild attack who initially require only conservative care
2. Early recognition and appropriate treatment of biliary obstruction and potentially severe attacks to reduce morbidity and mortality caused by infection, organ failure, or pancreatic fluid collections
3. Manage complications of severe acute pancreatitis
4. Direct therapy to prevent recurrent attacks

Multidisciplinary collaboration often is required, and the endoscopist plays a central role. At present, urgent endoscopic treatment of acute pancreatitis is only considered when there is causal evidence of biliary pancreatitis.

CLINICAL FEATURES AND SIGNIFICANCE

It is usually not difficult to diagnose acute pancreatitis. It requires at least 2 of 3 criteria: (1) abdominal pain, typically located in the upper abdomen and often radiating to the back; (2) serum amylase and/or lipase increased 3 times greater than the upper limit of normal (lipase is more sensitive, specific, and remains increased longer than amylase); and/or (3) radiographic evidence of pancreatitis.[1] Gallstones are considered the most common single cause of acute pancreatitis, being responsible for at least half of all cases. About 5% of those with symptomatic gallstones develop acute biliary pancreatitis (ABP), and there is a 1% annual incidence of acute pancreatitis among those with gallstones.[2,3] Most ABP attacks are not severe, and full recovery without recurrence can be expected with conservative care and directed therapy to prevent future attacks. However, the overall mortality for an initial attack of ABP is at least 10%.[4,5] Up to 25% of ABP attacks are severe, carrying a significant risk for multiorgan system failure, long-term medical disability, and a mortality up to 30%.[6] Without definitive treatment, the risk of a recurrent attack within the next several months is about 30% to 50%.[7-11] Even after a mild attack, cholecystectomy and/or biliary sphincterotomy must be considered within weeks.[12,13] A large retrospective cohort study of more than 5000 patients with ABP emphasized the importance of early biliary intervention either with cholecystectomy or endoscopic retrograde cholangiopancreatography (ERCP) during index admission. Hospital readmission rates for ABP within 12 months were significantly reduced with cholecystectomy (14.0%–5.6%) or ERCP (13.1% vs 5.1%).[14]

The important questions an endoscopist must consider when caring for a patient with acute pancreatitis are:

- Is the cause of pancreatitis related to gallstones?
- Is there evidence of ongoing biliary obstruction?
- How severe is the attack?
- When should urgent ERCP be considered?
- What endoscopic therapy should be performed during urgent ERCP?
- When should elective ERCP be considered?

To address these questions, it is helpful to review the pathophysiologic factors of ABP and the clinical experiences that have provided historical insight regarding treatment principles.

PATHOPHYSIOLOGY

Pertinent factors related to the pathophysiology of ABP are (1) bile duct stones or crystals, (2) pancreatic duct obstruction, (3) common pancreaticobiliary channel, and (4) nonpatent accessory papilla.

Since the autopsy report in 1901 by Opie[15] of a gallstone impaction at the papilla, numerous surgical series have implicated bile duct stone impaction and/or passage as a cause of pancreatitis. Bile duct stone impaction was found in 26% to 72% of patients who had ABP when surgery was performed soon after an attack compared with less than 10% for patients undergoing elective surgery.[16–18] Out of 19 fatal cases of ABP that underwent autopsy, nearly half had a stone impacted at the papilla.[4] To implicate transpapillary stone passage, 2 studies in the 1970s reported that fecal stones were discovered in about 90% of patients who had suspected ABP compared with only about 10% of controls.[18,19] Biliary crystals or small stones are perhaps more prone to negotiate cystic duct and papillary migration and are considered to be more likely to cause ABP.[17,20–24]

Pancreatic duct obstruction may occur after stone impaction or sphincter of Oddi spasm. Distal bile duct stone impaction may obstruct the pancreatic duct orifice by compressing the pancreaticobiliary septum. Stone impaction at the papillary orifice also may cause pancreatic duct obstruction when there is a common pancreaticobiliary channel. Increased amylase levels were found in biliary T-tube fluid from a patient who had ABP that decreased promptly after sphincterotomy and removal of an impacted stone.[25] In addition, sphincter of Oddi spasm and a common pancreaticobiliary channel may cause functional papillary obstruction in patients with ABP who have passed bile duct stones. Compared with patients who had biliary stones and no history of pancreatitis, increased amylase levels were found in biliary T-tube fluid from patients with ABP who had documented transpapillary stone migration.[26] As an indication of sphincter spasm and a common channel, reflux of contrast into the pancreatic duct is observed in about two-thirds of intraoperative cholangiograms.[17,18,24,27,28] Compared with controls, basal sphincter of Oddi pressures were increased significantly in 30 consecutive patients with mild ABP when measured within 24 hours of admission.[29] Impaired drainage by means of the accessory papilla also contributes to promoting pancreatic ductal obstruction. The accessory papilla is patent in 30% to 70% from normal anatomic studies. Nowak and colleagues[30] reported that only 17% of patients with ABP had a patent accessory papilla compared with 69% of patients for controls.

Experimental studies have provided important information regarding mechanisms and timing of pancreatitis and subsequent organ injury. Pancreatic and biliary duct obstruction in animals causes pancreatitis, whereby the extent of histologic injury is related directly to duration of duct obstruction (up to 5 days), but progression of injury is prevented when duct obstruction is relieved.[31,32] Early pancreatic injury occurs within hours of duct obstruction, and necrotizing acinar injury is observed within 24 hours.[33,34] Data pertaining to the timing of duct obstruction and organ injury also are derived from studies of cytokines, the mediators of systemic inflammation, and distant organ dysfunction.[35,36] Cytokine production begins early and peaks about 24 to 36 hours after onset of symptoms. Inflammatory cytokine levels are increased significantly after severe attacks and organ dysfunction occurs between 36 and 72 hours after symptom onset.

LESSONS FROM SURGICAL EXPERIENCE

Three important principles regarding the treatment of ABP were learned from surgical studies:

1. There is benefit with early relief of ductal obstruction.
2. Benefit only occurs after surgical procedures that promote ductal drainage.
3. Early surgery without augmenting drainage is detrimental.

In the late 1970s, Acosta and colleagues[16] reported a case series of 132 patients who had ABP to compare outcomes for patients treated differently during 2 time periods. From 1964 to 1972, most patients were operated on for biliary tract disease electively or earlier only if there were absolute indications. During 1972 to 1975, patients underwent early surgery (14 of 46 having surgical sphincteroplasty) within 48 hours of symptom onset. There was only 2% mortality for the group that underwent early surgery compared with 16% for those undergoing elective or indicated surgery. The investigators concluded that "treatment given for acute gallstone pancreatitis in hopes of avoiding pancreatic necrosis must relieve obstruction quickly."[16] In a separate report by Acosta and colleagues,[37] the extent of pancreatic damage (interstitial to necrosis) correlated with duration of ampullary obstruction, and relief of obstruction was associated with remission of symptoms. Similar outcomes with an overall 5% mortality for ABP were reported by Stone and colleagues[38] from a randomized controlled trial comparing early (within 72 hours) versus delayed (3 months) surgery. Surgical procedures included sphincteroplasty and septotomy, after which a "sudden gush of clear pancreatic juice"[38] was observed when performed during the early operations.

A later randomized controlled trial concluded that early (≤48 hours) cholecystectomy was associated with increased mortality (15%) compared with when it was performed electively (2%).[39] However, procedures to augment ductal drainage (sphincteroplasty) were not done. A retrospective study also reported increased mortality (31%) in patients undergoing immediate surgery for ABP.[8]

CONCLUSIONS FROM PROSPECTIVE ENDOSCOPIC TRIALS

Although debates regarding the role of early surgery for ABP were escalating, the first endoscopic treatments for ABP were being reported. Van der Spuy[40] performed biliary sphincterotomy to promote spontaneous bile duct stone migration in 10 patients who had gallstone pancreatitis. Safrany and Cotton[41] performed ERCP with biliary sphincterotomy and stone extraction in 11 patients who had severe ABP; 9 patients had endoscopic therapy within 24 hours of hospital admission. Dramatic improvement was observed with respect to laboratory (liver and pancreas chemistries, white blood cell counts) and clinical symptoms. Rosseland and Solhaug[42] reported good outcomes after endoscopic therapy in 15 patients within 48 hours of symptom onset. From these early reports, it was concluded that ERCP was safe and effective in the setting of ABP.

Prospective trials have compared early ERCP with conservative therapy for ABP. However, it is difficult to draw firm conclusions because these studies lack congruency with respect to inclusion criteria, the timing of ERCP after onset of symptoms, and endoscopic intervention. Clinical outcomes for urgent ERCP in ABP may not be different from an elective ERCP strategy when a significant minority of elective ERCP patients undergo clinically indicated ERCP. Studies in which ERCP is not performed early enough may not prove beneficial. Any benefit for early ERCP may be negated unless all patients undergo sphincterotomy to augment ductal drainage. In addition, no studies have evaluated endoscopic expertise; an important factor because ERCP in the setting of acute pancreatitis can be more difficult. Nevertheless, these studies provide useful data.

An early meta-analysis concluded that early ERCP significantly reduces morbidity (25% vs 38%) and mortality (5% vs 9%) in ABP.[43] Two later meta-analyses evaluated 3 trials that excluded patients with cholangitis.[44,45] They concluded that early ERCP with or without endoscopic sphincterotomy in patients with either mild or severe pancreatitis does not lead to significant reduction in overall risk of complications or mortality. There was a suggestion that it may even lead to higher mortality. The definitions of early ERCP were defined differently in each study; some defined early as within 72 hours of admission and others defined it as within 72 hours of symptom onset. Also, endoscopic sphincterotomy was only performed when common bile duct stones were visualized during ERCP. There were also variation in definitions of overall complications.

The most recent meta-analysis, by Tse and Yuan,[46] evaluated 7 trials that compared early ERCP versus early conservative management for acute gallstone pancreatitis. The general definition of early in the meta-analysis was within 72 hours of admission. Overall, they did not find significant improvement in mortality and local or systemic complications of pancreatitis with early ERCP strategy compared with early conservative management; this conclusion was independent of whether patients had predicted mild or severe pancreatitis. Their results did support the empirical evidence of the benefits of early ERCP in patients with cholangitis.

It is instructive to carefully evaluate some of the individual endoscopic studies and focus on the important details such as whether ERCP was performed early (eg, within 24–48 hours of symptom onset), whether endoscopic therapy with sphincterotomy was performed, and the frequency of crossover endotherapy in conservative groups. **Table 1** summarizes these parameters for each study and more specific details of each study are discussed later.

Neoptolemos and colleagues[47] reported the first endoscopic randomized controlled trial in ABP comparing urgent ERCP (within 72 hours of hospital admission) in ABP with conservative care that only allowed ERCP after 5 days if indicated. Urgent ERCP was performed successfully in 88% of patients, but success was less likely if pancreatitis was severe (80%) versus mild (94%). Biliary sphincterotomy was performed in about one-third of patients (those found to have bile duct stones). Of patients confirmed to have gallstones, bile duct stones were discovered significantly more often in severe (63%) versus mild (25%) attacks. The study design does not strictly compare early versus clinically indicated ERCP, because ERCP was delayed by at least 72 hours in the urgent ERCP group, and ERCP in the conservative group was delayed for 5 days even when there was a need for ERCP. Significant differences were found only in patients predicted to have severe attacks; early ERCP was associated with lower overall complications (24% vs 61%) and a shorter hospital stay (9.5 days vs 17.0 days).

In the randomized trial reported by Fan and colleagues,[48] urgent ERCP was performed earlier, within 24 hours of hospital admission. Similar to the report by Neoptolemos and colleagues, early ERCP was performed successfully in 90% of patients, and biliary sphincterotomy was done only in the 38% of patients found to have ampullary or bile duct stones. Patients in the conservative group underwent selective ERCP at any time there were indications to proceed. Of the patients randomized to initial conservative care, 28% underwent ERCP, and 37% of these had treatment of ampullary or bile duct stones, usually within 3 days of admission when there was evidence of cholangitis, sepsis, shock, or other organ system failure. Further, of the patients in the

Table 1
Summary of prospective endoscopic trials for ERCP and ABP

Study	Trial Design	ERCP Group	Timing of ERCP	Sphincterotomy (%)	Conservative Group ERCPs (%)
Neoptolemos et al,[47] 1988	RCT	59 (34 mild, 25 severe)	≤72 h of admission	19/59 (32)	14/62 (23)
Fan et al,[48] 1993	RCT	97 (56 mild, 41 severe)	≤24 h of admission	37/97 (38)	27/98 (28)
Folsch et al,[49] 1997	RCT	126 (84 mild, 26 severe, 16 undefined)	≤72 h of symptoms	58/126 (46)	22/112 (20)
Zhou et al,[50] 2002	RCT	20 (13 mild, 7 severe)	≤24 h of admission	12/20 (60)	0/25 (0)
Oría et al,[51] 2007	RCT	51 (34 mild, 17 severe)	≤24–48 h of symptoms (46) 48–72 h of symptoms (5)	38/51 (75) —	2/52 (4) —
Van Santvoort et al,[52] 2009	Prospective observational	81 (all severe)	<24 h of symptoms (17) 24–48 h of symptoms (53) 48–72 h of symptoms (11)	69/81 (85) — —	7/72 (10) — —
Chen et al,[53] 2010	RCT	21 (all severe)	<24 h of symptoms (5) 24–48 h symptoms (10) >48 h of symptoms (6)	17/21 (81) — —	0/32 (0) — —

Abbreviation: RCT, randomized controlled trial.

conservative group with a predicted severe attack, almost half (45%) underwent selective ERCP. This study design decreases the ability to show benefit with early ERCP, because the ratio of patients who underwent sphincterotomy and treatment of stones was virtually identical in both groups. A significant minority (35%) of patients was discovered not to have a biliary cause for pancreatitis. Thus, benefit for urgent ERCP was only found in those proved to have gallstones. Compared with selective ERCP, urgent ERCP significantly reduced morbidity (33%–16%) and biliary sepsis (12%–0%), and there was a trend toward lower mortality (8%–2%).

Folsch and colleagues[49] compared early ERCP, defined as within 72 hours of symptom onset, with a conservative approach in a randomized controlled trial for patients who had suspected ABP, but excluded those with bilirubin levels of at least 5 mg/dL. ERCP was successful in 96% of patients in the early group, and biliary sphincterotomy was performed only in the 46% found to have bile duct stones. Selective ERCP was performed within 3 weeks of randomization on 20% of patients in the conservative treatment group if there was evidence of cholangitis or biliary colic. A lower success rate for selective ERCP (86%) was attributed to ampullary edema or periampullary diverticula. Similar overall morbidity and mortality were observed between the two groups.

A small trial by Zhou and colleagues[50] involving 45 patients evaluated the role of ERCP in patients with ABP within 24 hours of admission. Patients were randomly divided into ERCP and supportive treatment groups and then subdivided into mild or severe pancreatitis. Twenty patients in the ERCP group all received ERCP within 24 hours of admission. Twelve of the patients had a sphincterotomy for either stones or stenosis, and the remaining 8 patients had a nasobiliary drain placed for large stones or duodenal edema. None of the patients in the conservative management group underwent ERCP. There was a statistically significant decrease in complications and length of hospitalization in the ERCP group compared with the non-ERCP group only in patients with severe ABP.

Oría and colleagues[51] concluded that early endoscopic intervention failed to reduce systemic and local inflammation in patients with ABP. This randomized controlled trial compared ERCP (with endotherapy if evidence of bile duct stones) to conservative management. Some patients presented nearly 20 hours after onset of symptoms. ERCP was performed within 48 to 72 hours after symptom onset and only about three-fourths of patients in the ERCP group underwent sphincterotomy. Two patients in the conservative arm eventually had ERCP because of cholangitis or progressive jaundice. Measured outcomes included changes in organ failure score and computed tomography (CT) severity index during the first week of admission, incidence of local complications, and overall morbidity and mortality. There were no statistically significant differences between the ERCP and conservative management patient groups in these outcome measures.

Van Santvoort and colleagues[52] conducted a prospective observational multicenter study that evaluated a subset of patients with predicted severe ABP but without evidence of cholangitis. The decision to perform ERCP with or without sphincterotomy was left to the discretion of the treating physician. Patients who had an ERCP within 72 hours of symptom onset were classified as the early ERCP group and almost all (86%) underwent ERCP within 48 hours. Most patients (85%) in the ERCP group underwent therapy that included a biliary sphincterotomy. Patients who did not undergo ERCP or had ERCP later than 72 hours after onset of symptoms were in the conservative treatment group. Seven patients in the conservative group underwent an elective ERCP at a median of 5 days after symptoms (range 4–18 days). In patients with predicted severe ABP and concurrent cholestasis, early ERCP was associated with significantly fewer complications including pancreatic necrosis. Despite the study not being a randomized controlled trial, it still provides favorable observational data for the role of early ERCP in patients with severe ABP.

Chen and colleagues[53] evaluated the efficacy of early endoscopic intervention without fluoroscopy for severe ABP in the intensive care unit. More than 70% of patients randomized to the endoscopic intervention arm underwent ERCP within 48 hours of symptoms; cannulation was reported to be more difficult when performed later. Biliary sphincterotomy with stone removal was completed in 80%. The remaining patients had suppurative cholangitis and were treated initially with nasobiliary drainage only. No patients in the conservative arm received ERCP. Patients in the endoscopic intervention group had a significant decrease in severity score at day 10; quicker relief of clinical symptoms including temperature, abdominal pain, and peritoneal irritation; and no mortality. There were 2 deaths in the conservative arm.

The available published randomized controlled trials for ABP performed sphincterotomy only if there was evidence of bile duct or ampullary stones. Also, the existing controlled studies do not provide data to compare outcomes of those who did or did not undergo sphincterotomy. Biliary sphincterotomy likely augments pancreatic drainage and bile flow, particularly for patients who have a common pancreaticobiliary channel. An abstract by Nowak and colleagues[54] compared outcomes in a consecutive series of 280 patients with ABP. Duodenoscopy was performed within 24 hours of admission to assess for stone impaction. Seventy-five patients (27%) who had stone impaction underwent urgent treatment with sphincterotomy. The remaining patients with a normal papilla were randomized to urgent sphincterotomy (n = 103) or conservative treatment (n = 102). Patients who underwent urgent sphincterotomy (impacted stones plus randomized patients) had significantly fewer complications (17%) and lower mortality (2%) compared with those treated conservatively (36% and 13%, respectively). Another abstract by Nowak and colleagues[55] reported outcomes after biliary sphincterotomy within 24 hours of admission in 307 consecutive patients who had ABP treated over 10 years. Outcomes were analyzed according to predicted severity and interval between sphincterotomy and onset of pain. The best outcomes (7% complications, 0% mortality) were observed when sphincterotomy was performed before 24 hours elapsed after onset of pain, despite 31% of these patients having a predicted severe attack. For patients who underwent sphincterotomy more than 72 hours after symptom onset, outcomes were worse (20% complications, 13% mortality), even though only 18% had predicted severe attacks.

INITIAL CLINICAL EVALUATION

Clinical evaluation of a patient with ABP (**Box 1**) should be directed to answer the following questions:

1. Is the cause of pancreatitis related to gallstones?
2. Is there evidence of ongoing biliary obstruction?
3. How severe is the attack?

Is the Cause of Pancreatitis Related to Gallstones?

Establishing the cause of acute pancreatitis is important when developing a treatment algorithm. If ABP is not diagnosed in a timely fashion, the potential for benefit with endoscopic therapy may be lost. Further, recurrent pancreatitis may result without appropriate treatment when gallstones are not recognized as the cause of pancreatitis.

Box 1
Important clinical evaluation of patients with suspected acute biliary pancreatitis
Evidence for biliary cause
Female
History of biliary colic
Age greater than 50 years
Alanine aminotransferase greater than or equal to 3 times normal
Dilated bile duct
Evidence of ongoing biliary obstruction
Cholangitis
Unrelenting pain
Laboratory trend of increasing liver tests
Factors associated with severe attack
Age greater than 55 years
Body mass index greater than 30
Organ system dysfunction
Baseline Acute Physiology and Chronic Health Evaluation (APACHE)-II score 8 and/or increasing score during initial 24 hours
Hematocrit greater than or equal to 44% and/or failure to decrease during initial 24 hours
Bedside Index for Severity in Acute Pancreatitis (BISAP) score of greater than or equal to 3 within 24 hours of presentation
Systemic Inflammatory Response Syndrome

Women older than 50 years are more likely to have gallstones as the cause of pancreatitis.[56] A history of antecedent biliary colic may suggest a biliary cause, but laboratory studies and imaging are most helpful to establish the diagnosis of ABP. Serum alanine aminotransferase increase of at least 3 times the upper limit of normal has been shown to have a positive predictive value of 95% for ABP.[57] Serum calcium and triglycerides are additional laboratory tests that should be obtained at admission to exclude other causes of pancreatitis.

Transabdominal ultrasound generally is considered the best initial imaging study to establish a cause for pancreatitis. Ultrasound is highly specific for diagnosing cholelithiasis and has been shown to be about 90% accurate in patients who have gallstone pancreatitis.[58,59] CT of the abdomen with contrast generally has a limited role in the initial evaluation of patients who have acute pancreatitis. However, CT may be helpful to rule out other important causes of abdominal pain and to identify mass and cystic lesions of the pancreas. Magnetic resonance cholangiopancreatography and endoscopic ultrasound may be helpful in some cases to diagnose choledocholithiasis but are of limited benefit for showing gallstones in the absence of choledocholithiasis.

Is there Evidence of Ongoing Biliary Obstruction?

Whether there is ongoing biliary obstruction is of central importance to determine whether ERCP is likely to benefit a patient with acute pancreatitis. As discussed earlier, bile obstruction and pancreatic duct obstruction are paramount to the pathophysiology and treatment of ABP. Cholangitis with symptoms of abdominal pain, fever, and jaundice is not difficult to recognize. Otherwise, clinical and biochemical trends are most useful for identifying ongoing biliary obstruction. Unrelenting pain and increasing liver function test abnormalities may indicate ongoing obstruction caused by an impacted stone. Acosta and colleagues[60] reported that decreasing severity of abdominal pain, decreasing serum bilirubin, and presence of bile in a nasogastric tube aspirate strongly suggested ampullary stone decompression.

Diagnosis of choledocholithiasis (without ampullary stone impaction) is important but not with respect to the potential need for urgent intervention. Endoscopic ultrasonography has a high sensitivity for diagnosis of bile duct stones.[61,62] Okan and colleagues[63] reported results of magnetic resonance cholangiopancreatography in 81 patients with nonsevere ABP and found a low false-negative rate of 7.4% for diagnosing choledocholithiasis. ERCP should not be considered as a diagnostic test in this setting.

How Severe is the Attack?

Persistent organ dysfunction (circulatory, respiratory, and renal failure) and infected pancreatic necrosis portend increased mortality. However, such events often occur after a missed opportunity to intervene in hopes of preventing them. Baseline patient factors (age older than 55 years and body mass index greater than 30) and early clinical evidence for organ dysfunction have been shown to predict the severity of acute pancreatitis.[64]

Acute pancreatitis generally has a biphasic clinical course. The first phase, within 2 weeks of the attack, is characterized by the patient's clinical course and the inflammatory immune response. The severity of this phase is related to presence of one or more organ system dysfunctions, which can occur in up to 40% of severe cases with a mortality of 30%. The second phase occurs after 2 weeks of symptoms when patients are more susceptible to infectious complications, and the assessment involves a morphologic evaluation of the pancreas. About three-fourths of cases have an edematous pancreas that resolves without serious sequelae. The remaining quarter of cases develop necrosis with mortality related to infection and independent of the extent of necrosis. The most severe complication is infected pancreatic or peripancreatic necrosis, which occurs in about one-third of patients; the remaining two-thirds of patients have sterile necrosis. The greatest risk for infection is about 2 to 4 weeks after presentation.[1]

The Ranson score,[65] the most recognized prognostic method, and the Glasgow modification of the Imrie score,[66] are of limited use, because they require 48 hours of clinical data. A large meta-analysis concluded that the Ranson score is a poor predictor of severity and offers no advantage compared with clinical judgment.[67]

The APACHE-II (Acute Physiology and Chronic Health Evaluation II) and serum hematocrit both remain valid for assessment of severity at presentation.[64] The APACHE-II is calculated easily after entering patient parameters such as age, vital signs, hematocrit, leukocyte count, sodium, potassium, creatinine, cardiopulmonary, and neurologic parameters to generate a composite score. Combining an obesity score with the APACHE-II seems to improve accuracy for prediction of severe or mild acute pancreatitis.[68] Serum hematocrit as an indicator of third spacing and volume depletion has proved to be useful in predicting the clinical course of acute pancreatitis. Hematocrit of at least 44% at presentation and a failure to decrease during the first 24 hours seems to correlate with pancreatic necrosis and development of organ failure.[69,70] Further, hematocrit less than 44% seems to predict a more benign course of acute pancreatitis.[71] None of the prognostic scoring methods are specific for ABP.

Singh and colleagues[72] generated a scoring system to use as a bedside index for severity in acute pancreatitis (BISAP). The BISAP score includes 5 variables: blood urea nitrogen greater than 25 mg/dL, presence or absence of impaired mental status, systemic inflammatory response syndrome, age greater than 60 years, and pleural effusion on imaging. One point is given for each variable and 3 or more points within 24 hours of presentation is associated with a greater mortality, increased risk of organ failure, and pancreatic necrosis.

Another classification for severity of pancreatitis is the Atlanta criteria, which was first instituted in the early 1990s.[73] Numerous pancreas experts convened in Atlanta, Georgia, to establish a clinically based classification system for acute pancreatitis. They came to a consensus for standardized definitions, clinical manifestations, pathologic findings for degrees of pancreatitis, and certain complications such as fluid collections, pancreatic necrosis, pseudocysts, and abscesses. The Atlanta criteria have recently been revised to reflect substantial advances in understanding of acute pancreatitis.[74] Severity is classified into mild, moderate, or severe depending on presence and duration of organ failure and local and/or systemic complications (**Box 2**).

ROLE OF ERCP

Questions regarding the role for ERCP in the setting of ABP are:

- When should urgent ERCP be considered?
- What endoscopic therapy should be performed during urgent ERCP?
- When should elective ERCP be considered?

Suggested indications and timing for ERCP in ABP are shown in **Box 3**.

When Should Urgent ERCP be Considered?

ERCP is indicated in the setting of ABP when there is evidence of acute cholangitis, and when there is evidence of ongoing biliary obstruction. This view is supported by the Tse and Yuan[46] meta-analysis and the International Association of Pancreatology evidence-based guidelines for management of acute biliary pancreatitis.[75]

Existing experimental data and clinical insights from surgical and endoscopic experience all suggest that procedures to augment ductal drainage must be accomplished

---

Box 2
Classification of acute pancreatitis severity

Mild acute pancreatitis

No organ failure

No local or systemic complications

Moderately severe acute pancreatitis

Organ failure that resolves within 48 hours (transient organ failure) and/or

Local or systemic complications without persistent organ failure

Severe acute pancreatitis

Persistent organ failure greater than 48 hours

From Banks PA, Bollen TL, Dervenis C, et al. Classification of acute pancreatitis–2012: revision of the Atlanta classification and definitions by international consensus. Gut 2013;62:108; with permission.

> **Box 3**
> **Indications and timing for ERCP in acute biliary pancreatitis**
>
> *Urgent (within 48 hours of symptom onset)*
> Cholangitis
> Ongoing biliary obstruction
> *Elective*
> Jaundice or imaging shows choledocholithiasis
> Abnormal intraoperative cholangiography
> Biliary sphincterotomy as primary therapy in poor operative candidates
> Biliary sphincterotomy as temporary therapy during pregnancy

early in the course of ABP to be of benefit. However, there is no clear definition of what is early. Radiological evidence suggests that pancreatic necrosis occurs within 4 days.[76] Surgeons may discover pancreatic necrosis about 48 hours after onset of symptoms.[37] A case-control study compared extent of pancreatic injury at laparotomy between patients with ongoing ampullary obstruction with those with spontaneous ampullary stone clearance.[77] Pancreatic injury was similar between the two groups if ampullary obstruction was cleared within 48 hours, but more than 80% of patients with ampullary obstruction for more than 48 hours developed pancreatic necrosis. A randomized controlled trial comparing early (24–48 hours) versus delayed (after 48 hours) ERCP and sphincterotomy for ABP and evidence of ampullary obstruction found significantly less morbidity for those treated within 48 hours of symptom onset.[78] Thus, benefit is likely if ductal drainage is achieved within the first 2 days. The clinical situation also dictates whether an early ERCP is indicated. For example, ERCP is indicated whenever there is evidence of symptomatic biliary obstruction, independently of when the attack started. However, there may be limited benefit, if any, even after a severe attack when ERCP is performed several days after onset of significant symptoms. Delay between clinical symptoms and presentation for medical attention is a potential uncontrollable limitation of an urgent ERCP strategy. One prospective study found that only two-thirds of patients present within 24 hours of symptom onset.[79] A retrospective study reported that 70% of patients presented for clinical attention after delay of more than 2 days.[11] Differentiating between milder initial symptoms of biliary colic and more significant pancreatic symptoms may explain this discrepancy.

What Endoscopic Therapy Should be Performed during Urgent ERCP?

There are several arguments that support doing a biliary sphincterotomy in all cases of ABP whenever urgent ERCP is done. First, most studies of ERCP in patients with ABP report that about 50% have bile duct or ampullary stones.[49,80–82] Second, biliary sphincterotomy augments pancreatic drainage in addition to ensuring bile drainage. Third, sphincter of Oddi dysfunction may contribute to the pathophysiology of ABP even after bile duct stone migration. From a retrospective study, ERCP with biliary sphincterotomy was performed in 24 of 35 patients with severe ABP even though 10 (42%) did not have bile duct stones.[82] A significantly lower incidence of pancreatic necrosis (8% vs 64%) and mortality (4% vs 36%) was observed in those who were treated with sphincterotomy compared with those who were not. Fourth, biliary sphincterotomy may protect against further attacks.[12] A retrospective study reported that patients undergoing sphincterotomy after ABP were significantly less likely to have recurrent pancreatitis independently of whether cholecystectomy was done.[83] Fifth, sphincterotomy may be adequate therapy and may delay, and perhaps obviate, cholecystectomy (discussed later). Any potential for benefit of biliary sphincterotomy must be weighed against the risk of postprocedure complications.

Different techniques in performing a sphincterotomy may be required in the setting of ABP. If there is evidence of ampullary obstruction caused by an impacted stone, a needle-knife precut sphincterotomy may need to be performed before stone extraction (Video 1). Otherwise, standard sphincterotomy techniques can be used (Video 2). Bile duct stenting without sphincterotomy may impair pancreatic drainage further, and this should be avoided unless there is evidence of life-threatening cholangitis in the setting of coagulopathy or other contraindication to sphincterotomy.

There may be some rationale for considering pancreatic drainage procedures in addition to biliary sphincterotomy at the time of urgent ERCP. Pancreatic sphincterotomy and/or stenting might augment pancreatic drainage and favorably affect the course of severe ABP. Two studies reported that main pancreatic duct disruptions are found in 30% to 44% of patients with ABP with pancreatic necrosis when ERCP is performed within 1 week of an attack.[84,85] However, early ERCP (within several days) rarely shows a pancreatic duct disruption even when there is extensive pancreatic necrosis.[84] Therefore, the decision of whether to proceed with pancreatic endotherapy cannot be made based on early pancreatography findings. Also, pancreatic instrumentation and stenting generally introduce bacterial colonization and potentially lead to infection of sterile necrosis.[86]

Recent studies have evaluated the safety of pancreatic duct stents in patients with ABP. None of the studies reported increased infections or complications after temporary pancreatic duct placement. However, the risk is primarily in patients with severe necrotizing pancreatitis, and there were limited numbers of such patients in these studies.

Fejes and colleagues[87] evaluated the feasibility and safety of urgent ERCP, defined as within 48 hours of symptom onset, and pancreatic duct stenting with short ($\leq$5 cm) small-caliber (3 or 4 F) stents as a bridging procedure in ABP. Pancreatic stents were placed if biliary cannulation was difficult or failed and/or if sphincterotomy was contraindicated. Consecutive patients (n = 87) with severe ABP had emergency ERCP; 60 underwent ERCP with sphincterotomy and stone extraction (if necessary) without pancreatic duct stenting. The remaining 27 patients had a small-caliber pancreatic stent placed. In the patients who had a pancreatic stent placed, selective biliary access, sphincterotomy, and stone extraction were difficult but successful in 14 of the 27 patients. Cannulation was unsuccessful despite needle-knife precut in 8 patients. The remaining 5 patients had successful cannulation but no sphincterotomy because of poor blood coagulation status. The stents were removed an average of 10 days after the initial ERCP procedure. Patients who had a pancreatic duct stent had a lower overall complication rate (7.4% vs 25%) and fewer complications in those with predicted severe attacks (13% vs 40%).

Another study also suggested that pancreatic duct stenting can be safe and effective in ABP to reduce the incidence of complications.[88] In a nonrandomized fashion, outcomes after pancreatic duct stenting and biliary sphincterotomy were compared with sphincterotomy alone. Patients had ERCP performed within 72 hours from onset of pain. Half the patients had a pancreatic stent insertion (5 Fr, 3–5 cm), with the main indication being a difficult cannulation. All pancreatic duct stents were removed within 10 days after ERCP. The overall complication rate in the stent group (10%) was significantly lower than in the no-stent group (31%).

Guoqian and colleagues[89] reported results from the study of patients with ABP and difficult biliary sphincterotomy who were randomly assigned to a pancreatic stent group or a no-stent group. The stents had internal flanges and were 3 to 5 Fr, and 5 to 7 cm long. All the stents were removed within 1 to 2 weeks. They reported that pancreatic duct stenting in patients with ABP lowered the overall complication rate (8% vs 32%).

Preliminary data on pancreatic duct stenting in ABP suggest that pancreatic duct placement might lead to a decrease the overall complication rate. However, the patients in these studies who received a pancreatic duct stent also had a difficult or failed biliary cannulation and/or sphincterotomy, and thus there may have been indications for prophylactic pancreatic duct stenting. In addition, the numbers of patients with severe necrotizing pancreatitis who have a high risk of introducing infection by placement of a pancreatic stent were limited. More prospective randomized trials to evaluate pancreatic duct stenting in ABP are needed, ideally in patients without difficult ERCP.

When Should Elective ERCP be Considered?

As mentioned earlier, most patients who have ABP have a mild attack that resolves with conservative care. Thus, whether to proceed with cholecystectomy and a preoperative ERCP become common questions. The important variables to consider are the patient's operative risk, the likelihood for choledocholithiasis, and the success and complication profiles of the endoscopist.

Most patients undergo cholecystectomy after recovering from ABP. Intraoperative cholangiography can be performed to determine whether postoperative ERCP is needed, so, in general, there is a limited role for preoperative ERCP. A randomized controlled trial found that selective postoperative ERCP (after positive intraoperative cholangiogram) was more cost-effective than preoperative ERCP in patients with increased risk for bile duct stones who had recovered from mild to moderate ABP.[90] However, it is reasonable to consider preoperative ERCP when a need for endoscopic therapy is strongly suspected based on clinical criteria or imaging studies. Patients who have jaundice might benefit from ERCP to diagnose and treat choledocholithiasis or other biliary tract disorders such as Mirizzi syndrome or ampullary, bile duct, or pancreatic neoplasia. In patients without jaundice, it is helpful to consider the likelihood for a retained common bile duct stone. Multivariate analysis from a prospective study on patients who had ABP found that abnormal total bilirubin on the second hospital day was the best predictor of choledocholithiasis.[91] Choledocholithiasis is uncommon (20%–30%) following a mild attack of ABP.[92,93] A decision analysis compared strategies of intraoperative cholangiography, endoscopic ultrasound, magnetic resonance cholangiopancreatography, and ERCP in patients who had mild ABP.[94] Simple observation and elective cholecystectomy with intraoperative cholangiography was the least expensive option when the probability of choledocholithiasis was less than 15%. EUS was cost-effective for an intermediate probability of choledocholithiasis, whereas ERCP was cost-effective when the probability of choledocholithiasis was greater than 45%.

Cholecystectomy after recovery from ABP remains the standard of care for patients who are good candidates for surgery. However, common sense and existing literature support the practice of sphincterotomy as primary therapy in elderly patients and those who are otherwise unfit to undergo cholecystectomy.[95–97] Outcomes after ERCP with sphincterotomy from case series of patients with ABP are notable for most patients remaining symptom free without the need for cholecystectomy.[80,98,99] A recent large retrospective study compared outcomes for patients treated with cholecystectomy with or without ERCP versus those treated with ERCP alone. The risk of recurrent pancreatitis after long-term follow-up (6%) was similar for both groups but mean age was 20 years older in the ERCP-alone group. The investigators concluded that ERCP with endoscopic therapy was an appropriate alternative to cholecystectomy in elderly (>75 years old) and in those unfit for surgery.[100]

There are scenarios in which it might be reasonable to consider elective ERCP with endopancreatic therapy in the setting of ABP.[101] Refractory symptoms or smoldering pancreatitis characterized by pain or inability to advance diet may indicate impaired pancreatic ductal drainage caused by duct disruption and/or sphincter of Oddi dysfunction. Imaging studies can be used to diagnose symptomatic acute pancreatic fluid collections or other conditions that may indicate a pancreatic duct disruption such as pleural effusion or pancreatic ascites. There is some promise for secretin-stimulated magnetic resonance cholangiopancreatography for diagnosis of pancreatic duct disruptions.[102] Transpapillary techniques have been used successfully to treat acute pancreatic duct disruptions.[103] However, pancreatic stenting to treat duct disruptions from acute pancreatitis is successful in less than 50% of cases, and may lead to infection of otherwise sterile necrosis in patients with necrotizing pancreatitis.[104]

SUMMARY

Acute pancreatitis is considered an endoscopic emergency when a biliary cause is likely and there is acute cholangitis or ongoing biliary obstruction. Biliary sphincterotomy should be considered in all patients who undergo urgent ERCP for severe ABP, preferably within 48 hours of symptom onset. Elective ERCP should be considered when there is jaundice or proven choledocholithiasis by noninvasive imaging or intraoperative cholangiography. There remains some debate regarding the role of early ERCP in the setting of ABP without evidence of biliary obstruction. Further studies should better establish the indicators for ampullary obstruction and predictors for severe attacks. Additional prospective endoscopic trials are still needed to clarify the optimal timing of biliary intervention, the potential benefit of biliary sphincterotomy in all cases independent of biliary obstruction, and the usefulness of pancreatic stenting.

SUPPLEMENTARY DATA

Supplementary data related to this article can be found online at http://dx.doi.org/10.1016/j.giec.2013.06.002.

REFERENCES

1. Van Brunschot S, Bakker O, Besselink M, et al. Treatment of necrotizing pancreatitis. Clin Gastroenterol Hepatol 2012;10:1190–201.
2. Curran FT, Neoptolemos JP. Acute biliary pancreatitis. Ann Ital Chir 1995;66(2):197–202.
3. Moreau JA, Zinsmeister AR, Melton LJ, et al. Gallstone pancreatitis and the effect of cholecystectomy: a population-based cohort study. Mayo Clin Proc 1988;63:466–73.
4. Mayer AD, McMahon MJ, Benson EA, et al. Operations upon the biliary tract in patients with acute pancreatitis: aims, indications, and timing. Ann R Coll Surg Engl 1984;66:179–83.
5. Bhatia V, Garg PK, Tandon RK, et al. Endoscopic retrograde cholangiopancreatography induced pancreatitis often has a benign outcome. J Clin Gastroenterol 2006;40:726–31.

6. Mayerle J, Simon P, Lerch MM. Medical treatment of acute pancreatitis. Gastroenterol Clin North Am 2004;33:855–69.

7. Ranson JH. The timing of biliary surgery in acute pancreatitis. Ann Surg 1979; 189:654–62.

8. Tondelli P, Harder F, Schuppisser JP, et al. Acute gallstone pancreatitis: best timing for biliary surgery. Br J Surg 1982;69:709–10.

9. Delorio AV, Vitale GC, Reynolds M, et al. Acute biliary pancreatitis: the roles of laparoscopic cholecystectomy and endoscopic retrograde cholangiopancreatography. Surg Endosc 1995;9:392–6.

10. Paloyan D, Simonowitz D, Skinner DB. The timing of biliary tract operations in patients with pancreatitis associated with gallstones. Surg Gynecol Obstet 1975;141:737–9.

11. Frei GJ, Frei VT, Thirlby RC, et al. Biliary pancreatitis: clinical presentation and surgical management. Am J Surg 1986;151:170–4.

12. Hernandez V, Pascual I, Almela P, et al. Recurrence of acute gallstone pancreatitis and relationship with cholecystectomy or endoscopic sphincterotomy. Am J Gastroenterol 2004;99:2417–23.

13. Johnson CD, Charnley R, Rowlands B, et al. UK guidelines for the management of acute pancreatitis. Gut 2005;54:iii1–9.

14. Nguyen G, Rosenberg M, Chong R, et al. Early cholecystectomy and ERCP are associated with reduced readmissions for acute biliary pancreatitis: a nationwide, population-based study. Gastrointest Endosc 2012;75(1):47–55.

15. Opie EL. The etiology of acute hemorrhagic pancreatitis. Bull Johns Hopkins Hosp 1901;12:182–8.

16. Acosta JM, Rossi R, Galli OM, et al. Early surgery for acute gallstone pancreatitis: evaluation of a systematic approach. Surgery 1978;83(4):367–70.

17. Armstrong CP, Taylor TV, Jeacock J, et al. The biliary tract in patients with acute gallstone pancreatitis. Br J Surg 1985;72:551–5.

18. Kelly TR. Gallstone pancreatitis: pathophysiology. Surgery 1976;80(4):488–92.

19. Acosta JM, Ledesma CL. Gallstone migration as a cause of acute pancreatitis. N Engl J Med 1974;290:484–7.

20. Houssin D, Castaing D, Lemoine J, et al. Microlithiasis of the gallbladder. Surg Gynecol Obstet 1983;157:20–4.

21. Diehl AK, Holleman DR, Chapman JB, et al. Gallstone size and risk of pancreatitis. Arch Intern Med 1997;157:1674–8.

22. Venneman NG, Buskens E, Besselink MG, et al. Small gallstones are associated with increased risk of acute pancreatitis: potential benefits of prophylactic cholecystectomy? Am J Gastroenterol 2005;100:2540–50.

23. Venneman NG, Renooij W, Rehfeld JF, et al. Small gallstones, preserved gallbladder motility, and fast crystallization are associated with pancreatitis. Hepatology 2005;41:738–46.

24. Jones BA, Salsberg BB, Mehta MH, et al. Common pancreaticobiliary channels and their relationship to gallstone size in gallstone pancreatitis. Ann Surg 1987; 205(2):123–5.

25. Lerch MM, Weidenbach H, Hernandez CA, et al. Pancreatic outflow obstruction as the critical event for human gallstone-induced pancreatitis. Gut 1994;35: 1501–3.

26. Hernandez CA, Lerch MM. Sphincter stenosis and gallstone migration through the biliary tract. Lancet 1993;341:1371–3.

27. Armstrong CP, Taylor TV. Pancreatic duct reflux and acute gallstone pancreatitis. Ann Surg 1986;204(1):59–64.

28. Oria A, Alvarez J, Chiappetta L, et al. Risk factors for acute pancreatitis in patients with migrating gallstones. Arch Surg 1989;124:1295–6.
29. Krusyna T, Zajac A, Karcz D. Sphincter of Oddi manometry in patients with acute biliary pancreatitis: evidence for sphincter of Oddi dysfunction in acute biliary pancreatitis. Scand J Gastroenterol 2004;39:696–7.
30. Nowak A, Nowakowska-Dutawa E, Rybicka J. Patency of the Santorini duct and acute biliary pancreatitis. A prospective ERCP study. Endoscopy 1990;22:124–6.
31. Kueppers PM, Russell DH, Moody FG. Reversibility of pancreatitis after temporary pancreaticobiliary duct obstruction in rats. Pancreas 1993;8:632–7.
32. Runzi M, Saluja A, Lerch MM. Early ductal decompression prevents the progression of biliary pancreatitis: an experimental study in the opossum. Gastroenterology 1993;105:157–64.
33. Lerch MM, Saluja AK, Runzi M, et al. Pancreatic duct obstruction triggers acute necrotizing pancreatitis in the opossum. Gastroenterology 1993;104:853–61.
34. Lerch MM, Saluja AK, Dawra R, et al. Acute necrotizing pancreatitis in the opossum: earliest morphological changes involve acinar cells. Gastroenterology 1992;103:205–13.
35. Norman J. The role of cytokines in the pathogenesis of acute pancreatitis. Am J Surg 1998;175:76–83.
36. Norman JG. New approaches to acute pancreatitis: role of inflammatory mediators. Digestion 1999;60(Suppl 1):57–60.
37. Acosta JM, Pellegrini CA, Skinner DB. Etiology and pathogenesis of acute biliary pancreatitis. Surgery 1980;88:118–23.
38. Stone HH, Fabian TC, Dunlop WE. Gallstone pancreatitis: biliary tract pathology in relation to time of operation. Ann Surg 1981;194(3):305–10.
39. Kelly TR, Wagner DS. Gallstone pancreatitis: a prospective randomized trial of the timing of surgery. Surgery 1988;104:600–5.
40. Van der Spuy S. Endoscopic sphincterotomy in the management of gallstone pancreatitis. Endoscopy 1981;13:25–6.
41. Safrany L, Cotton PB. A preliminary report: urgent duodenoscopic sphincterotomy for acute gallstone pancreatitis. Surgery 1981;89:424–8.
42. Rosseland AR, Solhaug JH. Early or delayed endoscopic papillotomy in gallstone pancreatitis. Ann Surg 1984;199(2):165–7.
43. Sharma VK, Howden CW. Meta-analysis of randomized controlled trials of endoscopic retrograde cholangiography and endoscopic sphincterotomy for the treatment of acute biliary pancreatitis. Am J Gastroenterol 1999;94(11):3211–4.
44. Petrov M, van Santvoort H, Besselink M, et al. Early endoscopic retrograde cholangiopancreatography versus conservative management in acute biliary pancreatitis without cholangitis: a meta-analysis of randomized trials. Ann Surg 2008;247(2):250–7.
45. Uy M, Daez M, Sy P, et al. Early ERCP in acute gallstone pancreatitis without cholangitis: a meta-analysis. JOP 2009;10(3):299–305.
46. Tse F, Yuan Y. Early routine endoscopic retrograde cholangiopancreatography strategy versus early conservative management strategy in acute gallstone pancreatitis. Cochrane Database Syst Rev 2012;(5):CD009779.
47. Neoptolemos JP, Carr-Locke DL, London NJ, et al. Controlled trial of urgent endoscopic retrograde cholangiopancreatography and endoscopic sphincterotomy versus conservative treatment for acute pancreatitis due to gallstones. Lancet 1988;2:979–83.
48. Fan ST, Lai EC, Mok FP, et al. Early treatment of acute biliary pancreatitis by endoscopic papillotomy. N Engl J Med 1993;328:228–32.

49. Folsch UR, Nitsche R, Ludtke R, et al. Early ERCP and papillotomy compared with conservative treatment for acute biliary pancreatitis. N Engl J Med 1997; 336(4):237–42.

50. Zhou M, Li N, Lu R. Duodenoscopy in treatment of acute gallstone pancreatitis. Hepatobiliary Pancreat Dis Int 2002;1(4):608–10.

51. Oría A, Cimmino D, Ocampo C, et al. Early endoscopic intervention versus early conservative management in patients with acute gallstone pancreatitis and biliopancreatic obstruction: a randomized clinical trial. Ann Surg 2007;245(1):10–7.

52. Van Santvoort HC, Besselink M, Vries A, et al. Early endoscopic retrograde cholangiopancreatography in predicted severe acute biliary pancreatitis: a prospective multicenter study. Ann Surg 2009;250(1):68–75.

53. Chen P, Hu B, Wang C, et al. Pilot study of urgent endoscopic intervention without fluoroscopy on patients with severe acute biliary pancreatitis in the intensive care unit. Pancreas 2010;39(3):398–402.

54. Nowak A, Nowakowska-Dulawa E, Marek TA, et al. Final results of the prospective, randomized, controlled study on endoscopic sphincterotomy versus conventional management in acute biliary pancreatitis. Gastroenterology 1995; 108(4):A380.

55. Nowak A, Nowakowska-Dulawa E, Marek TA, et al. Timing of endoscopic sphincterotomy for acute biliary pancreatitis: a prospective study. Gastrointest Endosc 1996;43(4):391.

56. French Consensus Conference on Acute Pancreatitis: conclusions and recommendations. Eur J Gastroenterol Hepatol 2001;13(Suppl 4):S3–13.

57. Tenner S, Dubner H, Steinberg W. Predicting gallstone pancreatitis with laboratory parameters: a meta-analysis. Am J Gastroenterol 1994;89:1863–6.

58. Neoptolemos JP, Hall AW, Finlay DF, et al. The urgent diagnosis of gallstones in acute pancreatitis: a prospective study of three methods. Br J Surg 1984;71:230–3.

59. Wang SS, Lin XZ, Tsai YT, et al. Clinical significance of ultrasonography, computed tomography, and biochemical tests in the rapid diagnosis of gallstone-related pancreatitis: a prospective study. Pancreas 1988;3:153–8.

60. Acosta JM, Ronzano GD, Pellegrini CA. Ampullary obstruction monitoring in acute gallstone pancreatitis: a safe, accurate, and reliable method to detect pancreatic ductal obstruction. Am J Gastroenterol 2000;95:122–7.

61. Scheiman JM, Carlos RC, Barnett JL, et al. Can endoscopic ultrasound or magnetic resonance cholangiopancreatography replace ERCP in patients with suspected biliary disease? A prospective trial and cost analysis. Am J Gastroenterol 2001;96:2900–4.

62. Canto MI, Chak A, Stellato T, et al. Endoscopic ultrasonography versus cholangiography for the diagnosis of choledocholithiasis. Gastrointest Endosc 1998; 47:439–48.

63. Okan I, Bas G, Sahin M, et al. Diagnostic value of MRCP in biliary pancreatitis: results of long-term follow up. Acta Chir Belg 2012;112:359–64.

64. Banks PA, Freeman ML. Practice guidelines in acute pancreatitis. Am J Gastroenterol 2006;101:2379–400.

65. Ranson JH. Etiologic and prognostic factors in human acute pancreatitis: a review. Am J Gastroenterol 1982;77:633–8.

66. Blamey SL, Imrie CW, O'Neill J, et al. Prognostic factors in acute pancreatitis. Gut 1984;25:1340–6.

67. De Bernardinis M, Violi V, Roncoroni L, et al. Discriminant power and information content of Ranson's prognostic signs in acute pancreatitis: a meta-analytic study. Crit Care Med 1999;10:2272–83.

68. Johnson CD, Toh SK, Campbell MJ. Combination of APACHE-II score and an obesity score (APACHE-O) for the prediction of severe acute pancreatitis. Pancreatology 2004;4:1–6.
69. Brown A, Orav J, Banks PA. Hemoconcentration is an early marker for organ failure and necrotizing pancreatitis. Pancreas 2000;20:367–72.
70. Brown A, Baillargeon JD, Hughes MD, et al. Can fluid resuscitation prevent pancreatic necrosis in severe acute pancreatitis? Pancreatology 2002;2:104–7.
71. Lankisch PG, Mahlke R, Blum T, et al. Hemoconcentration: an early marker of severe and/or necrotizing pancreatitis? A critical appraisal. Am J Gastroenterol 2001;96:2081–5.
72. Singh V, Wu B, Bollen T, et al. A prospective evaluation of the bedside index for severity in acute pancreatitis score in assessing mortality and intermediate markers of severity in acute pancreatitis. Am J Gastroenterol 2009;104: 966–71.
73. Bradley EL 3rd. A clinically based classification system for acute pancreatitis. Summary of the International Symposium on Acute Pancreatitis, Atlanta, GA, September 11 through 13, 1992. Arch Surg 1993;128:586–90.
74. Banks PA, Bollen TL, Dervenis C, et al. Classification of acute pancreatitis–2012: revision of the Atlanta classification and definitions by international consensus. Gut 2013;62:102–11.
75. Uhl W, Warshaw A, Imrie C, et al. IAP guidelines for the surgical management of acute pancreatitis. Pancreatology 2002;2(6):565–73.
76. Isenmann R, Buchler M, Waldemar U, et al. Pancreatic necrosis: an early finding in severe acute pancreatitis. Pancreas 1993;8:358–61.
77. Acosta JM, Rubio Galli OM, Rossi R, et al. Effect of duration of ampullary gallstone obstruction on severity of lesions of acute pancreatitis. J Am Coll Surg 1997;184:499–505.
78. Acosta JM, Katkhouda N, Debian KA, et al. Early ductal decompression versus conservative management for gallstone pancreatitis with ampullary obstruction: a prospective randomized clinical trial. Ann Surg 2006;243:33–40.
79. Levy P, Borouchowicz A, Hastier P, et al. Diagnostic criteria in predicting a biliary origin of acute pancreatitis in the era of endoscopic ultrasound: multicenter prospective evaluation of 213 patients. Pancreatology 2005;5:450–6.
80. Liu CL, Lo CM, Fan ST, et al. Acute biliary pancreatitis: diagnosis and management. World J Surg 1997;21:149–54.
81. Gislason H, Vetrhus M, Horn A, et al. Endoscopic sphincterotomy in acute gallstone pancreatitis: a prospective study of the late outcome. Eur J Surg 2001; 167:204–8.
82. Besselink MG, Van Minnen LP, Bosscha K, et al. Beneficial effects of ERCP and papillotomy in predicted severe biliary pancreatitis. Hepatogastroenterology 2005;52:37–9.
83. Hammarstrom LE, Stridbeck H, Ihse I. Effect of endoscopic sphincterotomy and interval cholecystectomy on late outcome after gallstone pancreatitis. Br J Surg 1988;85:333–6.
84. Neoptolemos JP, London NJ, Carr-Locke DL. Assessment of main pancreatic duct integrity by endoscopic retrograde pancreatography in patients with acute pancreatitis. Br J Surg 1993;80:94–9.
85. Uomo G, Molino D, Visconti M, et al. The incidence of main pancreatic duct disruption in severe biliary pancreatitis. Am J Surg 1998;176:49–52.
86. Kozarek R, Hovde O, Attia F, et al. Do pancreatic duct stents cause or prevent pancreatic sepsis? Gastrointest Endosc 2003;58(4):505–9.

87. Fejes R, Kurucsai G, Szekely A, et al. Feasibility and safety of emergency ERCP and small-caliber pancreatic stenting as a bridging procedure in patients with acute biliary pancreatitis but difficult sphincterotomy. Surg Endosc 2010;24:1878–85.

88. Dubravcsik Z, Hritz I, Fejes R, et al. Early ERCP and biliary sphincterotomy with or without small-caliber pancreatic stent insertion in patients with acute biliary pancreatitis: better overall outcome with adequate pancreatic drainage. Scand J Gastroenterol 2012;47:729–36.

89. Guoqian D, Mingfang Q, Wang C, et al. The safety and utility of pancreatic duct stents in the emergency ERCP of acute biliary pancreatitis but difficult sphincterotomy. Hepatogastroenterology 2012;59(120):2374–6.

90. Chang L, Lo S, Stabile BE, et al. Preoperative versus postoperative endoscopic retrograde cholangiopancreatography in mild to moderate gallstone pancreatitis: a prospective randomized trial. Ann Surg 2000;231:82–7.

91. Chang L, Lo SK, Stabile BE, et al. Gallstone pancreatitis: a prospective study on the incidence of cholangitis and clinical predictors of retained common bile duct stones. Am J Gastroenterol 1998;93(4):527–31.

92. Neoptolemos JP. The theory of persisting common bile duct stones in severe gallstone pancreatitis. Ann R Coll Surg Engl 1989;71:326–31.

93. Hallal AH, Amortegui JD, Jeroukhimov IM, et al. Magnetic resonance cholangiopancreatography accurately detects common bile duct stones in resolving gallstone pancreatitis. J Am Coll Surg 2005;200:869–75.

94. Arguedas MR, Dupont AW, Wilcox CM. Where do ERCP, endoscopic ultrasound, magnetic resonance cholangiopancreatography, and intraoperative cholangiography fit in the management of acute biliary pancreatitis? A decision analysis model. Am J Gastroenterol 2001;96:2892–9.

95. Siegel JH, Veerappan A, Cohen SA, et al. Endoscopic sphincterotomy for biliary pancreatitis: an alternative to cholecystectomy in high-risk patients. Gastrointest Endosc 1994;40:573–5.

96. Welbourn CR, Beckly DE, Eyre-Brook IA. Endoscopic sphincterotomy without cholecystectomy for gallstone pancreatitis. Gut 1995;37:119–20.

97. Uomo G, Manes G, Laccetti M, et al. Endoscopic sphincterotomy and recurrence of acute pancreatitis in gallstone patients considered unfit for surgery. Pancreas 1997;14(1):28–31.

98. Vazquez-Iglesias JL, Gonzalez-Conde B, Lopez-Roses L, et al. Endoscopic sphincterotomy for prevention of the recurrence of acute biliary pancreatitis in patients with gallbladder in situ. Surg Endosc 2004;18:1442–6.

99. Kaw M, Al-Antably Y, Kaw P. Management of gallstone pancreatitis: cholecystectomy or ERCP and endoscopic sphincterotomy. Gastrointest Endosc 2002; 56(1):61–5.

100. Bignell M, Dearing M, Hindmarsh A, et al. ERCP and endoscopic sphincterotomy (ES): a safe and definitive management of gallstone pancreatitis with the gallbladder left in situ. J Gastrointest Surg 2011;15:2205–10.

101. Lau ST, Simchuk EJ, Kozarek RA, et al. A pancreatic ductal leak should be sought to direct treatment in patients with acute pancreatitis. Am J Surg 2001;181:411–5.

102. Arvanitakis M, Delhaye M, De Maertelaere V, et al. Computed tomography and magnetic resonance imaging in the assessment of acute pancreatitis. Gastroenterology 2004;126:715–23.

103. Kozarek R. Role of ERCP in acute pancreatitis. Gastrointest Endosc 2002; 56(Suppl 6):S231–6.

104. Telford JJ, Farrell JJ, Saltzman JR, et al. Pancreatic stent placement for duct disruption. Gastrointest Endosc 2002;56(1):18–24.

Preventing Pancreatitis after Endoscopic Retrograde Cholangiopancreatography

Nisa M. Kubiliun, MD, B. Joseph Elmunzer, MD*

KEYWORDS

- Endoscopic retrograde cholangiopancreatography • ERCP • Pancreatitis
- Post-ERCP pancreatitis • Complications

KEY POINTS

- Risk stratification and thoughtful patient selection are critical in preventing post-ERCP pancreatitis; in this era of highly accurate diagnostic alternatives, ERCP should be a near-exclusively therapeutic procedure.
- In the case of difficult cannulation, alternate techniques, such as double-wire cannulation and precut sphincterotomy, should be implemented early.
- Contrast-facilitated cannulation, aggressive/repeated pancreatic injection, dilation of an intact biliary sphincter, and sphincter of Oddi manometry without aspiration should be avoided.
- Prophylactic pancreatic stents should be placed in all high-risk cases.
- Rectal nonsteroidal antiinflammatory drugs should be administered in all high-risk cases and based on a very favorable risk-benefit ratio, should be considered in all patients undergoing ERCP.

OVERVIEW

Post–endoscopic retrograde cholangiopancreatography (ERCP) pancreatitis (PEP) is defined as new or increased abdominal pain that is clinically consistent with a syndrome of acute pancreatitis, pancreatic enzyme elevation at least 3 times the upper limit of normal 24 hours after the procedure, and resultant hospitalization (or prolongation of existing hospitalization) by more than 1 night.[1] Pancreatitis is still the most common complication of ERCP, occurring in 2% to 10% of cases and accounting for substantial morbidity, occasional mortality, and health care expenditures in excess of $150 million annually in the United States.[2–4] Despite substantial advances over

The authors have no conflicts of interest to disclose.
Division of Gastroenterology, University of Michigan Medical Center, 3912 Taubman Center, Ann Arbor, MI 48109, USA
* Corresponding author.
E-mail address: badihe@umich.edu

the last several decades in patient selection, equipment, procedural technique, and prophylactic interventions, PEP remains a serious health problem, and its prevention remains a major clinical and research priority. Herein is an evidence-based review of approaches to prevent pancreatitis after ERCP, as well as suggestions for necessary research objectives in this important area.

RECOGNIZING PATIENTS AT INCREASED RISK FOR PEP

PEP prevention begins with recognition of patients at increased risk, because a high index of suspicion for and early identification of post-ERCP pancreatitis are critically important in ensuring favorable clinical outcomes. The ability to risk stratify patients based on well-established clinical characteristics can concretely influence the decision-making process that surrounds PEP prevention and the management of its potentially devastating sequelae. Armed with the risk assessment information outlined later in the discussion, clinicians can tailor costly and potentially dangerous risk-reducing strategies. For example, prophylactic pancreatic stent placement (PSP) and consideration of post-procedure hospital observation are appropriate for a patient predicted to be at high risk for PEP but are not justified in low-risk cases.

A substantial amount of research over the last 2 decades has contributed to the understanding of the independent risk factors for post-ERCP pancreatitis. These risk factors, listed in **Table 1**, are divided into patient-related and procedure-related characteristics. The definite and probable patient-related risk factors that predispose to PEP are a clinical suspicion of sphincter of Oddi dysfunction (SOD) (regardless of whether or not sphincter of Oddi manometry is performed)[3,5–10]; a history of prior PEP[5,11–13]; and a history of recurrent pancreatitis,[6] normal bilirubin,[5,14] younger age,[11,15,16] and female gender.[5,6,16] The definite and probable procedure-related risk factors for PEP are difficult cannulation,[3,5,13] precut (access) sphincterotomy,[3,6,13] pancreatic sphincterotomy,[5,11] ampullectomy,[17,18] repeated or aggressive pancreatography,[3,5,6,15] balloon dilation of an intact biliary sphincter,[19–21] and possibly passage of a guidewire deep into the pancreatic duct (PD).[22] An important risk-stratification principle is that predictors of PEP appear synergistic in nature.[5] For example, a widely referenced multicenter study by Freeman and colleagues,[5] predating prophylactic PSP, showed that a young woman with a clinical suspicion of SOD, normal bilirubin, and a difficult cannulation has a risk of PEP in excess of 40%. Of note, biliary sphincterotomy and Billroth 2 anatomy do not appear to predispose to PEP.

Patient-related characteristics are not modifiable but can be used (at least in part) to predict the risk of PEP before ERCP, allowing appropriate case selection and a meaningful discussion with the patient regarding the risk-benefit ratio of the procedure. For

Table 1
Independent risk factors for post-ERCP pancreatitis

Patient-related Factors	Procedure-related Factors
Suspected sphincter of Oddi dysfunction (SOD)	Difficult cannulation
Prior post-ERCP pancreatitis	Precut (access) sphincterotomy
Normal bilirubin	Pancreatic sphincterotomy
Younger age	Ampullectomy
Female gender	Repeated or aggressive pancreatography
History of recurrent pancreatitis	Balloon dilation of an intact biliary sphincter

example, a young woman with suspected biliary SOD but moderate symptoms that are partially responsive to pain-modulating therapy may elect to forgo ERCP after understanding her elevated risk of severe PEP.

Procedural risk factors may occasionally be modified during the case (see later discussion) but in combination with patient-related factors, allow a global assessment of a patient's overall risk profile, guiding the implementation of appropriate prophylactic interventions, such as aggressive intravenous fluid administration, rectal indomethacin, PSP, and a lower threshold for hospital observation after the procedure.

Operator (endoscopist)-dependent characteristics have also been implicated in the risk of PEP. Endoscopist procedure volume is suggested to be a risk factor for PEP, although multicenter studies have not confirmed this trend, presumably because low-volume endoscopists tend to perform lower-risk cases.[3,5,15,23] Nevertheless, potentially dangerous cases (based on either patient-related factors or anticipated high-risk interventions) are best referred to expert medical centers where a high-volume endoscopist with expertise in prophylactic PSP can perform the case and where more experience with rescue from serious complications may improve clinical outcomes.[24,25] Similarly, trainee involvement in ERCP is a possible independent risk factor for PEP, although results of existing multivariable analyses are conflicting.[5,10] It stands to reason that inexperienced trainees may augment procedure-related risk factors, such as prolonging a difficult cannulation or delivering excess electrosurgical current during an inefficient pancreatic sphincterotomy, etc. Therefore, an improved understanding of the process of ERCP training is necessary to minimize the contribution of trainee involvement to the development of PEP. Future research focused on defining ERCP training metrics and developing an evidence-based list of appropriate fellow cases based on stage of training and skill level is needed. Further, defining the optimal parameters that guide trainee-attending scope exchange during any particular case or intervention is necessary to maximize learning potential while minimizing patient risk.

Several additional points regarding clinical risk stratification are worth considering. First, patients with a clinical suspicion of SOD, particularly women, are not only at increased risk for PEP in general, but are also more likely to develop severe pancreatitis and death.[3,5,26] When considering the risk-benefit ratio of ERCP in this patient population, not only should the patient's overall risk of PEP be assessed, but their probability of experiencing a more dramatic clinical course should also be considered and discussed. An additional consideration is that several clinical characteristics are thought to significantly reduce the risk of PEP. First, biliary interventions in patients with a preexisting biliary sphincterotomy probably confer a very low risk of PEP. Prior sphincterotomy will have generally separated the biliary and pancreatic orifices (**Fig. 1**), allowing avoidance of the pancreas and making pancreatic sphincter or duct trauma unlikely. Further, patients with chronic pancreatitis, in particular those with calcific pancreatitis, are at low risk for PEP because of gland atrophy, fibrosis, and consequent decrease in exocrine enzymatic activity.[5] Similarly, the progressive decline in pancreatic exocrine function associated with aging may protect older patients from pancreatic injury.[27] Lastly, perhaps because of post-obstructive parenchymal atrophy, patients with pancreatic head malignancy appear to be relatively protected as well.[28]

Although understanding these aforementioned risk factors and incorporating them into clinical decision-making are important aspects of preventing PEP, additional research focused on developing more robust risk-stratification tools based on existing literature and future multicenter studies is important. Such risk stratification instruments are unlikely to be developed using conventional statistical models (ie, multivariable

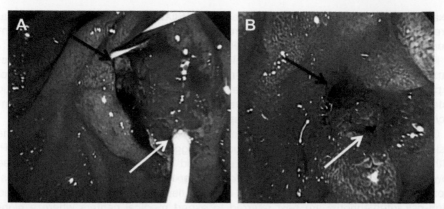

Fig. 1. Endoscopic images demonstrating the separation between biliary orifice (*black arrow*) and pancreatic orifice (*white arrow*) that results from biliary sphincterotomy, during the procedure (*A*) and 6 weeks after sphincterotomy (*B*; different patient).

regression analysis) but may require the use of novel, more advanced prediction methods involving artificial intelligence, such as machine learning, a technique that has already been successfully utilized in both business and medicine.[29] In addition, a more specific understanding of how these tools' output should concretely direct clinical management is necessary.

PATIENT SELECTION

Thoughtful patient selection before ERCP remains a fundamental strategy for preventing pancreatitis. Endoscopic ultrasound (EUS) and magnetic resonance cholangio-pancreatography (MRCP) allow highly accurate pancreaticobiliary imaging while avoiding the significant risks of ERCP.[30–32] Two large meta-analyses have demonstrated that EUS is highly sensitive and specific in the detection of bile duct stones (sensitivity 89%–94%; specificity 94%–95%).[33,34] Similarly, MRCP has a sensitivity of 85% to 92% and a specificity of 93% to 97% for the same indication,[32,35] although magnetic resonance imaging (MRI) appears less sensitive than EUS for stones smaller than 6 mm.[36,37] Additionally, EUS, MRI, and other noninvasive modalities such as radionucleotide-labeled scan and percutaneous drain fluid analysis are very accurate in diagnosing a multitude of other pancreaticobiliary processes (eg, chronic pancreatitis, malignancy, and leaks), often obviating the need for ERCP.[38–40]

Indeed, the utilization of ERCP as a diagnostic procedure has steadily declined in favor of less invasive but equally accurate alternative tests, and ERCP has appropriately become a near-exclusively therapeutic procedure reserved for patients with a high pretest probability of intervention.[41,42] This trend is consistent with recent clinical practice guidelines on the role of endoscopy in the evaluation of choledocholithiasis and the National Institutes of Health consensus statement on ERCP for diagnosis and therapy, both favoring less-invasive tests over ERCP in the *diagnosis* of biliary disease.[43,44]

An exception to the widespread practice of reserving ERCP for patients with a high likelihood of therapeutic intervention is the evaluation of patients with suspected SOD, for which an accurate, less-invasive alternative to ERCP-guided sphincter of Oddi manometry (SOM) remains elusive.[45,46] Even when considering patients for SOM, however, thoughtful clinical judgment is necessary to select those who are most likely to benefit from the procedure. An ongoing multicenter clinical trial (the EPISOD study) evaluating the role of ERCP in patients with suspected SOD but no laboratory or radiographic abnormalities will help clarify the risk-benefit ratio of ERCP for this population and hopefully allow improved patient selection in this challenging context.[47] Another possible exception to the therapeutic ERCP trend may be the evaluation of biliary complications in liver transplant recipients, for whom a recent retrospective study suggested that *diagnostic* ERCP is a reasonable and efficient clinical approach in this patient population based on a high likelihood of therapeutic intervention and a very low rate of complications, in particular PEP.[48]

PROCEDURE TECHNIQUE

Efficient and atraumatic technical practices during ERCP are central to minimizing the risk of pancreatitis. Many of the procedure-related risk factors listed earlier, while predisposing to PEP, are mandatory elements of a successful case. Even though these high-risk interventions are unavoidable for execution of the clinical objective, certain strategies can be utilized to minimize procedure-related risk.

As mentioned, difficult cannulation and PD injection are both independent risk factors for PEP. As such, interventions that improve the efficiency of cannulation and limit injection of contrast into the pancreas are likely to decrease the risk of pancreatitis. Guidewire-assisted cannulation accomplishes both, representing a major paradigm shift in ERCP practice. In contrast to conventional contrast-assisted cannulation, which may lead to inadvertent injection of the PD or contribute to papillary edema, guidewire-assisted cannulation uses a small-diameter wire with a hydrophilic tip that is initially advanced into the duct, subsequently guiding passage of the catheter. Because the wire is thinner and more maneuverable than the cannula, it is easier to advance across a potentially narrow and off-angle orifice. Moreover, this process limits the likelihood of an inadvertent pancreatic or intramural papillary injection. A recent Cochrane Collaboration meta-analysis, which included 12 randomized controlled trials (RCTs) involving 3450 subjects, indeed confirms that guidewire-assisted cannulation reduces the risk of PEP by approximately 50% (relative risk [RR] 0.51, 95% confidence interval [CI] 0.32–0.82).[49] A more recent prospective cohort study enrolling a mix of high-risk and low-risk subjects revealed no difference in PEP between the contrast and guidewire-assisted groups[50]; however, the results of this study have been questioned for a multitude of reasons, including the selection bias introduced by the nonrandomized design of the study.[51] When wire cannulation is used for biliary access, it is important to advance the guidewire cautiously in the event in case it is actually in the PD where forceful advancement of the wire may induce pancreatitis by perforating a sidebranch.

When initial cannulation attempts are unsuccessful, several alternative techniques are available to facilitate biliary access. The double wire technique is a common second-line approach when initial cannulation attempts result in repeated unintentional passage of the wire into the pancreas. The wire can be left in the PD, thereby straightening the common channel and partially occluding the pancreatic orifice, allowing subsequent biliary cannulation alongside the existing pancreatic wire. The double wire technique has been shown to improve cannulation success compared with standard methods,[52] although some data suggest a higher incidence of PEP with this technique or when a wire is passed inadvertently into the PD.[22,53] Furthermore, a recent RCT of difficult-cannulation cases requiring double wire technique demonstrated that prophylactic PSP reduced the incidence of PEP by approximately 90% in this patient population.[54] On this basis, some experts believe that a prophylactic pancreatic stent should be placed in all patients requiring double wire cannulation or when the wire inadvertently passes more than once into the pancreas. Others, including the authors, however, believe that placement of a wire in the pancreas does not independently predispose to PEP and that pancreatitis in this context is generally related to the preceding difficult cannulation. If the double wire technique is used early in a low-risk patient (within 2–3 cannulation attempts) and the wire advances seamlessly into the PD in a typical pancreatic trajectory, PSP may not be necessary.

Additional alternative cannulation techniques include wire cannulation alongside a pancreatic stent, precut sphincterotomy, septotomy, and needle-knife fistulotomy.[55,56] Although these techniques are immensely helpful in gaining biliary access during challenging cases, some have been implicated as procedure-related risk factors for PEP. In many cases, however, the risk of PEP is actually driven by the preceding prolonged cannulation time that leads to increasing papillary trauma/edema. Therefore, implementing alternate cannulation techniques early in the case and in rapid succession is an important aspect of reducing PEP. This principle is best demonstrated by a recent meta-analysis of 6 randomized trials, which showed that early precut sphincterotomy significantly reduced the risk of PEP when compared with repeated standard cannulation attempts (2.5% vs 5.3%, odds ratio 0.47).[57] However, the studies included in this meta-analysis were conducted in mostly low-risk patients, often with favorable anatomy for precut sphincterotomy. Further studies are needed to define the exact point at which the risk-benefit ratio favors precut sphincterotomy over repeated cannulation attempts, although the natural tendency to continue standard cannulation attempts beyond 5 to 10 minutes should be controlled, and alternative strategies should be attempted early in a difficult case.

Other technical strategies that reduce the risk of PEP include avoiding the frequency and vigor of PD injection, performing SOM using the aspiration technique[58] and avoiding balloon dilation of an intact biliary sphincter, especially without prophylactic PSP. In coagulopathic patients with choledocholithiasis and native papillae, balloon dilation can be avoided by providing real-time decompression with a bile duct stent and repeating the ERCP with sphincterotomy and stone extraction when coagulation parameters have been restored. If this is not possible, and balloon dilation is mandatory, longer duration dilation (2–5 minutes) appears to result in lower rates of pancreatitis compared with 1-minute dilation.[59] Of note is that balloon dilation *after* biliary sphincterotomy to facilitate large-stone extraction does not appear to increase the risk of PEP.[60,61] All these factors are modifiable and should be considered during every ERCP.

PROCEDURE EQUIPMENT

Recent advances in ERCP equipment have increased technical success rates but have unfortunately not reduced the risk of post-ERCP pancreatitis.[62] In particular, the use of a sphincterotome or a steerable catheter has been shown to improve cannulation success compared with a standard cannula but does not result in lower PEP rates.[63] Similarly, comparative effectiveness studies evaluating sphincterotomes of various diameters have shown no difference in the risk of PEP.[64,65] There are no comparative effectiveness data evaluating the effect of various guidewires on the risk of pancreatitis.[66]

Along these same lines, the type of contrast medium used during pancreatography does not appear to affect the incidence of PEP,[67] and it remains unclear (but unlikely) that the now commonly used automated electrosurgical current delivery systems offer any protection over the previously popular pure-cut current for thermal injury–induced pancreatitis.[68]

Overall, it appears that equipment has little to no impact on post-ERCP pancreatitis. Therefore, practitioners should use the devices with which they are most comfortable for any particular indication to maximize technical success and efficiency, the latter of which is likely inversely related to the risk of PEP.

PROPHYLACTIC PANCREATIC STENT PLACEMENT

One of many proposed mechanisms of PEP implicates impaired PD drainage caused by trauma-induced edema of the papilla. PSP is therefore thought to reduce the risk of PEP by relieving PD hypertension that develops as a result of transient procedure–induced stenosis of the pancreatic orifice. Eight RCTs (>650 subjects) and at least 10 nonrandomized trials have consistently demonstrated that PSP reduces the risk of PEP by approximately 60% to 80%.[69,70] In the most recently published meta-analysis of RCTs, PSP resulted in an absolute PEP risk reduction of 13.3% (95% CI, 8.8%–17.8%) with a number needed to treat to prevent 1 episode of 8 (95% CI, 6–11).[69] Equally importantly, prophylactic pancreatic stents appear to profoundly reduce the likelihood of severe and necrotizing pancreatitis.[69,70]

It is important to keep in mind that the demonstrated benefits of PSP must be weighed against several potential disadvantages. First, attempting to place a PD stent with subsequent failure actually increases the risk of PEP above baseline by inducing injury to the pancreatic orifice but providing no subsequent ductal decompression.[71,72] Second, significant nonpancreatitis complications induced by PSP, such as stent migration and duct perforation, occur in 4.4% of cases.[70] Further, prolonged stent retention may induce ductal changes that resemble chronic pancreatitis,[73] although the long-term clinical relevance of these changes remains unclear. PSP is associated with some patient inconvenience and increased costs by mandating follow-up abdominal radiography to ensure spontaneous passage of the stent and additional upper endoscopy to retrieve retained stents in 5% to 10% of cases.[74,75]

Despite these considerations, PSP is widely regarded as an effective means of preventing PEP, is commonly used in academic medical centers in the United States,[76] and is recommended by the European Society of Gastrointestinal Endoscopy.[17] In light of the aforementioned concerns and the associated costs, however, PSP should be reserved for high-risk cases.[17,77] Based on the known independent patient and procedure-related risk factors for PEP, experts have suggested that the following cases are appropriate for prophylactic PD stent placement: (1) clinical suspicion of SOD (whether or not manometry or therapeutic intervention performed), (2) prior PEP, (3) difficult cannulation, (4) precut (access) sphincterotomy, (5) pancreatic sphincterotomy (major or minor papilla), (6) endoscopic ampullectomy, (7) aggressive instrumentation or injection of the PD, and (8) balloon dilation of an intact biliary sphincter.[76,78] Furthermore, a preliminary study has suggested that "salvage" PSP may be beneficial early in the course of PEP for patients who did not originally receive a stent or in the case of early stent dislodgement.[79] Additional studies are necessary to fully evaluate PSP for this indication.

Several questions regarding optimization of the PSP process remain. First, there is limited consensus regarding the optimal stent length and caliber.[76] An early study suggested improved outcomes with 3-F or 4-F stents[80]; however, a subsequent RCT showed no difference in PEP rates but a higher insertion success rate with the 5-F stents.[75] Similarly, there is little consensus regarding optimal stent length. Most experts agree that the intrapancreatic tip of the stent should not rest at the pancreatic genu (**Fig. 2**)[78]; however, whether short stents (ending in the pancreatic head) or

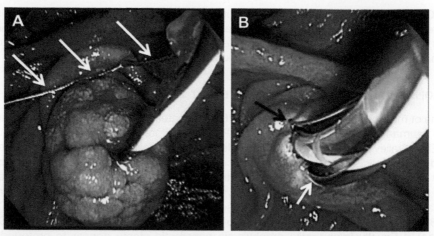

Fig. 2. Endoscopic images demonstrating secure guidewire access to the pancreas (for subsequent prophylactic stent placement) before therapeutic intervention. (*A*) A guidewire is advanced through an ampullary adenoma into the pancreatic duct before ampullectomy (snare – *white arrows*). (*B*) A guidewire (*white arrow*) is secured in the pancreatic duct before biliary sphincterotomy (*black arrow*).

longer stents (ending in the body or tail) are preferable is unknown, and comparative effectiveness studies in this area are needed.

Another important question regarding PSP is the acceptable amount of time that is spent on the insertion process in cases of difficult pancreatic access. Although the merits of PSP have been clearly presented earlier, if achieving pancreatic access proves difficult, there is presumably a point of diminishing returns when the risk of additional attempts outweighs the benefit of stent placement, especially if insertion eventually proves unsuccessful. Future clinical studies are unlikely to answer this question in a methodologically rigorous fashion; therefore, endoscopists should be aware of this important clinical balance and use their best judgment regarding the acceptable duration of time for stent insertion. One potential approach to circumvent this problem in cases of anticipated stent placement (for example ampullectomy or SOD cases) is to place and maintain a guidewire in the PD early in the case to guarantee PD access later on, avoiding the occasional phenomenon of failing to identify the pancreatic orifice due to the anatomic distortion that develops as a consequence of edema, sphincterotomy, or ampullectomy (**Fig. 3**). Another approach is to place the prophylactic pancreatic stent before therapeutic intervention.

PHARMACOPREVENTION

Historically, pharmacoprevention for PEP has been a disappointing enterprise. In excess of 35 pharmacologic agents have been studied for the prophylaxis of pancreatitis, and more than 60 prospective clinical trials addressing chemoprevention have been published since the year 2000. Until recently, however, no medication had proved consistently effective in preventing PEP on the basis of high-quality clinical trial data, and no pharmacologic prophylaxis for PEP had been adopted into widespread clinical use. Traditionally, clinical trials in this area have suffered from inadequate sample sizes and/or conflicting results. Moreover, the pessimism surrounding PEP pharmacoprevention had been amplified by prior positive meta-analyses that were

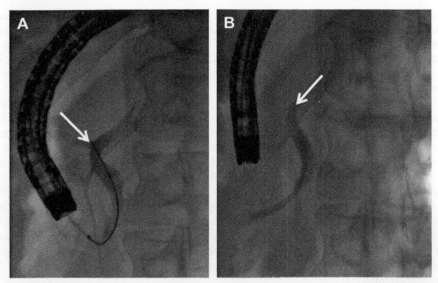

Fig. 3. Fluoroscopic images depicting the pancreatic genu (*white arrow*) (*A*) and a prophylactic/ therapeutic pancreatic stent ending immediately at the genu (*white arrow*) (*B*). This patient developed significant epigastric abdominal pain (without pancreatitis) for 48 hours after the procedure that resolved on replacing the stent with a shorter one.

subsequently disproved by further clinical investigation.[81,82] Recently, however, research focusing on nonsteroidal antiinflammatory drugs (NSAIDs) has provided renewed hope for pharmacoprevention by demonstrating that a medication can indeed be meaningfully effective in preventing post-ERCP pancreatitis.

Nonsteroidal Antiinflammatory Drugs

NSAIDs are potent inhibitors of phospholipase A2, cyclooxygenase, and neutrophil–endothelial interactions, all believed to play an important role in the pathogenesis of acute pancreatitis.[83,84] NSAIDs are inexpensive, widely available, easily administered, and have a favorable risk profile when given as a single dose, making them an attractive option in the prevention of PEP. Four initial studies evaluating the protective effects of single-dose rectal indomethacin or diclofenac were conducted between 1998 and 2005, and demonstrated conflicting, but generally encouraging results.[85–88] In 2008, a meta-analysis of these RCTs, involving 912 patients, demonstrated a robust 64% reduction in PEP associated with rectal NSAIDs (RR 0.34, 95% CI 0.22–0.60) and no increase in associated adverse events.[89]

Despite this meta-analysis, however, NSAIDs were seldom used in clinical practice due to the absence of conclusive RCT evidence.[90] Moreover, it remained unclear whether NSAIDs provide incremental benefit over temporary PSP. Therefore, a large-scale multicenter methodologically rigorous RCT was conducted to definitively evaluate the efficacy of prophylactic rectal indomethacin for preventing PEP in high-risk cases.[91] After enrolling 602 subjects, more than 80% of who received a prophylactic pancreatic stent, the study was terminated prematurely because of the clear benefit of indomethacin. In this study, rectal indomethacin was associated with a 7.7% absolute risk reduction (number needed to treat = 13) and a 46% relative risk reduction in PEP ($P = .005$). Further, indomethacin reduced the incidence of moderate-severe PEP by 50% ($P = .03$) and the median hospital length of stay in those who developed pancreatitis (*P*<.001). The main limitation of this study is that more than 80% of enrolled subjects had suspected SOD, although subgroup analysis revealed a clear trend toward benefit in subjects without SOD who received indomethacin (8.5% vs 20.0%, *P* = .11). Also important to note is that indomethacin appeared effective in both subjects who received a prophylactic pancreatic stent and those who did not.

On the basis of these data, it is appropriate to recommend rectal NSAIDs to patients undergoing high-risk ERCP and strong consideration should be given to including rectal NSAIDs administration in future quality measure statements. Controversy remains, however, within the advanced endoscopy community, regarding the role of NSAIDs in low-risk cases. Unfortunately, an adequately powered clinical trial in low-risk subjects would necessitate 2000 to 3000 subjects (depending on baseline risk), requiring many years to complete and incurring substantial costs. In light of the very low cost of a single dose of NSAIDs, its highly favorable safety profile, and a prior meta-analysis suggesting that it is equally effective in low-risk subjects,[89] the time and resources necessary to conduct a definitive RCT may not be justified. The European Society of Gastrointestinal Endoscopy recommends rectal indomethacin or diclofenac for *all* patients undergoing ERCP as a grade A recommendation.[17]

Nitroglycerin and Glyceryl Trinitrate

The data for nitroglycerin and its analogues remain conflicting. Glyceryl trinitrate (GTN) is a smooth muscle relaxant, which may lower sphincter of Oddi pressures, thereby reducing post-procedure intraductal hypertension. Eight RCTs have been conducted evaluating the role of GTN in PEP prevention; 3 of these studies demonstrated a significant reduction in PEP,[92–94] whereas the remaining 5 showed no benefit. Nevertheless, the 4 published meta-analyses of nitroglycerin suggest benefit, particularly for the sublingual form, although the results are tempered by a significant incidence in headache and hypotension.[95–98] Furthermore, it is unclear whether nitroglycerin would provide incremental benefit over PSP and rectal indomethacin. An adequately powered, methodologically rigorous RCT evaluating the sublingual route of GTN in addition to indomethacin and PSP is worth considering.

Nafamostat

Nafamostat mesylate is a low–molecular weight protease inhibitor that inhibits trypsin, a proteolytic enzyme considered to play an initial role in the pathogenesis of pancreatitis. Nafamostat has a 20-time longer half-life and is 10 to 100 times more potent than gabexate mesylate, another protease inhibitor that has been the focus of much prior research and is utilized in clinical practice in certain parts of the world.[17] Three recent RCTs have identified a significant reduction in PEP associated with nafamostat: Yoo and colleagues[99] 2011, n = 266 (2.8% nafamostat group vs 9.1% control group, *P* = .03); Choi and colleagues[100] 2009, n = 704 (3.3% nafamostat vs 7.4% control, *P* = .018); and Park and colleagues[101] 2011 n = 608 (3 arms: 13.0% PEP in control group vs 4.0% in 20 mg nafamostat group vs 5.1% in 50 mg nafamostat group, *P*<.0001). Unfortunately, none of the RCTs detected a difference in PEP rates in high-risk patients, and the low-risk subgroups are underpowered. A major concern related to the use of nafamostat is its prolonged duration of intravenous infusion; the aforementioned studies initiated administration of the drug 1 hour before the ERCP and continued for 6 to 24 hours after the procedure. Although nafamostat may hold promise in preventing PEP, particularly in low-risk patients, it likely represents an impractical and perhaps prohibitively costly approach in this era of rising health care expenditures.

Somatostatin and Octreotide

Somatostatin and its long-acting synthetic analogue, octreotide, have been studied extensively as preventive agents for PEP, with data available from close to 30 RCTs. Both are potent inhibitors of pancreatic exocrine activity and may therefore prevent or mitigate the pathophysiologic process that leads to pancreatitis. Unfortunately, the overwhelming majority of data pertaining to octreotide have failed to demonstrate a prophylactic benefit. One bright spot in the octreotide story is 2 recent meta-analyses in which subgroup analysis suggests that a dose of at least 0.5 mg may reduce the rate of PEP compared with placebo.[102,103] No benefit was associated with lower doses (<0.5 mg), consistent with the previously existing body of literature.[104]

The data for somatostatin have been somewhat more encouraging. The most recent meta-analysis, including 10 RCTs, concluded that somatostatin significantly reduces the risk of PEP, particularly when delivered in high doses infused for more than 12 hours or bolused.[104] Additionally, a recent RCT evaluating combination therapy with diclofenac (100 mg rectally before ERCP) plus somatostatin (0.25 mg/h for 6 hours) significantly reduced the frequency of PEP (4.7% vs 10.4%; $P = .015$) in subjects at elevated risk.[105]

On the basis of existing data, octreotide and somatostatin cannot be recommended in clinical practice. More definitive RCTs are necessary to elucidate the roles of high-dose octreotide, high-dose somatostatin in bolus or infusion form, and these agents in combination with NSAIDs.

Secretin

A large single-center RCT revealed that a single dose of secretin administered immediately before ERCP reduced the risk of PEP in a mixed population of subjects.[106–108] The applicability of these results is limited because the study predated prophylactic PSP, did not standardize the definition of PEP or the routine measurement of pancreatic enzymes, and did not use the intention-to-treat principle. This study remains hypothesis generating, and the utility of a contemporary methodologically rigorous trial should be discussed.

Antibiotics

In a single RCT of low methodologic quality, ceftazidime was found to reduce PEP.[107] Because an infectious mechanism for PEP is biologically plausible, the results of this pilot study should be verified in larger trials.

Drugs that are Likely to be Ineffective

Agents with predominantly negative study results, which are unlikely to have a future role in PEP prevention include interleukin 10, corticosteroids, allopurinol, heparin, gabexate, ulinastatin, nifedipine, pentoxifylline, N-acetylcysteine, and topical lidocaine sprayed on the papilla.

As mentioned previously, PEP pharmacoprevention research has suffered from weaknesses in methodologic quality, primarily due to inadequate sample sizes, inconsistent definitions of PEP, and failure to analyze data according to the intention-to-treat principle. Additional resources used to conduct clinical trials in this important area should be justified by enrolling an adequate sample size, using the accepted definition of PEP, and adhering to fundamental RCT principles.

FUTURE DIRECTIONS

Despite the approaches outlined earlier, up to 10% of high-risk patients will still develop PEP. Appropriate patient selection, sound procedural technique, NSAIDs, and pancreatic stents have been effective in *improving* the problem; however, additional research in multiple areas is necessary to achieve the goal of *solving* PEP.

In addition to the research questions presented throughout this article, several ongoing or soon to be initiated studies are worth noting. There are 4 enrolling pharmacoprevention RCTs registered on the ClinicalTrials.gov website. These studies are evaluating intramuscular diclofenac, somatostatin, and topical PD lidocaine. In addition, a randomized study comparing standard dose rectal indomethacin (100 mg at the time of ERCP) with an intensive dose regimen (150 mg at time of the ERCP, followed by 50 mg 4 hours later) will begin enrolling patients in early 2013.

Regarding future research involving PSP, a *post hoc* analysis of the large, recently published indomethacin RCT[91] suggested that a prevention strategy involving rectal indomethacin alone is more effective and substantially less costly than a strategy of PSP alone or the combination of both.[108] Although current data suggest that rectal indomethacin is effective *in addition* to PSP, this hypothesis-generating analysis suggests that prophylactic rectal indomethacin could *replace* PSP in clinical practice. Because PSP is technically challenging, time consuming, and costly, a comparative effectiveness study evaluating indomethacin alone versus the combination of indomethacin and PSP appears justified and is in the planning phase.

SUMMARY

a. Pancreatitis is an important and potentially preventable complication of ERCP.
b. Patients can be risk-stratified for PEP according to patient and procedure-related characteristics, guiding prophylactic interventions and allowing early detection of the complication.
c. Thoughtful patient selection is critical in preventing PEP; in this era of highly accurate diagnostic alternatives, ERCP should be a near-exclusively therapeutic procedure.
d. In the case of difficult cannulation, alternate techniques, such as double-wire cannulation and precut sphincterotomy, should be implemented early.
e. Contrast-facilitated cannulation, aggressive/repeated pancreatic injection, dilation of an intact biliary sphincter, and sphincter of Oddi manometry without aspiration should be avoided.
f. Prophylactic pancreatic stents should be placed in all high-risk cases.
g. Rectal NSAIDs should be administered in all high-risk cases, and based on a very favorable risk-benefit ratio, should be considered in all patients undergoing ERCP.
h. Ongoing and upcoming pharmacoprevention trials, as well as a comparative effectiveness study of indomethacin versus prophylactic PSP will further improve the endoscopists' ability to efficiently and effectively prevent PEP.

REFERENCES

1. Cotton PB, Lehman G, Vennes J, et al. Endoscopic sphincterotomy complications and their management: an attempt at consensus. Gastrointest Endosc 1991;37:383–93.
2. Freeman ML, Guda NM. Prevention of post-ERCP pancreatitis: a comprehensive review. Gastrointest Endosc 2004;59:845–64.
3. Freeman ML, Nelson DB, Sherman S, et al. Complications of endoscopic biliary sphincterotomy. N Engl J Med 1996;335:909–18.

4. Healthcare Cost and Utilization Project. 2012. Available at: http://hcupnet.ahrq.gov. Accessed April 6, 2012.
5. Freeman ML, DiSario JA, Nelson DB, et al. Risk factors for post-ERCP pancreatitis: a prospective, multicenter study. Gastrointest Endosc 2001;54:425–34.
6. Masci E, Mariani A, Curioni S, et al. Risk factors for pancreatitis following endoscopic retrograde cholangiopancreatography: a meta-analysis. Endoscopy 2003;35:830–4.
7. Cotton PB, Garrow DA, Gallagher J, et al. Risk factors for complications after ERCP: a multivariate analysis of 11,497 procedures over 12 years. Gastrointest Endosc 2009;70:80–8.
8. Singh P, Gurudu SR, Davidoff S, et al. Sphincter of Oddi manometry does not predispose to post-ERCP acute pancreatitis. Gastrointest Endosc 2004;59:499–505.
9. Fogel EL, Eversman D, Jamidar P, et al. Sphincter of Oddi dysfunction: pancreaticobiliary sphincterotomy with pancreatic stent placement has a lower rate of pancreatitis than biliary sphincterotomy alone. Endoscopy 2002;34:280–5.
10. Maldonado ME, Brady PG, Mamel JJ, et al. Incidence of pancreatitis in patients undergoing sphincter of Oddi manometry (SOM). Am J Gastroenterol 1999;94:387–90.
11. Cheng CL, Sherman S, Watkins JL, et al. Risk factors for post-ERCP pancreatitis: a prospective multicenter study. Am J Gastroenterol 2006;101:139–47.
12. Friedland S, Soetikno RM, Vandervoort J, et al. Bedside scoring system to predict the risk of developing pancreatitis following ERCP. Endoscopy 2002;34:483–8.
13. Vandervoort J, Soetikno RM, Tham TC, et al. Risk factors for complications after performance of ERCP. Gastrointest Endosc 2002;56:652–6.
14. Mehta SN, Pavone E, Barkun JS, et al. Predictors of post-ERCP complications in patients with suspected choledocholithiasis. Endoscopy 1998;30:457–63.
15. Loperfido S, Angelini G, Benedetti G, et al. Major early complications from diagnostic and therapeutic ERCP: a prospective multicenter study. Gastrointest Endosc 1998;48:1–10.
16. Williams EJ, Taylor S, Fairclough P, et al. Risk factors for complication following ERCP; results of a large-scale, prospective multicenter study. Endoscopy 2007;39:793–801.
17. Dumonceau JM, Andriulli A, Deviere J, et al. European Society of Gastrointestinal Endoscopy (ESGE) Guideline: prophylaxis of post-ERCP pancreatitis. Endoscopy 2010;42:503–15.
18. Patel R, Varadarajulu S, Wilcox CM. Endoscopic ampullectomy: techniques and outcomes. J Clin Gastroenterol 2012;46:8–15.
19. Disario JA, Freeman ML, Bjorkman DJ, et al. Endoscopic balloon dilation compared with sphincterotomy for extraction of bile duct stones. Gastroenterology 2004;127:1291–9.
20. Baron TH, Harewood GC. Endoscopic balloon dilation of the biliary sphincter compared to endoscopic biliary sphincterotomy for removal of common bile duct stones during ERCP: a metaanalysis of randomized, controlled trials. Am J Gastroenterol 2004;99:1455–60.
21. Weinberg B, Shindy W, Lo S. Endoscopic balloon sphincter dilation (sphincteroplasty) versus sphincterotomy for common bile duct stones. Cochrane Database Syst Rev 2006;(4):CD004890.
22. Wang P, Li ZS, Liu F, et al. Risk factors for ERCP-related complications: a prospective multicenter study. Am J Gastroenterol 2009;104:31–40.

23. Rabenstein T, Schneider HT, Bulling D, et al. Analysis of risk factors of endoscopic sphincterotomy techniques: preliminary results of a prospective study with emphasis on the reduced risk of acute pancreatitis under low-dose anticoagulation. Endoscopy 2000;32:10–9.

24. Ghaferi AA, Birkmeyer JD, Dimick JB. Variation in hospital mortality associated with inpatient surgery. N Engl J Med 2009;361(14):1368–75.

25. Ghaferi AA, Birkmeyer JD, Dimick JB. Hospital volume and failure to rescue with high-risk surgery. Med Care 2011;49(12):1076–81.

26. Trap R, Adamsen S, Hart-Hansen O, et al. Severe and fatal complications after diagnostic and therapeutic ERCP: a prospective series of claims to insurance covering public hospitals. Endoscopy 1999;31:125–30.

27. Laugier R, Bernard JP, Berthezene P, et al. Changes in pancreatic exocrine secretion with age: pancreatic exocrine secretion does decrease in the elderly. Digestion 1991;50:202–11.

28. Banerjee N, Hilden K, Baron TH, et al. Endoscopic biliary sphincterotomy is not required for transpapillary SEMS placement for biliary obstruction. Dig Dis Sci 2011;56:591–5.

29. Waljee AK, Higgins PD. Machine learning in medicine: a primer for physicians. Am J Gastroenterol 2010;105:1224–6.

30. Hawes RH. The evolution of endoscopic ultrasound: improved imaging, higher accuracy for fine needle aspiration and the reality of endoscopic ultrasound-guided intervention. Curr Opin Gastroenterol 2010;26:436–44.

31. Petrov MS, Savides TJ. Systematic review of endoscopic ultrasonography versus endoscopic retrograde cholangiopancreatography for suspected choledocholithiasis. Br J Surg 2009;96:967–74.

32. Romagnuolo J, Bardou M, Rahme E, et al. Magnetic resonance cholangiopancreatography: a meta-analysis of test performance in suspected biliary disease. Ann Intern Med 2003;139:547–57.

33. Garrow D, Miller S, Sinha D, et al. Endoscopic ultrasound: a meta-analysis of test performance in suspected biliary obstruction. Clin Gastroenterol Hepatol 2007;5:616–23.

34. Tse F, Liu L, Barkun AN, et al. EUS: a meta-analysis of test performance in suspected choledocholithiasis. Gastrointest Endosc 2008;67:235–44.

35. Verma D, Kapadia A, Eisen GM, et al. EUS vs MRCP for detection of choledocholithiasis. Gastrointest Endosc 2006;64:248–54.

36. Boraschi P, Neri E, Braccini G, et al. Choledocholithiasis: diagnostic accuracy of MR cholangiopancreatographyd3 year experience. Magn Reson Imaging 1999; 17:1245–53.

37. Zidi SH, Prat F, Le Guen O, et al. Use of magnetic resonance cholangiography in the diagnosis of choledocholithiasis: prospective comparison with a reference imaging method. Gut 1999;44:118–22.

38. Gardner TB, Levy MJ. EUS diagnosis of chronic pancreatitis. Gastrointest Endosc 2010;71:1280–9.

39. Lambie H, Cook AM, Scarsbrook AF, et al. Tc99m-hepatobiliary iminodiacetic acid (HIDA) scintigraphy in clinical practice. Clin Radiol 2011;66:1094–105.

40. Darwin P, Goldberg E, Uradomo L. Jackson Pratt drain fluid-to-serum bilirubin concentration ratio for the diagnosis of bile leaks. Gastrointest Endosc 2010; 71:99–104.

41. Mazen Jamal M, Yoon EJ, Saadi A, et al. Trends in the utilization of endoscopic retrograde cholangiopancreatography in the United States. Am J Gastroenterol 2007;102:966–75.

42. Coté GA, Sherman S. Advances in pancreatobiliary endoscopy. Curr Opin Gastroenterol 2010;26:429–35.
43. ASGE Standards of Practice Committee. The role of endoscopy in the evaluation of suspected choledocholithiasis. Gastrointest Endosc 2010;71:1–9.
44. NIH state-of-the-science statement on endoscopic retrograde cholangiopancreatography (ERCP) for diagnosis and therapy. NIH Consens State Sci Statements 2002;19(1):1–26.
45. Rosenblatt ML, Catalano MF, Alcocer E, et al. Comparison of sphincter of Oddi manometry, fatty meal sonography, and hepatobiliary scintigraphy in the diagnosis of sphincter of Oddi dysfunction. Gastrointest Endosc 2001;54:697–704.
46. Di Francesco V, Brunori MP, Rigo L, et al. Comparison of ultrasound-secretin test and sphincter of Oddi manometry in patients with recurrent acute pancreatitis. Dig Dis Sci 1999;44:336–40.
47. Cotton PB, Durkalski V, Orrell KB, et al. Challenges in planning and initiating a randomized clinical study of sphincter of Oddi dysfunction. Gastrointest Endosc 2010;72:986–91.
48. Elmunzer BJ, Debenedet AT, Volk ML, et al. Clinical yield of diagnostic endoscopic retrograde cholangiopancreatography in orthotopic liver transplant recipients with suspected biliary complications. Liver Transpl 2012;18:1479–84.
49. Tse F, Yuan Y, Moayyedi P, et al. Guidewire-assisted cannulation of the common bile duct for the prevention of post-endoscopic retrograde cholangiopancreatography (ERCP) pancreatitis. Cochrane Database Syst Rev 2012;(12): CD009662.
50. Mariani A, Giussani A, Di Leo M, et al. Guidewire biliary cannulation does not reduce post-ERCP pancreatitis compared with the contrast injection technique in low-risk and high-risk patients. Gastrointest Endosc 2012;75:339–46.
51. Bassan MS, Holt BA, Mahady S, et al. Guidewire biliary cannulation does not reduce post-ERCP pancreatitis compared with the contrast injection technique in low-risk and high-risk patients. Gastrointest Endosc 2012;76:229–30.
52. Ito K, Fujita N, Noda Y, et al. Pancreatic guidewire placement for achieving selective biliary cannulation during endoscopic retrograde cholangiopancreatography. World J Gastroenterol 2008;14:5595–600.
53. Herreros de Tejada A, Calleja JL, Diaz G, et al. Double-guidewire technique for difficult bile duct cannulation: a multicenter randomized, controlled trial. Gastrointest Endosc 2009;70:700–9.
54. Ito K, Fujita N, Noda Y, et al. Can pancreatic duct stenting prevent post-ERCP pancreatitis in patients who undergo pancreatic duct guidewire placement for achieving selective biliary cannulation? A prospective randomized controlled trial. J Gastroenterol 2010;45:1183–91.
55. Testoni PA, Testoni S, Giussani A. Difficult biliary cannulation during ERCP: how to facilitate biliary access and minimize the risk of post-ERCP pancreatitis. Dig Liver Dis 2011;43:596–603.
56. Bourke MJ, Costamagna G, Freeman ML. Biliary cannulation during endoscopic retrograde cholangiopancreatography: core technique and recent innovations. Endoscopy 2009;4:612–7.
57. Cennamo V, Fuccio L, Zagari RM, et al. Can early precut implementation reduce endoscopic retrograde cholangiopancreatography-related complication risk? Meta-analysis of randomized controlled trials. Endoscopy 2010;42:381–8.
58. Sherman S, Troiano FP, Hawes RH, et al. Sphincter of Oddi manometry: decreased risk of clinical pancreatitis with use of a modified aspirating catheter. Gastrointest Endosc 1990;36:462.

59. Liao WC, Tu YK, Wu MS, et al. Balloon dilation with adequate duration is safer than sphincterotomy for extracting bile duct stones: a systematic review and meta-analyses. Clin Gastroenterol Hepatol 2012;10(10):1101–9.

60. Misra SP, Dwivedi M. Large-diameter balloon dilation after endoscopic sphincterotomy for removal of difficult bile duct stones. Endoscopy 2008;40:209–13.

61. Heo JH, Kang DH, Jung HJ, et al. Endoscopic sphincterotomy plus large balloon dilation versus endoscopic sphincterotomy for removal of bile-duct stones. Gastrointest Endosc 2007;66:720–6.

62. Freeman ML, Guda NL. Cannulation techniques for ERCP: a review of reported techniques. Gastrointest Endosc 2005;61:112–25.

63. Schwacha H, Allgaier HP, Deibert P, et al. A sphincterotome-based technique for selective transpapillary common bile duct cannulation. Gastrointest Endosc 2000;52:387–91.

64. Abraham NS, Williams SP, Thompson K, et al. 5F sphincterotomes and 4F sphincterotomes are equivalent for the selective cannulation of the common bile duct. Gastrointest Endosc 2006;63:615–21.

65. Garcia-Cano J, Gonzalez-Martin JA. Bile duct cannulation: success rates for various ERCP techniques and devices at a single institution. Acta Gastroenterol Belg 2006;69:261–7.

66. Somogyi L, Chuttani R, Croffie J, et al. Guidewires for use in GI endoscopy. Gastrointest Endosc 2007;65:571–6.

67. George S, Kulkarni AA, Stevens G, et al. Role of osmolality of contrast media in the development of post-ERCP pancreatitis: a metanalysis. Dig Dis Sci 2004;49: 503–8.

68. Freeman ML. Complications of endoscopic retrograde cholangiopancreatography: avoidance and management. Gastrointest Endosc Clin N Am 2012;22:567–86.

69. Choudhary A, Bechtold ML, Arif M, et al. Pancreatic stents for prophylaxis against post-ERCP pancreatitis: a meta-analysis and systematic review. Gastrointest Endosc 2011;73:275–82.

70. Mazaki T, Masuda H, Takayama T. Prophylactic pancreatic stent placement and post-ERCP pancreatitis: a systematic review and meta-analysis. Endoscopy 2010;42:842–5.

71. Freeman ML, Overby C, Qi D. Pancreatic stent insertion: consequences of failure and results of a modified technique to maximize success. Gastrointest Endosc 2004;5:8–14.

72. Freeman ML. Role of pancreatic stents in prevention of post-ERCP pancreatitis. JOP 2004;5:322–7.

73. Bakman YG, Safdar K, Freeman ML. Significant clinical implications of prophylactic pancreatic stent placement in previously normal pancreatic ducts. Endoscopy 2009;41:1095–8.

74. Zolotarevsky E, Fehmi SM, Anderson MA, et al. Prophylactic 5-Fr pancreatic duct stents are superior to 3-Fr stents: a randomized controlled trial. Endoscopy 2011;43:325–30.

75. Chahal P, Tarnasky PR, Petersen BT, et al. Short 5Fr vs long 3Fr pancreatic stents in patients at risk for post-endoscopic retrograde cholangiopancreatography pancreatitis. Clin Gastroenterol Hepatol 2009;7:834–9.

76. Brackbill S, Young S, Schoenfeld P, et al. A survey of physician practices on prophylactic pancreatic stents. Gastrointest Endosc 2006;64(1):45–52.

77. Das A, Singh P, Sivak MV Jr, et al. Pancreatic-stent placement for prevention of post-ERCP pancreatitis: a cost-effectiveness analysis. Gastrointest Endosc 2007;65(7):960–8.

78. Freeman ML. Pancreatic stents for prevention of post-endoscopic retrograde cholangiopancreatography pancreatitis. Clin Gastroenterol Hepatol 2007;5: 1354–65.
79. Madacsy L, Kurucsai G, Joo I, et al. ERCP and insertion of a small-caliber pancreatic stent to prevent the evolution of severe post-ERCP pancreatitis: a case-controlled series. Surg Endosc 2009;23:1887–93.
80. Rashdan A, Fogel EL, McHenry L Jr, et al. Improved stent characteristics for prophylaxis of post-ERCP pancreatitis. Clin Gastroenterol Hepatol 2004;2: 322–9.
81. Andriulli A, Leandro G, Niro G, et al. Pharmacologic treatment can prevent pancreatic injury after ERCP: a meta-analysis. Gastrointest Endosc 2000;51:1–7.
82. Andriulli A, Leandro G, Federici T, et al. Prophylactic administration of somatostatin or gabexate does not prevent pancreatitis after ERCP: an updated meta-analysis. Gastrointest Endosc 2007;65:624–32.
83. Gross V, Leser HG, Heinisch A, et al. Inflammatory mediators and cytokines — new aspects of the pathophysiology and assessment of severity of acute pancreatitis? Hepatogastroenterology 1993;40:522–30.
84. Makela A, Kuusi T, Schrader T. Inhibition of serum phospholipase-A2 in acute pancreatitis by pharmacologic agents in vitro. Scand J Clin Lab Invest 1997; 57:401–8.
85. Murray B, Carter R, Imrie C, et al. Diclofenac reduces the incidence of acute pancreatitis after endoscopic retrograde cholangiopancreatography. Gastroenterology 2003;124:1786–91.
86. Sotoudehmanesh R, Khatibian M, Kolahdoozan S, et al. Indomethacin may reduce the incidence and severity of acute pancreatitis after ERCP. Am J Gastroenterol 2007;102:978–83.
87. Khoshbaten M, Khorram H, Mamad L, et al. Role of diclofenac in reducing post-endoscopicretrograde cholangiopancreatography pancreatitis. J Gastroenterol Hepatol 2008;23:e11–6.
88. Montaño Loza A, Rodriguez Lomeli X, Garcia Correa J, et al. Effect of rectal administration of indomethacin on amylase serum levels after endoscopic retrograde cholangiopancreatography, and its impact on the development of secondary pancreatitis episodes. Rev Esp Enferm Dig 2007;99:330–6.
89. Elmunzer B, Waljee A, Elta G, et al. A meta-analysis of rectal NSAIDs in the prevention of post-ERCP pancreatitis. Gut 2008;57:1262–7.
90. Dumonceau J, Rigaux J, Kahaleh M, et al. Prophylaxis of post-ERCP pancreatitis: a practice survey. Gastrointest Endosc 2010;71:934–9.
91. Elmunzer BJ, Scheiman JM, Lehman GA, et al. A randomized trial of rectal indomethacin to prevent post-ERCP pancreatitis. N Engl J Med 2012;366:1414–22.
92. Hao JY, Wu DF, Wang YZ, et al. Prophylactic effect of glyceryl trinitrate on post-endoscopic retrograde cholangiopancreatography pancreatitis: a randomized placebo-controlled trial. World J Gastroenterol 2009;15:366–8.
93. Moreto M, Zaballa M, Casado I, et al. Transdermal glyceryl trinitrate for prevention of post-ERCP pancreatitis: a randomized doubleblind trial. Gastrointest Endosc 2003;57:1–7.
94. Sudhindran S, Bromwich E, Edwards PR. Prospective randomized double-blind placebo-controlled trial of glyceryl trinitrate in endoscopic retrograde cholangiopancreatography-induced pancreatitis. Br J Surg 2001;88:1178–82.
95. Bai Y, Xu C, Yang X, et al. Glyceryl trinitrate for prevention of pancreatitis after endoscopic retrograde cholangiopancreatography: a meta-analysis of randomized, double-blind, placebo-controlled trials. Endoscopy 2009;41:690–5.

96. Chen B, Fan T, Wang CH. A meta-analysis for the effect of prophylactic GTN on the incidence of post-ERCP pancreatitis and on the successful rate of cannulation of bile ducts. BMC Gastroenterol 2010;10:85.

97. Bang UC, Nojgaard C, Andersen PK, et al. Meta-analysis: Nitroglycerin for prevention of post-ERCP pancreatitis. Aliment Pharmacol Ther 2009;29:1078–85.

98. Shao LM, Chen QY, Chen MY, et al. Nitroglycerin in the prevention of post-ERCP pancreatitis: a meta-analysis. Dig Dis Sci 2010;55:1–7.

99. Yoo KS, Huh KR, Kim YJ, et al. Nafamostat mesilate for prevention of post-endoscopic retrograde cholangiopancreatography pancreatitis a prospective, randomized, double-blind, controlled trial. Pancreas 2011;40:181–6.

100. Choi CW, Kang DH, Kim GH, et al. Nafamostat mesylate in the prevention of post-ERCP pancreatitis and risk factors for post-ERCP pancreatitis. Gastrointest Endosc 2009;69:e11–8.

101. Park KT, Kang DH, Choi CW, et al. Is high-dose nafamostat mesilate effective for the prevention of post-ERCP pancreatitis, especially in high-risk patients? Pancreas 2011;40:1215–9.

102. Zhang Y, Chen QB, Gao ZY, et al. Meta-analysis: octreotide prevents post-ERCP pancreatitis, but only at sufficient doses. Aliment Pharmacol Ther 2009;29: 1155–64.

103. Omata F, Deshpande G, Tokuda Y, et al. Meta-analysis: somatostatin or its long-acting analogue, octreotide, for prophylaxis against post-ERCP pancreatitis. J Gastroenterol 2010;45:885–95.

104. Bai Y, Gao J, Zou D-W, et al. Prophylactic octreotide administration does not prevent post-endoscopic retrograde cholangiopancreatography pancreatitis. Pancreas 2008;37:241–6.

105. Katsinelos P, Fasoulas K, Paroutoglou G, et al. Combination of diclofenac plus somatostatin in the prevention of post-ERCP pancreatitis: a randomized, double-blind, placebo-controlled trial. Endoscopy 2012;44:53–9.

106. Jowell PS, Branch MS, Fein SH, et al. Intravenous synthetic secretin reduces the incidence of pancreatitis induced by endoscopic retrograde cholangiopancreatography. Pancreas 2011;40:533–9.

107. Raty S, Sand J, Pulkkinen M, et al. Post-ERCP pancreatitis: reduction by routine antibiotics. J Gastrointest Surg 2001;5:339–45.

108. Elmunzer BJ, Higgins PD, Saini SD, et al. Does rectal indomethacin eliminate the need for prophylactic pancreatic stent placement in patients undergoing high-risk ERCP? Post hoc efficacy and cost-benefit analyses using prospective clinical trial data. Am J Gastroenterol 2013;108(3):410–5.

Endoscopic Therapy of Necrotizing Pancreatitis and Pseudocysts

Jessica M. Fisher, MD[a], Timothy B. Gardner, MD[b],*

KEYWORDS

- Therapeutic endoscopy • Pancreatitis • Pancreatic fluid collection
- Necrotizing pancreatitis • Walled off necrosis • Pancreatic pseudocyst
- Endoscopic ultrasound

KEY POINTS

- In the last several years, endoscopic management of pancreatic pseudocysts and walled-off necrosis has come to serve as an important primary interventional technique for therapeutic gastroenterologists.
- Although a primary means of treatment at many centers, it additionally serves as an adjunct to other minimally invasive interventional techniques, such as percutaneous drainage or laparoscopic necrosectomy and video-assisted retroperitoneal debridement.
- Endoscopic drainage and debridement are most clearly indicated in patients with well-encapsulated pancreatic or peripancreatic collections of fluid or necrotic debris with signs of infection and clinical deterioration, luminal or biliary obstruction, or severe pain.
- To ensure optimal patient outcomes, the use of periprocedural antibiotics, endoscopic ultrasonography guidance for localization of puncture site, multiple pigtail drains or enteral stents at the fistula site, serial direct endoscopic necrosectomy as needed, and serial imaging is recommended.
- The endoscopist should be prepared to repeat procedures as needed depending on the patient's clinical status and imaging results.
- Although more prospective comparative trials are needed to refine future practice guidelines, endoscopic management of pancreatic pseudocysts and walled-off necrosis is a safe and effective therapeutic option in the appropriate patient population.

INTRODUCTION

The endoscopic management of pancreatic fluid collections (PFC) and walled-off necrosis (WON) has become increasingly common and frequently within the capability of the therapeutic endoscopist.[1–6] New tools, such as linear-array endoscopic

[a] Division of Gastroenterology, Department of Medicine, University of Washington, 1959 Northeast Pacific Street, Box 356424, Seattle, WA 98195, USA; [b] Section of Gastroenterology, Department of Medicine, Dartmouth-Hitchcock Medical Center, One Medical Center Drive, Lebanon, NH 03756, USA
* Corresponding author.
E-mail address: timothy.b.gardner@hitchcock.org

Gastrointest Endoscopy Clin N Am 23 (2013) 787–802
http://dx.doi.org/10.1016/j.giec.2013.06.013
1052-5157/13/$ – see front matter © 2013 Elsevier Inc. All rights reserved.

ultrasonography (EUS), retroperitoneal sinus tract endoscopy, and video-assisted retroperitoneal debridement (VARD), have revolutionized retroperitoneal access to treat PFCs and WON.[7–11] Based on mounting evidence, a recent international consensus of leading surgeons, interventional endoscopists, interventional endoscopists, and pancreatologists concluded that minimally invasive routes of necrosectomy, and especially endoscopic transluminal necrosectomy, is now the procedure of choice for the management of WON in most circumstances.[12]

Although therapeutic endoscopists have been performing these procedures for 2 decades, there are several issues that still need to be addressed before these procedures are widely adapted and accepted.[13] Although progress has been made with the more appropriate definitions for pancreatic collections per the recently published revised Atlanta Classification of acute pancreatitis, these definitions have yet to be adapted universally.[14] In addition, the timing and indications for intervention are not universally defined and agreed on. Furthermore, it is unclear if formal therapeutic endoscopic training is necessary to credential providers or whether these procedures should be offered by the general gastroenterologist or surgeon. Finally, although there have now been 2 prospective trials comparing single-modality endoscopic techniques (one retroperitoneal as an adjunct to VARD, and the other transluminal direct endoscopic necrosectomy) with surgical techniques, these have yet to be comprehensively evaluated outside the Dutch Pancreatitis Study Group.[8,9]

This article highlights the techniques used for endoscopic management of PFC and WON. It provides information regarding patient selection criteria, indications and timing of interventions, procedural technique, periprocedural management, and review of potential complications of endoscopic management. It is hoped that the reader will be left with both an understanding of the benefits of minimally invasive techniques and an appreciation and respect for the potential risk and complications inherent in these procedures.

PATIENT EVALUATION OVERVIEW
Patient Selection

It is essential to have standard definitions of WON and PFCs to select patients appropriately for this procedure. For example, it is no longer acceptable to use the term "pseudocyst" to describe the entire spectrum of PFC, which is a common practice among radiologists, surgeons, and gastroenterologists. PFC by definition occur when there is fluid leakage from the pancreas or liquefaction of pancreatic necrosis as a result of some type of pancreatic injury or damage. The new Atlanta Classification, listed as follows, provides characterization of PFCs in standardized fashion based on the presence or absence of necrosis and the time from injury.[14]

- Acute fluid collection: interstitial pancreatitis; less than 4 weeks since injury; no encapsulated wall
- Acute necrotic collection: necrotic pancreatitis; less than 4 weeks since injury; no encapsulated wall
- Pseudocyst: interstitial pancreatitis; greater than 4 weeks since injury; encapsulated wall; no solid debris. Usually extrapancreatic, but can occasionally be intrapancreatic as a result of "disconnected pancreatic duct, especially after surgical debridement"
- Walled-off necrosis: necrotic pancreatitis; greater than 4 weeks since injury; encapsulated wall; solid debris. Can be pancreatic and/or extrapancreatic, extending far into the pelvis or elsewhere in the abdomen.

When there is acute pancreatic injury and leakage from the pancreatic duct, that injury can be caused by either necrotic or interstitial disease. If interstitial, the resulting fluid collection is termed an acute fluid collection, which can be peripancreatic or pancreatic. If necrotic, this collection is termed an acute necrotic collection. Most acute fluid and acute necrotic collections will resolve spontaneously. However, if they do not resolve after 4 weeks, the acute fluid collection will be labeled a pseudo-cyst as long as there is no evidence of solid debris. The acute necrotic collection will be termed walled-off necrosis if the collection develops an encapsulated wall and con-tains solid debris. WON may involve the pancreas only (rarely), pancreas plus extrap-ancreatic tissues (most commonly), or extrapancreatic tissues alone (uncommonly). It is important therefore to recognize and define properly the collection so that the appropriate intervention can then be performed. **Fig. 1** demonstrates representative computed tomographic (CT) scan images of the 4 types of collections.

It should also be noted that it is critical to make sure that all fluid collections are in-flammatory in nature. Patients with fluid collections thought secondary to inflammation should have an antecedent history of pancreatic injury. Unfortunately, patients are sometimes misdiagnosed with inflammatory collections when in fact they actually have premalignant or malignant cystic pancreatic lesions, such as mucinous cystic neoplasms, islet cell neoplasms with cystic degeneration, or intraductal papillary mucinous neoplasms.[15–18]

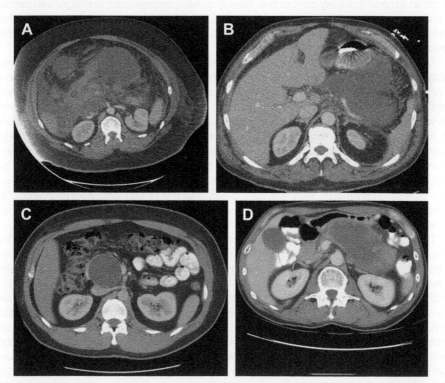

Fig. 1. Representative examples of postacute pancreatitis fluid collections as defined by the revised Atlanta classification. (*A*) Acute fluid collection. (*B*) Acute necrotic collection. (*C*) Pancreatic pseudocyst. (*D*) WON.

Therefore, in summary, patients on whom endoscopic therapy is being considered must have a PFC that arises from pancreatic duct injury and not a spontaneous premalignant or malignant lesion. The collection should have an encapsulated wall and therefore ideally should have resulted from an injury at least 4 weeks before the planned intervention, although that may not be feasible in some cases. As discussed later, the patient should also have an appropriate indication and an experienced provider performing the proposed procedure.

Indication and Timing of Intervention

There are usually several interventional methods for the management of pancreatic pseudocysts and WON that can be used effectively. Therefore, coordination among the surgeon, gastroenterologist, and interventional radiologist is critical to a positive outcome for the patient. It is imperative to choose the technique that is not only the most appropriate for that particular patient's clinical situation but also with which the treating institution has the most familiarity and past success.

In addition to classifying fluid collections and necrosis accurately, it is also critical to define the indication for and timing of endoscopic intervention.[19–21] Without exception, the most important urgent indication for treating a pseudocyst or WON is the presence, or suspected presence, of infection, especially those with systemic clinical deterioration despite maximal medical support. Although the case is sometimes made that infected pancreatic necrosis can be treated with antibiotics and supportive care alone, removal of infected tissue is still often required.[22] In addition, other indications, such as luminal or biliary obstruction from external compression, undiagnosed sepsis syndrome, persistent pain requiring narcotics, or recurrent acute pancreatitis, can also drive the need for drainage or debridement.[13] The algorithm in **Fig. 2** displays this treatment modality.

The goals of treatment might also determine which type of procedure is required and generally focus on the need to either *control* or *remove* the source of infection. For example, the need to control the source of infection, rather than complete removal, may be important in a hospitalized patient with a known sepsis syndrome in which the infected pancreatic necrosis is not well encapsulated. In this situation, it may be safer and more efficacious to debride the collection percutaneously. Conversely, in an ambulatory patient with a symptomatic gastric outlet obstruction from WON, the goal may be to remove this tissue completely and this can likely be accomplished with a single endoscopic modality. Not only will goals of care influence the type of intervention, they will also determine the timing and aggressiveness of treatment. Location of the collection—extension into the pelvis, for example—may also determine the type of therapy.

Time to treatment has been an important controversy in the evaluation of endoscopic efficacy.[12,22–24] Interventions within the first few weeks for necrotizing pancreatitis, especially single-modality endoscopic techniques, are generally associated with poor outcomes and should be reserved for infected necrosis in a severely ill patient with clinical deterioration. Poorly organized or liquefaction necrosis is more difficult to manage by any method compared with necrosis containing a well-encapsulated rim. Therefore, the guiding principle for timing of debridement is to delay, if at all possible, any intervention until the collection has become encapsulated. Although encapsulation can occur in some patients as early as 1 week after the onset of acute pancreatitis, this is unusual, and typically encapsulation does not occur until at least 4 weeks after the initial injury.[23]

Ample literature supports the importance of timing.[12] In a retrospective series from the Mayo Clinic Rochester, 138 patients with pancreatic necrosis, acute pseudocysts,

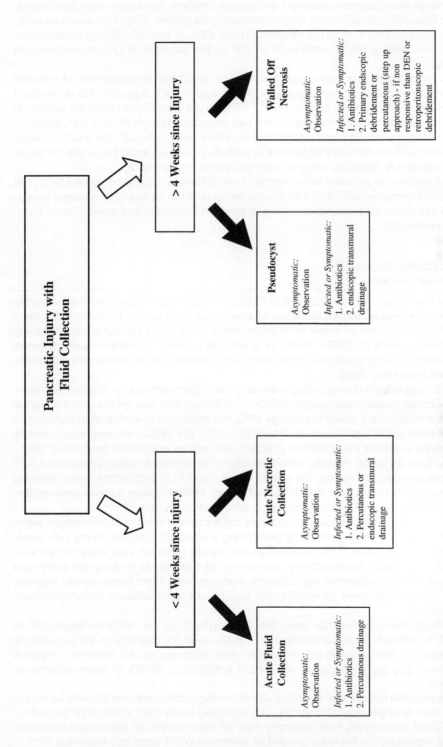

Fig. 2. Treatment modality as determined by type of pancreatic injury.

Pancreatic Injury with Fluid Collection

< 4 Weeks since injury

Acute Fluid Collection

Asymptomatic: Observation

Infected or Symptomatic:
1. Antibiotics
2. Percutanous drainage

Acute Necrotic Collection

Asymptomatic: Observation

Infected or Symptomatic:
1. Antibiotics
2. Percutanous or endoscopic transmural drainage

> 4 Weeks since Injury

Pseudocyst

Asymptomatic: Observation

Infected or Symptomatic:
1. Antibiotics
2. endoscopic transmural drainage

Walled Off Necrosis

Asymptomatic: Observation

Infected or Symptomatic:
1. Antibiotics
2. Primary endoscopic debridement or percutaneous (step up approach) - if non responsive than DEN or retroperitonscopic debridement

or chronic pseudocysts underwent endoscopic therapy. Resolution was significantly more frequent in patients with chronic pseudocysts (59/64, 92%) than acute pseudo-cysts (23/31, 74%, P = .02) or necrosis (31/43, 72%, P = .006). Waiting for encapsu-lation, or "walling off," therefore, is critical to the success of primary endoscopic therapy.[25,26]

As increasingly it is being reported that nonoperative management of infected pancreas necrosis is not only feasible, but also appropriate, it is critical to understand the nuances of indication and timing.[27–29] The single-modality endoscopic approach is best reserved for patients who have a well-encapsulated rim around the collection, which usually occurs several weeks after the initial insult. Although the degree of solid debris should not generally dictate the approach, having an appropriate site for fistula tract creation is critical to using endoscopic therapy (see **Fig. 2**).

The decision to proceed with a certain type of therapy should be guided by (1) the goals of therapy (ie, control of infection vs removal of the cavity), (2) the proper proce-dural indication, (3) preservation of organ function (pancreas and spleen), and (4) pa-tient preference.

PROCEDURAL TECHNIQUE
Historical Context

Since the 1970s, the management of PFCs and WON has transitioned from a purely surgical technique, to percutaneous interventional techniques, to endoscopic ther-apy.[30–33] With each of these techniques, there have been permutations, including the development of VARD, which is a technique used to perform percutaneous debridement using a retroperitoneal approach in which both laparoscopes and endo-scopes have been used.

PFC were initially drained using a transpapillary approach during endoscopic retro-grade cholangiopancreatography (ERCP).[34] Although this was an important advance in the endoscopist's ability to manage PFC, the revolution in endoscopic drainage of PFCs really came with the development of EUS in the 1980s, allowing endoscopists the ability to define the collection precisely, as well as outline the associated struc-tures, such as blood vessels, which needed to be avoided during intervention.[35,36] The breakthrough came with the advent of the linear EUS endoscope, which allowed drainage of PFCs via the gastrointestinal lumen. Multiple series subsequently estab-lished EUS-guided pseudocyst drainage as a firstline therapy.[37–40]

In 1996, Baron and colleagues reported the first experience with endoscopic man-agement of WON in 11 patients by performing a standard cystgastrotomy with naso-scystic tube irrigation.[15] Subsequent endoscopists reported their experiences with direct endoscopic necrosectomy, consisting of transmural endoscopic entry into the cavity and debridement with a variety of accessories. From those reports, multiple case series have been generated, but few comparative efficacy trials have been performed.

A major development has been the development of the "step-up approach" in which a minimally invasive technique is initially used for drainage of WON, which is definitive in about one-third of cases, with progression to minimally invasive necrosectomy (by endoscopic, sinus tract endoscopy, VARD, or open surgery) as needed.[41]

It is possible but not well studied that combining techniques may achieve better re-sults than a single approach alone. For example, sinus tract endoscopy combined with direct endoscopic necrosectomy may be more beneficial than single strategies alone, especially for the management of extensive WON deep into the pelvis.[42–45]

Preparation

Before the endoscopic drainage of a PFC or WON, the following issues should be addressed by the treating endoscopist:

- Define whether the procedure is being performed for source control or removal of the collection. The goals of therapy will undoubtedly drive which intervention is selected.
- Make sure the timing of intervention is appropriate. For example, has the wall of the collection been allowed enough time to mature if endoscopic transmural drainage is being considered?
- Be clear that the patient does not have any obvious medical contraindications to the procedure—coagulopathy, for example.
- Be certain that the procedure is within the realm of the endoscopist's, and the facility's, realm of expertise. In addition, all assisting nurses and technicians should have experience with the procedure.
- Make sure the collection is an inflammatory collection and not a premalignant condition, such as a mucinous cystic neoplasm or intraductal papillary mucinous neoplasm.
- Clearly define the risks and benefits of the procedure with the patient and take time obtaining and documenting the patient's informed consent.
- Discuss with colleagues in surgery and interventional radiology the plans for the procedure and make sure appropriate backup is available.
- Be certain that an anesthesia team generally is managing the patients with appropriate airway protection because there is the potential for extensive reflux and subsequent aspiration of fluid following initial cavity puncture.
- Be certain to have availability of appropriate endoscopic expertise following the procedure (ie, planning to leave town in the period following the procedure is not advised in case there are complications that need to be managed).

Patient Positioning

Positioning of the patient should generally be determined based on the clinical scenario. In hemodynamically unstable patients, supine positioning is generally safer. In stable patients, prone positioning may allow for better gravitational drainage from posteriorly located collections and decrease the incidence of fluid reflux and aspiration. All patients should have general endotracheal intubation for airway protection.

Technique

Although the endoscopic technique for management is fairly standardized, there are several variations at each stage of the procedure. Presented are the standard means by which drainage is performed, with variations highlighted at each step where applicable (**Fig. 3**).

1. Initial endoscopy: Initial endoscopy is performed using a therapeutic, side-viewing video duodenoscope, gastroscope, or echoendoscope. Although not every provider uses EUS to puncture the cavity initially and create the fistula tract, there is evidence that EUS-guided drainage of PFCs is substantially more effective and less prone to complications than "conventional" techniques.[46,47]
2. Procedural considerations:
   a. Routine antibiotic use is recommended for those not already receiving broad-spectrum antibiotics for presumed or documented infection.

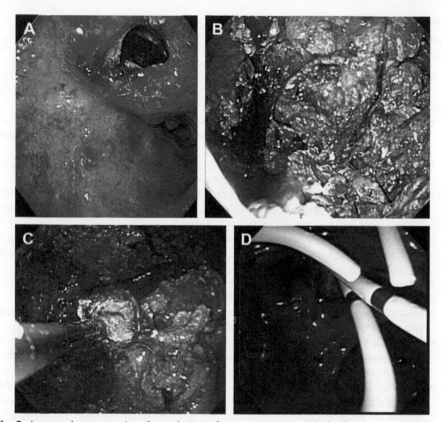

Fig. 3. Images demonstrating the technique for necrosectomy. (*A*) The fistula tract following creation of the cystenterostomy. (*B*) Inside the cavity demonstrating necrotic debris. (*C*) Debriding the cavity with a snare. (*D*) Stents in place into the cystenterostomy following debridement.

    b. If possible, CO_2 insufflation should be used to help minimize the risk of air embolism, a rare but potentially catastrophic complication.[13]

3. Assessment of the pancreatic duct: Integrity of the pancreatic duct can be assessed by CT, magnetic resonance cholangiopancreatography, EUS, or ERCP. Whether to perform direct pancreatography using ERCP at the time of initial drainage is subject to variable opinion, but does require a subsequent endoscopy for transpapillary stenting if the duct is later found to have a persistent leak. In general, though, in ill patients with infected necrosis, ERCP should generally be avoided at the initial intervention and postponed until after the infection is controlled. If evidence of a disconnected duct is found on ERCP, an attempt should be made to stent across the site of disruption (see below).

4. Identification of the fistula site: Localization of the most appropriate access site from within the gastric or duodenal lumen should be performed under EUS, because there is considerable agreement that, at least in PFCs, EUS allows for higher success rates and trends toward less complications, especially for non-bulging collections, collections in the tail, and those patients with varices.[46,47]

    a. With EUS: Endosonography is used to identify the appropriate site of transmural puncture. It is important to ensure that the cyst lumen is well approximated against the luminal gastroinestinal tract; the most appropriate site of transmural puncture should ideally be through a combined wall of 10 mm or less in thickness, although in some circumstances up to 20 mm may be acceptable.

b. Without EUS: External compression of the gastric or duodenal wall is determined endoscopically while referencing the most recent cross-sectional imaging.[48]

5. Puncture: When the appropriate site of puncture is identified, the gastric or duodenal walls are targeted and punctured. The choice of instrument to puncture is at the discretion of the endoscopist, and multiple sites of puncture can be performed for certain large collections.[49]

a. With EUS: Transmural puncture is performed under direct EUS guidance, with use of color-flow to avoid disruption of mural blood vessels at the time of wall puncture.[13] Most endoscopists use a 19-gauge fine-needle aspiration needle for puncture, and subsequently the needle sheath for initial dilation. Aspiration of cavity contents and/or demonstration of contrast injection into the cavity under fluoroscopic guidance confirms cavity access and allows collection of liquid for microbial culture. Recently, many endoscopists have been using a nonbeveled needle to avoid shearing of the hydrophilic coating that is present on many wires.

6. Fistula tract creation: Once the collection is accessed, any standard-sized guidewire (as small as 0.018 inch) is advanced into the collection under fluoroscopic guidance. Care should be used with a 0.035-inch guidewire, as these are fairly tight in a 19-gauge needle and can easily shear. Enlarging the fistula tract can be accomplished with several devices—simple low-profile dilating balloon, dilating catheter, or if resistant to those techniques, a wire-guided needle knife, fistulotome, or Soehendra screw-type stent retriever to act as a dilator. The entire sequence of procedures can be performed entirely through a therapeutic EUS scope, or, once the fistula and wire are in place, after exchange for a therapeutic duodenoscope.

7. Fistula tract dilation: Next, the tract is dilated to at least 10 mm in size using sequentially larger hydrostatic balloons. If purely liquid pseudocyst drainage is the goal, further dilation is not generally necessary. However, if endoscopic debridement is to be performed, the fistula tract must be dilated to at least 12 mm to allow passage of the endoscope into the collection. Therefore, as long as there is no contraindication—bleeding, disrupted fistula tract, patient instability, etc—generally the goal is to dilate the fistula tract fully to 20 mm at the time of the first endoscopy.

a. If bleeding occurs during fistula puncture or dilation from the fistulous tract, bleeding can be controlled by prolonged balloon tamponade, epinephrine injection, or rarely, thermocoagulation or clip placement. Immediate bleeding from within the cavity, as a result of a pseudoaneurysm, which can be more easily identified during EUS puncture of a cavity, is more difficult to manage, sometimes requiring cavity entry and direct hemostasis, or even angiographic embolization.

8. Stent placement for drainage: If draining a pseudocyst, the next step is to place stents to maintain the patency of the fistula tract and not necessarily act as a conduit for drainage. Current stenting practices vary, but the standard use of at least 2 parallel double-pigtail stents allow the fistula tract to drain even if the stents become occluded due to the space between the round catheters. Placement of one stent is fraught with occlusion risk and increases the risk of treatment failure. It is important that the fistula tract be kept patent so that fluid can escape from the

collection, pus can be released into the lumen, and the collection can be allowed to collapse. The authors generally recommend 10-F double-pigtail stents of 2 to 4 cm length, preferably of soft material to minimize trauma to the back wall of the cavity or intestinal obstruction if the stents migrate spontaneously. Alternatives are placement of a fully covered biliary type metallic stent, or even various forms of larger enteral or esophageal metallic stents to create a larger fistula.[50]

    a. Recently, a single-step system called the NAVIX system (Xlumena, Mountain View, CA) has been US Food and Drug Administration approved for chronic pseudocyst drainage. A fully integrated transluminal access device that creates and dilates an access tract, then facilitates placement of 2 guidewires, it is the first device specifically approved for pseudocyst drainage.

9. Debridement of WON: WON requires the additional step of debriding the intracavitary solid debris because the necrosis will often not resolve with the simple creation of a fistula tract.[13] Debridement of the intracavitary solid debris is performed by driving a gastroscope or duodenoscope through the dilated fistula tract into the necrotic cavity. The fluid contents within the necrotic cavity are then aspirated through the endoscope until dry, and devitalized necrotic tissue is then removed. The devitalized pancreatic tissue can be removed via a combination of several accessories including balloons, snares, waterjets, and baskets, and cap-suction techniques. The goal is to remove as much of the devitalized necrotic tissue as possible from the cavity, but without disrupting a major vessel or the wall of the cavity, potentially leading to perforation, bleeding, or air embolus.

    a. At the conclusion of each debridement session, stents must be left in place to allow the fistula tract to remain patent. Although the authors' choice is to use pigtail stents as with the pseudocyst drainage, many types of stents can be used per endoscopist preference, including fully covered metal stents, which may allow for dissolution of solid necrosis by gastric and bile acids over several weeks to months; the stent is subsequently removed once the collection has resolved.

10. Disconnected pancreatic duct: Most often, PFC arise in the context of some degree of pancreatic ductal disruption. Commonly, a disconnected duct will serve as a "feeding source" to the collection. Before effective endoscopic cystgastrotomy, endosocpists attempted to bridge the disruption with pancreatic duct stent placement. However, creating a cystenterotomy fistula tract will usually allow for adequate pancreatic drainage and general current practice it to leave the stents across the fistula tract permanently to allow for adequate pancreatic drainage proximal to the site of disruption.[51]

COMPLICATIONS AND MANAGEMENT

The interventional nature of endoscopic therapy for PFCs and necrosis does lend itself to potential complications. For example, the largest case series reported a major complication rate of 13%, including 5 patients with pneumoperitoneum/perforation (all of which were managed nonoperatively) and one periprocedural death, which was believed to be from an air embolism.[52] Eighteen percent of patients developed bleeding requiring endoscopic intervention and in 2 patients bleeding could not be controlled by endoscopic means and embolization by interventional radiology was necessary. Similar complication rates have been found in the other large series and generally the complication rate of transmural drainage is believed to be approximately 15% to 25%.[8,9,52–58]

It is imperative for endoscopists to recognize these life-threatening complications and to act accordingly. In the case of bleeding, every attempt should be made to control the bleeding endoscopically using closure devices, such as endoclips, and pharmacologic therapies, such as epinephrine. In the case of bleeding that is unable to be controlled endoscopically, interventional radiology should be consulted for embolization. Again, this underscores the importance of alerting the interventional radiologists before any attempt at drainage or debridement.

If pneumoperitoneum does occur, it is important to recognize the source immediately. In the case of fistula tract disruption, this can usually be managed nonoperatively with nasogastric tube suction, antibiotics, and conservative therapy. However, if the wall of the collection becomes disrupted (ie, during debridement) surgical intervention will usually be necessary.

As mentioned above, there is the potential for air embolism during these procedures and every attempt should be made to use CO_2 insufflation if possible. Although CO_2 does not reduce the risk of gas embolism per se, the rapidity at which CO_2 is cleared from the bloodstream, compared with oxygen, makes the hemodynamic effect of an air embolism with CO_2 generally less profound.

To prevent infection, broad-spectrum antibiotics should be given at least periprocedurally. Although there are limited data on whether long-term antibiotics are effective or appropriate, general consensus is that antibiotics should be prescribed for at least 2 to 3 days following the procedure.

Finally, it cannot be emphasized enough that before undertaking any definitive drainage of PFC or WON, the diagnosis should be firmly established as an inflammatory collection, and not intraductal papillary mucinous neoplasms or cystadenocarcinoma. Fine-needle aspiration of the collection with cytopathologic inspection can easily confirm this.

POSTOPERATIVE CARE

In an uncomplicated procedure, hospital admission is generally not necessary, even when performing an initial debridement for necrosis. Following an uncomplicated pseudocyst drainage, cross-sectional imaging should be repeated in 2 to 4 weeks to make sure resolution or near resolution of the cavity has occurred. If there has been complete resolution, no further treatment is necessary, including the removal of the plastic stents, which will typically migrate through the intestinal tract spontaneously without complication. If the collection recurs, consideration must be made for repeat transmural drainage, with possible transpapillary drainage as well if pancreatic ductal disruption is suspected.

Following an initial uncomplicated necrosectomy procedure, serial cross-sectional imaging with CT or magnetic resonance imaging every 1 to 2 weeks is performed to evaluate the status of the collection until resolution. Most often, repeat debridement will need to occur within 1 to 2 weeks after the initial cystenterostomy has been performed. At each debridement, the steps outlined above should be followed, as often there will need to be repeat dilation of the fistula tract. Each session should attempt to remove progressively more devitalized tissue.

One technique that the authors find especially helpful is to stop patients from taking any acid-suppressive therapy as the collection is resolving. Their belief is that gastric acid allows for further debridement of the collection, which in turn facilitates more rapid resolution. As with pseudocysts, plastic stents to do not need to be removed endoscopically on cavity resolution; they will usually migrate spontaneously.

In addition, if the collection fails to resolve or reaccumulates, alternative therapies, such as retroperitoneal catheter-based adjunctive techniques, such as sinus tract endoscopy, or VARD should be considered. Pancreatic ductal disruption should again always be considered as a cause of reaccumulating collections and dealt with accordingly.

OUTCOMES

There have been very few prospective, comparative effectiveness trials evaluating the success of minimally invasive approaches for PFCs and WON. In fact, effectiveness data for endoscopic therapy are limited to mostly single-center case series. However, in recent years, there have been a few trials that have laid the foundation for further endoscopic research in this field.

For pancreatic pseudocysts, the most robust study was a retrospective case-controlled study at a single center that matched 10 patients who underwent surgical cystgastrostomy with 20 patients who underwent an EUS-guided cystgastrostomy.[55] Although there were no significant differences in rates of treatment success (100% vs 95%, $P = .36$), procedural complications (none in either cohort), or reinterventions (10% vs 0%, $P = .13$) between surgery versus an EUS-guided cystgastrostomy, the mean length of a postprocedure hospital stay for an EUS-guided cystgastrostomy was significantly shorter than for surgical cystgastrostomy (2.65 vs 6.5 days, $P = .008$). In addition, the average direct cost per case for EUS-guided cystgastrostomy was significantly less when compared with surgical cystgastrostomy ($9077 vs $14,815, $P = .01$), which corresponded to a cost savings of $5738 per patient. A prospective, randomized trial comparing EUS-guided versus open surgical cystgastrostomy for the treatment of pseudocysts has been reported in abstract form and is in press (Varadarajulu). This study showed significant advantage of EUS-guided drainage over surgery with respect to cost, hospital stay and quality of life, with no differences in treatment success or recurrence.

The only randomized, prospective study comparing minimally invasive techniques with open necrosectomy is a study of 88 hospitalized patients from the Dutch Acute Pancreatitis Study Group.[8] In this multicenter study, 88 patients with pancreatic necrosis with suspected or confirmed infection were randomized to open necrosectomy or a step-up approach of percutaneous drainage followed by, if necessary, minimally invasive retroperitoneal necrosectomy. The authors found that in patients treated with the "step-up" approach, 35 were treated with percutaneous drainage only, new-onset multisystem organ failure occurred less often, and major complications and death were significantly lower (40% vs 69%, $P = .006$) compared with the open necrosectomy group.

The same group has also subsequently published the PENGUIN trial, a prospective, randomized trial of 22 patients hospitalized with infected pancreatic necrosis.[9] Patients underwent percutaneous catheter drainage, with a step-up approach, and if they failed to respond to simple catheter drainage, they were randomized to endoscopic transgastric or surgical necrosectomy. Endoscopic necrosectomy consisted of transgastric puncture, balloon dilatation, retroperitoneal drainage, and necrosectomy. Surgical necrosectomy consisted of VARD or, if not feasible, laparotomy. The authors found that endoscopic necrosectomy reduced the postprocedural proinflammatory response as measured by serum interleukin-6 levels and a predefined composite end point of major complications (new-onset multiple organ failure, intra-abdominal bleeding, enterocutaneous fistula, or pancreatic fistula) or death compared with the surgical group.

Given the small number of comparative effectiveness trials, it is critical for the endoscopic community to continue to collaborate on the design and implementation of more robust studies.

CURRENT CONTROVERSIES/FUTURE DIRECTIONS

Although the development of endoscopic therapies for PFCs and WON has revolutionized the care of patients, there still remain several controversies, questions, and limitations that need to be addressed because these techniques become more commonplace as detailed below:

- Robust comparative effectiveness studies evaluating the efficacy of transmural endoscopic techniques versus other minimally invasive techniques
- To what extent must providers be credentialed/trained
- Whether all facilities should be allowed to perform these procedures
- Improving on the debridement tools for necrosectomy
- The role of placing metallic stents and allowing natural debridement versus performing serial endoscopic necrosectomy
- Whether EUS localization needs to be used for every drainage procedure
- Should CO_2 be required to prevent air embolus during every procedure
- Further defining the role of pancreatic duct drainage in managing PFCs and WON
- How best to manage disconnected duct syndrome (ie, leaving cystgastrostomy stents in place indefinitely vs transpapillary pancreatic duct stenting).

SUMMARY

In the last 3 decades, the endoscopic management of pancreatic pseudocysts and necrosis has become increasingly common. Not only are therapeutic endoscopists draining simple collections but have recently begun extraluminal debridement of pancreatic necrosis with good success. Although these techniques are promising, further prospective trials are necessary to validate their effectiveness, cost, and safety when compared with standard operative and percutaneous techniques.

REFERENCES

1. Varadarajulu S, Bang JY, Phadnis MA, et al. Endoscopic transmural drainage of peripancreatic fluid collections: outcomes and predictors of treatment success in 211 consecutive patients. J Gastrointest Surg 2011;15(11):2080–8.
2. Baillie J. Pancreatic pseudocysts (part I). Gastrointest Endosc 2004;59:873–9.
3. Baillie J. Pancreatic pseudocysts (part II). Gastrointest Endosc 2004;60:105–13.
4. Binmoeller KF, Seifert H, Soehendra N. Endoscopic pseudocyst drainage: a new instrument for simplified cystoenterostomy. Gastrointest Endosc 1994;40:112.
5. Binmoeller KF, Seifert H, Walter A, et al. Transpapillary and transmural drainage of pancreatic pseudocysts. Gastrointest Endosc 1995;42:219–24.
6. Baron TH. Endoscopic drainage of pancreatic fluid collections and pancreatic necrosis. Gastrointest Endosc Clin N Am 2003;13:743–64.
7. Kozarek RA. Endoscopic treatment of pancreatic pseudocysts. Gastrointest Endosc Clin N Am 1997;7:271–83.
8. van Santvoort HC, Besselink MG, Bakker OJ, et al. A step-up approach or open necrosectomy for necrotizing pancreatitis. N Engl J Med 2010;362:1491–502.

9. Bakker OJ, van Santvoort HC, Burnschot S, et al. Endoscopic transgastric vs. surgical necrosectomy for infected necrotizing pancreatitis. J Am Med Assoc 2012;307:1053–61.

10. Papachristou GI, Takahashi N, Chahal P, et al. Peroral endoscopic drainage/debridement of walled-off pancreatic necrosis. Ann Surg 2007;245:943–51.

11. Seifert H, Wehrmann T, Schmitt T, et al. Retroperitoneal endoscopic debridement for infected peripancreatic necrosis. Lancet 2000;356:653–5.

12. Freeman ML, Werner J, van Santvoort HC, et al. Interventions for necrotizing pancreatitis: summary of a multidisciplinary consensus conference. Pancreas 2012;41(8):1176–94.

13. Gardner TB, Chahal P, Papachristou GI, et al. A comparison of direct endoscopic necrosectomy with transmural endoscopic drainage for the treatment of walled-off pancreatic necrosis. Gastrointest Endosc 2009;69:1085–94.

14. Banks PA, Bollen TL, Dervenis C, et al. Classification of acute pancreatitis 2012—revision of the Atlanta classification and definitions by international consensus. Gut 2013;62:102–11.

15. Baron TH, Thaggard WG, Morgan DE, et al. Endoscopic therapy for organized pancreatic necrosis. Gastroenterology 1996;111:755–64.

16. Brugge WR, Lewandrowski K, Lee-Lewandrowski E, et al. Diagnosis of pancreatic cystic neoplasms: a report of the cooperative pancreatic cyst study. Gastroenterology 2004;126:1330–6.

17. Bradley EL 3rd. A clinically based classification system for acute pancreatitis. Summary of the International Symposium on Acute Pancreatitis, Atlanta, GA, September 11 through 13, 1992. Arch Surg 1993;128:586–90.

18. Banks PA, Freeman ML. Practice guidelines in acute pancreatitis. Am J Gastroenterol 2006;101:2379–400.

19. Bollen TL, van Santvoort HC, Besselink MG, et al. The Atlanta Classification of acute pancreatitis revisited. Br J Surg 2008;95:6–21.

20. Talukdar R, Vege SS. Early management of severe acute pancreatitis. Curr Gastroenterol Rep 2011;13(2):123–30.

21. Hansen BØ, Schmidt PN. New classification of acute pancreatitis. Ugeskr Laeger 2011;173(1):42–4 [in Danish].

22. Garg PK, Sharma M, Madan K, et al. Primary conservative treatment results in mortality comparable to surgery in patients with infectedpancreatc necrosis. Clin Gastroenterol Hepatol 2010;8(12):1089–94.

23. Takahashi N, Papachristou GI, Schmit GD, et al. CT findings of walled-off pancreatic necrosis (WOPN): differentiation from pseudocyst and prediction of outcome after endoscopic therapy. Eur Radiol 2008;18:2522–9.

24. Baron TH, Harewood GC, Morgan DE, et al. Outcome differences after endoscopic drainage of pancreatic necrosis, acute pancreatic pseudocysts, and chronic pancreatic pseudocysts. Gastrointest Endosc 2002;56:7–17.

25. Charnley RM, Lochan R, Gray H, et al. Endoscopic necrosectomy as primary therapy in the management of infected pancreatic necrosis. Endoscopy 2006;38:925–8.

26. Escourrou J, Shehab H, Buscail L, et al. Peroral transgastric/transduodenal necrosectomy: success in the treatment of infected pancreatic necrosis. Ann Surg 2008;248:1074–80.

27. van Santvoort HC, Bakker OJ, Bollen TL, et al. A conservative and minimally invasive approach to necrotizing pancreatitis improves outcome. Gastroenterology 2011;141:1254–63.

28. van Santvoort HC, Besselink MG, Bakker OJ, et al. Endoscopic necrosectomy in necrotising pancreatitis: indication is the key. Gut 2010;59:1587.
29. Wilcox CM, Varadarajulu S, Morgan D, et al. Progress in the management of necrotizing pancreatitis. Expert Rev Gastroenterol Hepatol 2010;4:701–8.
30. Beger HG, Krautzberger W, Bittner R, et al. Results of surgical treatment of necrotizing pancreatitis. World J Surg 1985;9:972–9.
31. Branum G, Galloway J, Hirchowitz W, et al. Pancreatic necrosis: results of necrosectomy, packing, and ultimate closure over drains. Ann Surg 1998;227: 870–7.
32. Echenique AM, Sleeman D, Yrizarry J, et al. Percutaneous catheter-directed debridement of infected pancreatic necrosis: results in 20 patients. J Vasc Interv Radiol 1998;9:565–71.
33. Fotoohi M, D'Agostino HB, Wollman B, et al. Persistent pancreatocutaneous fistula after percutaneous drainage of pancreatic fluid collections: role of cause and severity of pancreatitis. Radiology 1999;213:573–8.
34. Barthet M, Sahel J, Bodiou-Bertei C, et al. Endoscopic transpapillary drainage of pancreatic pseudocysts. Gastrointest Endosc 1995;42(3):208–13.
35. Baron TH. Endoscopic drainage of pancreatic pseudocysts. J Gastrointest Surg 2008;12:369–72.
36. Hookey LC, Debroux S, Delhaye M, et al. Endoscopic drainage of pancreatic fluid collections in 116 patients: a comparison of etiologies, drainage techniques and outcomes. Gastrointest Endosc 2006;63:635–43.
37. Carter CR, McKay CJ, Imrie CW. Percutaneous necrosectomy and sinus tract endoscopy in the management of infected pancreatic necrosis: an initial experience. Ann Surg 2000;232:175–80.
38. Hawes RH. Endoscopic management of pseudocysts. Rev Gastroenterol Disord 2003;3:135–41.
39. Kozarek RA, Brayko CM, Harlan J, et al. Endoscopic drainage of pancreatic pseudocysts. Gastrointest Endosc 1985;31:322–7.
40. Cremer M, Deviere J, Engelholm L. Endoscopic management of cysts and pseudocysts in chronic pancreatitis: long-term follow-up after 7 years of experience. Gastrointest Endosc 1989;35:1–9.
41. Besselink MG. The 'step-up approach' to infected necrotizing pancreatitis: delay, drain, debride. Dig Liver Dis 2011;43:421–2.
42. Wiersema MJ, Baron TH, Chari ST. Endosonography-guided pseudocyst drainage with a new large-channel linear scanning echoendoscope. Gastrointest Endosc 2001;53:811–3.
43. Besselink MG, van Santvoort HC, Nieuwenhuijs VB, et al. Minimally invasive 'step-up approach' versus maximal necrosectomy in patients with acute necrotising pancreatitis (PANTER trial): design and rationale of a randomised controlled multicenter trial. BMC Surg 2006;6:6.
44. Gluck M, Ross A, Irani S, et al. Endoscopic and percutaneous drainage of symptomatic walled-off pancreatic necrosis reduces hospital stay and radiographic resources. Clin Gastroenterol Hepatol 2010;8:1083–8.
45. Ross A, Gluck M, Irani S, et al. Combined endoscopic and percutaneous drainage of organized pancreatic necrosis. Gastrointest Endosc 2010;71: 79–84.
46. Varadarajulu S, Christein JD, Tamhane A, et al. Prospective randomized trial comparing EUS and EGD for transmural drainage of pancreatic pseudocysts (with videos). Gastrointest Endosc 2008;68:1102–11.

47. Park DH, Lee SS, Moon SH, et al. Endoscopic ultrasound-guided versus conventional transmural drainage for pancreatic pseudocysts: a prospective randomized trial. Endoscopy 2009;41:842–8.
48. Sauer B, Kahaleh M. Prospective randomized trial comparing EUS and EGD for transmural drainage of pancreatic pseudocysts: a need for a large randomized study. Gastrointest Endosc 2010;71:432.
49. Varadarajulu S, Phadnis MA, Christein JD, et al. Multiple transluminal gateway technique for EUS-guided drainage of symptomatic walled-off pancreatic necrosis. Gastrointest Endosc 2011;74:74–80.
50. Antillon MR, Bechtold ML, Bartalos CR, et al. Transgastric endoscopic necrosectomy with temporary metallic esophageal stent placement for the treatment of infected pancreatic necrosis. Gastrointest Endosc 2009;69:178–80.
51. Shrode CW, Macdonough P, Gaidhane M, et al. Multimodality endosocpic treatment of pancreatic duct disruption with with stenting and pseudocyst drainage: how efficacious is it? Dig Dis Sci 2013;45(2):129–33.
52. Gardner TB, Coelho-Prabhu N, Gordon SR, et al. Direct endoscopic necrosectomy for the treatment of walled-off pancreatic necrosis: results from a multicenter U.S. series. Gastrointest Endosc 2011;73:718–26.
53. Raczynski S, Teich N, Borte G, et al. Percutaneous transgastric irrigation drainage in combination with endoscopic necrosectomy in necrotizing pancreatitis. Gastrointest Endosc 2006;64:420–4.
54. Talreja JP, Kahaleh M. Endotherapy for pancreatic necrosis and abscess: endoscopic drainage and necrosectomy. J Hepatobiliary Pancreat Surg 2009;16:605–12.
55. Varadarajulu S, Lopes TL, Wilcox CM, et al. EUS versus surgical cystgastrostomy for management of pancreatic pseudocysts. Gastrointest Endosc 2008;68:649–55.
56. Seewald S, Groth S, Omar S, et al. Aggressive endoscopic therapy for pancreatic necrosis and pancreatic abscess: a new safe and effective treatment algorithm. Gastrointest Endosc 2005;62:92–100.
57. Hocke M, Will U, Gottschalk P, et al. Transgastral retroperitoneal endoscopy in septic patients with pancreatic necrosis or infected pancreatic pseudocysts. Z Gastroenterol 2008;46:1363–8.
58. Seifert H, Biermer M, Schmitt W, et al. Transluminal endoscopic necrosectomy after acute pancreatitis: a multicentre study with long-term follow-up (the GEPARD Study). Gut 2009;58:1260–6.

Endoscopic Therapy for Acute Recurrent Pancreatitis

Jason R. Roberts, MD[a],*, Joseph Romagnuolo, MD, MSc[b]

KEYWORDS

- Acute recurrent pancreatitis • Endoscopic therapy • Idiopathic pancreatitis
- Endoscopic spincterotomy • Biliary pancreatitis • Relapsing pancreatitis
- Pancreas divisum • Sphincter of Oddi dysfunction

KEY POINTS

- Endoscopy plays an important role in both the diagnosis and the initial management of recurrent acute pancreatitis, as well as the investigation of refractory disease, but it has known limitations and risks.
- Sound selective use of these therapies, complemented with other lines of investigation such as genetic testing, can dramatically improve frequency of attacks and associated quality of life.
- Whether endoscopic therapy can reduce progression to chronic pancreatitis, or reduce the risk of malignancy, is debatable, and remains to be proven.

INTRODUCTION

Acute pancreatitis (AP) is a common disease, affecting 17 per 100,000 persons per year in the United States alone. Eighty percent of cases are uncomplicated and self-limited, whereby patients are expected to have a complete symptomatic and pathologic recovery. On the other hand, approximately 20% will go on to have subsequent attacks, which are described as recurrent acute pancreatitis (RAP), which is primarily dependent on whether the underlying cause is able to be treated or removed.[1-3] Although there is no formally agreed on definition, RAP is generally considered as 2 or more episodes of AP with or without complete or near-complete resolution of symptoms between episodes.[4] Occasionally, patients are labeled as having RAP but are not truly documented as meeting the standard definition of having admissions for bone fide pancreatitis as defined by 2 of 3 of the following: compatible pain, lipase and/or amylase more than 3 times normal, and/or imaging as supporting evidence. Patients with only mild pancreatic enzyme elevations

[a] Division of Gastroenterology, Hepatology, and Nutrition, University of Louisivlle School of Medicine, 550 South Jackson Street, Louisville, KY 40202, USA; [b] Division of Gastroenterology and Hepatology, Medical University of South Carolina, 25 Courtenay Drive, ART 7100A, MSC 290, Charleston, SC 29425, USA
* Corresponding author.
E-mail address: jason.roberts@louisville.edu

Gastrointest Endoscopy Clin N Am 23 (2013) 803–819
http://dx.doi.org/10.1016/j.giec.2013.06.006
1052-5157/13/$ – see front matter © 2013 Elsevier Inc. All rights reserved.

are better labeled as such—pain and hyperenzymemia of unclear significance. Before embarking on many of the expensive and/or invasive studies discussed in this article, it is important to ensure that one or more of the patient's pain admissions were, in fact, AP. Perhaps, however, abdominal pain only without documented pancreatitis is not a focus of this review for idiopathic RAP (IRAP). Certainly Sphincter of Oddi dysfunction (SOD) is a consideration in these patients and the ddx does overlap with that of IRAP, which also includes divisum, but the efficacy of sphincter of Oddi manometry (SOM)-guided sphincter treatment and minor papillotomy is less painful only in population without objective pathology.

The natural history of RAP is incompletely understood, with most data coming from population studies showing a 25% to 45% recurrence in alcohol-related AP.[5,6] Although only about 10% of individual AP attacks in RAP are severe, cumulative morbidity and mortality, as well as health care- and quality of life–related costs are substantial.[7] Most AP is due to gallstones or excessive alcohol; right upper quadrant ultrasound and a thorough history of alcohol use (past, present, and binge) are standard first-line investigations. Abstinence of alcohol significantly reduces the recurrence of alcohol-related pancreatitis, and cholecystectomy is effective at preventing recurrent biliary pancreatitis, thereby addressing the 2 most common causes of RAP. Smoking is a newly recognized risk factor, but the effect of smoking cessation on outcomes is not clear; it should lower the risk of chronic pancreatitis and cancer at the least.[8] Despite a thorough history, routine laboratory evaluation, and routine biliary/pancreatic imaging, 30% of RAP remains unexplained and is referred to as idiopathic (IRAP).[9–12]

DEFINING AND STUDYING IRAP

The incidence, natural history, and treatment of IRAP have been difficult to study because there has been some lack of consensus on a definition of "idiopathic." There are several diagnostic studies to investigate the remaining 30%, ranging from bile crystal analysis, pancreatic function testing, genetic testing for mutations associated with pancreatitis (secretin-stimulated), magnetic resonance cholangiopancreatography (MRCP), endoscopic ultrasound (EUS), ± secretin or elastography, and endoscopic retrograde cholangiopancreatography (ERCP) with SOM. Several of these investigations are invasive and are associated with morbidity, such as post-ERCP pancreatitis, and many are not readily available outside of tertiary care facilities; bile crystal analysis is done poorly and with inconsistent methods even in tertiary facilities and the relevance of microlithiasis is questionable, because of variability in interpretation and the small size of related studies.[13,14] The thresholds for alcohol intake and triglyceride levels to be deemed relevant can be variable. SOD as defined by SOM, findings suggestive of minimal change chronic pancreatitis, and presence of pancreas divisum (PD) are examples of findings that may simply be incidental; they play controversial roles as causes or explanations, and as such, they may or may not need to be "ruled out" before categorizing someone's pancreatitis as "unexplained."

For all of these reasons, studies evaluating endoscopic therapy in an IRAP population can involve a heterogeneous group. Furthermore, comparing studies from different institutions across different eras is problematic considering the changes to standard of care involved in setting the threshold of calling RAP "idiopathic." In a large single-center series involving 1241 patients with RAP, Fischer and colleagues[15] found that ERCP with SOM yielded a diagnosis in 65.8% of cases (40.8% SOD, 18.8% PD). Ninety-two percent of these cases were amenable to endoscopic therapy. However, the outcomes of intervention were not reported.

There is known overlap between RAP and chronic pancreatitis. It is likely that many patients in the alcoholic RAP studies who also had chronic pancreatitis actually were having flares of acute-on-chronic pancreatitis; although others may have begun with RAP, but accumulated damage, such that at the time of presentation, chronic pancreatitis changes were incidentally already present. This may also occur in young patients with presumed or proven genetic pancreatitis, and in other causes that are associated with both acute and chronic pancreatitis, such as hypertriglyceridemia. Using EUS to evaluate patients after a single episode of AP and those with RAP, Yusoff and colleagues[16] found significantly more chronic pancreatitis (usually of the small-duct or "minimal change" variety) in the RAP group than in the single-attack group (21% vs 42%), and in patients with, and without, an intact gallbladder (16% vs 39%). For EUS, one must be careful not to assess for chronic pancreatitis too close to the last acute attack, because lingering acute changes may be misinterpreted as chronic pancreatitis changes. The outcomes of RAP patients with and without chronic pancreatitis likely differ, yet the extent to which chronic pancreatitis in these studies was excluded varies from the use of inclusion criteria requiring no advanced morphologic (ductal or parenchymal) changes on cross-sectional imaging, to requiring a normal ERCP, to requiring normal pancreatic exocrine function testing. Furthermore, a substantial number of patients with acute recurrent pancreatitis suffer substantial interval chronic pain between overt attacks, some with and some without morphologic evidence of chronic pancreatitis. Conversely, other patients with clinical presentation of only RAP without interval pain have obvious calcific chronic pancreatitis. Thus the distinction between RAP and chronic pancreatitis may be clear only at either extreme.

RECURRENT PANCREATITIS WITH APPARENT OR POSSIBLE CAUSES
Biliary (Gallstone) Pancreatitis

Gallstones cause one of the most common, and treatable, forms of AP, accounting for 50% to 70% of cases.[17] Unlike most symptomatic choledocholithiasis with ongoing biliary obstruction in which a stone too large to pass through the sphincter of Oddi (SO) becomes lodged in the distal common bile duct, biliary pancreatitis is more likely to result from small stones that transiently obstruct the pancreas drainage at the SO before spontaneously passing—as such, even small stones and sludge are likely still relevant. The resultant edema/obstruction of the common channel presumably causes elevated intraductal pressure in the pancreas and/or reflux of bile into the duct leading to the activated enzymatic cascade of AP. Because most stones (80%) pass with the onset of the attack, the lack of imaging confirmation of a persistent bile duct stone after presentation cannot be considered as evidence against a biliary cause. RAP occurs very frequently (30%–90%) if cholelithiasis is present and the gallbladder is left in situ.[9,18–22] Cholecystectomy reduces the risk of biliary RAP to about 10%; this figure suggests that cholecystectomy is effective in preventing recurrent attacks of pancreatitis, while at the same time illustrating that cholelithiasis may be incidental in a small proportion of patients with RAP.

After endoscopic sphincterotomy became available in the 1970s, it became recognized as an effective primary therapy to prevent recurrent biliary pancreatitis in older patients, those unfit for cholecystectomy, and those who declined surgery. Laparoscopic cholecystectomy was associated with a decline in this practice. Recurrence of biliary pancreatitis with in situ gallbladder following endoscopic sphincterotomy ranged from 2% to 6% (median follow-up ranged from 12 to 51 months).[23–26] However, randomized trials have shown that unless life expectancy is less than a few years, laparoscopic cholecystectomy offers a lower rate of gallbladder-related biliary sepsis, even after biliary sphincterotomy. Contrary to the belief by some, occult choledocholithiasis as a cause of postcholecystectomy RAP is rare (0%, n = 57) and does not seem to justify empiric biliary sphincterotomy for presumed choledocholithiasis in the IRAP group, especially for those with normal or near-normal liver enzymes with their RAP attacks.[16] Even when liver enzymes are mildly abnormal, pancreatic edema and/or biliary SOD may be the more likely cause for the mild liver enzyme abnormalities.

Pancreas Divisum

PD is the most common congenital pancreatic ductal anomaly occurring in 2.7% to 22% of the Western populations; it is less common in Asians.[27,28] The clinical significance of PD is controversial as the majority of individuals with PD in the general population are asymptomatic; however, PD has been implicated by some as a cause of RAP, chronic pancreatitis, and chronic or recurrent epigastric pain. For proponents of the clinical significance of PD, the relatively smaller orifice of the minor papilla as compared with the major papilla results in increased intraductal pressures in the dorsal duct and interstitium in some patients,[29,30] and especially if genetically predisposed, this may result in RAP or chronic pancreatitis.

Endoscopic treatment of PD-related disease has consisted of ablation of the minor papilla via sphincterotomy or periods of stenting. The enthusiasm for these techniques has been tempered by the adverse events of stenting, and the lack of prospective controlled trials of minor papilla sphincterotomy. The only small randomized trial of PD in RAP used stenting; however, because of the risk for chronic stent-induced dorsal duct changes and need for repeat endoscopies to exchange/remove stents, minor papilla sphincterotomy has become the most widely used treatment.[31] Post-ERCP pancreatitis (5%–15%) and sphincter restenosis (20%–30%) are the most common adverse events.[32,33] Given the higher risks associated with therapy for the minor papilla compared with biliary sphincterotomy, it has become standard to routinely place a small-caliber (usually 3-Fr or 4-Fr) stent that either is without internal flanges or is made of soft material with an inner flange, and to administer 100 mg rectal indomethacin to reduce the risk of treatment-related pancreatitis.

One piece of evidence in favor of PD as a cause of RAP is its apparent concentration, or increase in prevalence, in IRAP patients who have had common causes excluded by a thorough history, routine laboratory testing, and pancreas/biliary imaging. In this group, the frequency of PD at ERCP ranges from 8% to 50% (commonly about 20%) compared with 3% to 12% in controls.[34–39] This apparent doubling of prevalence in patients with the outcome implies a possible doubling of risk by the presence of the PD factor.

It is well-recognized now that PD with RAP is associated with increased prevalence of genetic abnormalities. However, one should understand that this certainly does not necessarily mean the PD anatomy and intraductal pressure is not a cofactor in these patients.[40–43]

In fact, increased viscosity of secretions (due to genetic factors), in the presence of a small minor papilla orifice and PD anatomy, might explain increased penetrance of the phenotype in PD patients when they have cystic fibrosis transmembrane conductance regulator (CFTR) mutations. It is also not clear if those PD patients with genetic problems are less responsive to endoscopic therapy, or perhaps more responsive.[43]

Lans and colleagues[31] performed the only prospective randomized sham controlled study evaluating the efficacy of minor papilla therapy in RAP, consisting of mild bougie dilation with stenting. Nineteen patients with PD-associated RAP were randomized at the time of ERCP to papillary dilation with a graduated Soehendra catheter (4–7 Fr) and dorsal duct stenting (5 or 7 Fr) compared with sham. The stent group was followed with stent changes every 4 months for 1 year in parallel with the control group. After 1 year, the stents were removed and both groups were followed for 28 and 31 months, respectively, for the primary outcome (any RAP in follow-up). After randomization, no patients in the treatment group (n = 10) developed subsequent pancreatitis or required medical care for pain, versus 6 of the 9 patients in the control group, who experienced 7 episodes of pancreatitis during follow-up (P<.05). In addition, 5 patients in the control group were admitted to the hospital with 2 visiting the emergency room for pain. There was also a statistically significant reduction in pain for the stent group (P<.05) using a symptom questionnaire.

Studies of the more commonly used treatment, minor papilla sphincterotomy, have been confined to case series. In a retrospective study by Borak and colleagues,[29] 101 patients with PD were treated with minor papilla sphincterotomy for the indications of RAP, chronic pancreatitis, and abdominal pain without pancreatitis. Telephone questionnaire responses regarding narcotic dosage, symptom improvement (using a 5-point Likert scale), and need for repeat ERCP or acute medical care were used to assess treatment response with a median follow-up of 43 months (range 14–116). Success, defined as improvement or resolution of symptoms, without additional ERCP, and without requiring narcotics for pain control was achieved in 53.2% of RAP, 18.2% in chronic pancreatitis, and 41.4% with pain alone. Secondary success as defined by having 3 or fewer ERCPs with improved symptoms and no narcotic needs was seen in 71%, 45.5%, and 52.2%, respectively. Both needle-knife (usually over a pancreatic stent) and pull-type (traction) sphincterotomies (usually a miniature sphincterotome) appear safe; restenosis rates of the 2 techniques also appear similar.[44] Younger age may predict high restenosis after both endoscopic and surgical therapies.[44,45]

The pooled results of 14 studies evaluating endoscopic therapy success in the treatment of PD with RAP are shown in **Table 1**.[29,32,33,46–54] A total of 368 patients included in the studies were treated with minor papilla stenting or sphincterotomy and 316 (86%) of them were considered treatment successes. PD associated with chronic pancreatitis or pain alone had lower treatment response rates to endoscopic therapy at 51.3% and 44.4%, respectively. Most of these studies were retrospective, with variable definitions for treatment success, involved small patient numbers, had variable follow-up, and involved heterogeneity in therapies, including both sphincterotomy and stenting. The lack of a control group when the natural history is variable, as it is in RAP, is problematic, and the lack of blinding when looking at subjective outcomes like pain response is prone to bias. It is known that placebo responses in functional dyspepsia patients can be 30% to 40%. Blinding is less important to the more objective outcomes like documented hospitalization for biochemically proven RAP.[29]

It is clear that robust data are needed to assess the role of PD in RAP. The FRAMES (Frequency of Recurrent Acute pancreatitis after Minor papilla Endoscopic Sphincterotomy) study is a National Institutes of Health–funded pilot study. Romagnuolo and coinvestigators designed as a pilot a multicentered prospective series of sphincterotomy (with temporary small caliber duct stenting), and a critical step toward a multicentered randomized trial on this issue. Pain burden was carefully evaluated by a validated tool (the RAPID, Recurrent Abdominal Pain Intensity and Disability index), and blood was collected for genetic testing. The study demonstrated a low recurrence of pancreatitis 6 months after ERCP and a dramatic decrease in RAPID score after sphincterotomy from grade 4 of 4 to 1 of 4.[55] FRAMES also showed a very high minor papilla success rate in expert hands. The minor papilla is found proximally and to the

Table 1
Endoscopic therapy for PD associated with RAP

Author	Patients	Follow-up, mo	Response,[a] n (%)
Satterfield et al,[46] 1988	10	18	6 (60)
McCarthy et al,[47] 1988	19	14	17 (90)
Lans[b] et al,[31] 1992	10	28	10 (100)
Lehman et al,[33] 1993	17	20	13 (77)
Coleman et al,[48] 1994	9	23	7 (78)
Kozarek et al,[32] 1995	15	20	15 (100)
Jacob et al,[49] 1999	10	15	6 (60)
Ertan,[b,50] 2000	24	24	19 (79)
Heyries et al,[51] 2002	24	39	20 (83)
Linder[c] et al,[52] 2003	83	NA (3–36)	54 (66)
Linder[c] et al,[52] 2003	38	NA (1–120)	22 (58)
Borak et al,[29] 2009	62	44	44 (71)
Bierig[c] et al,[53] 2006	16	19	15 (94)
Kwan et al,[54] 2008	21	38	13 (62)
Overall	368	14–44	316 (86)

Abbreviation: NA, not available.
[a] Treatment response is defined as a reduction in symptoms, RAP, or hospitalizations.
[b] Indicates prospective trials.
[c] Presented as abstracts only.

right on the endoscopic screen of the major papilla, and the most stable approach position in most patients is a "long-scope" position, advancing the scope after "shortening" in front of the major papilla. Administering secretin intravenously has been shown to help in visualization of the minor papilla orifice and improve cannulation rates.[56] Despite the widely held concept that most patients with symptomatic PD have a prominent minor papilla, in the recent FRAMES study, half the minor papillas were very subtle, with greater than 10% of cases needing secretin just to find the minor papilla (Romagnuolo et al, Unpublished data, 2013). Methylene blue sprayed on the duodenal wall in the expected area of the minor papilla may help identify the orifice when clear pancreatic juice washes away the dye.[57–59] In comparison with the reasonably high success of free catheter cannulation in the major papilla, leading and cannulating the minor papilla with a wire is needed in most cases. The FRAMES study is intended as a pilot toward feasibility of a double-blind, randomized controlled trial comparing minor papillotomy with sham treatment in patients with PD and acute recurrent pancreatitis.

Sphincter of Oddi Dysfunction (SOD)

SOD is defined manometrically as sustained basal sphincter pressures greater than 40 mm Hg (30 seconds long monitoring, in 2 leads). SOD is a common finding in IRAP with an incidence ranging from 30% to 65%.[12,56,57,60] In addition, spasm of the SO is implicated as a mechanism for hypercalcemia-related pancreatitis, gallstone pancreatitis, post-ERCP pancreatitis, and perhaps some medication-induced pancreatitis. However, some authors have suggested that SOD may simply be a result of sphincter scarring from repeated pancreatitis and is not the cause of the disease.[61] Endoscopic biliary sphincterotomy alone or combined with pancreatic sphincterotomy has been used to treat SOD, but ERCP for this indication is associated with high reported rates of post-ERCP pancreatitis. In perfusion manometry catheter systems, aspirating while perfusing is critical to avoid increasing intraductal pressures; however, it is thought that the disease and the patient are the most important risk factors for post-ERCP pancreatitis, not the manometry. Skipping the manometry does not significantly reduce the risk.[62]

Hogan and colleagues[63] characterized patients meeting the Rome III criteria for SOD according to biliary/pancreatic ductal dilatation, elevated liver/pancreatic biomarkers, and pain. Type II pancreatic SOD is a heterogeneous group ranging from mild lipase elevations with pain to RAP, with an elevated basal sphincter pressure found in 58% (vs 92% in type 1 [more objective findings] and 35% in type 3 [no objective findings]).

In patients with well-documented RAP, where a thorough history, routine laboratory testing, and conventional imaging have not found a cause, abnormal SOM is found in 15% to 72%.[3,12,64–69] Surgical and endoscopic ablation of the biliary sphincter, pancreatic sphincter, or both have been shown to decrease future episodes of RAP.[60,65,68–76] **Table 2** summarizes endoscopic therapy for RAP in patients with documented SOD. The sphincter complex comprises a common sphincter and a biliary sphincter (both of which are cut when a biliary sphincterotomy is performed), and a pancreatic sphincter; as a result, depending on the relative contributions of the common versus the pancreatic sphincter to a person's manometric pancreatic sphincter hypertension, a simple biliary endoscopic sphincterotomy (BES) can reduce pancreatic sphincter pressures substantially in some patients.[77] In others, a dual (pancreatic and biliary) endoscopic sphincterotomy (DES) is needed to normalize the pancreatic sphincter pressures. Eversman and colleagues[78] showed these separate sphincter complexes clinically performing SOM in both sphincter segments in 593 patients referred for IRAP, AP, chronic pancreatitis, or unexplained abdominal pain. They reported a discordance rate of 26% to 35% between the 2 sphincter segments for biliary and pancreatic SOD, respectively. In patients with prior BES, with ongoing symptoms, there was residual pancreatic sphincter hypertension in 46%, compared with only 20% residual hypertension in patients with a previous DES.

Table 2				
Endoscopic therapy for sphincter of Oddi dysfunction associated with RAP				
Author	Patients, n	Design	Follow-up	Results/Recurrence
Kaw and Brodmerkel,[69] 2002	37	Prospective	29 mo (18–33)	29 (78%) no recurrence
Coyle et al,[60] 2002	21	Retrospective	Not given	Frequency dropped to <1/mo in 72%; pain severity decreased from 8.7 to 1.7 of 10
Wehrmann et al,[76] 2000	37	Prospective	32 mo (24–53)	32 (86%) no recurrence
Cote et al,[77] 2012	69 w/pSOD	Prospective, randomized to BES vs DES	78 mo (35–108)	BES: 17/33 (52%) no recurrence DES: 19/36 (53%) no recurrence
Cote et al,[77] 2012	20 w/normal SOM	Prospective, randomized to BES vs sham	78 mo (35–108)	BES: 8/11 (73%) no recurrence Sham: 8/9 (89%) no recurrence

It is not clear if biliary SOD in isolation is truly associated with RAP, or on a related note, whether BES alone can really reduce the risk of recurrence in RAP patients. Sherman and colleagues[68] showed no recurrence in 44% of RAP patients with SOD treated with BES alone over 5 years. A later study by Guelrud and colleagues[73] showed a lower rate of recurrence in pancreatic SOD RAP patients treated with DES, rather than BES, over 1 year. A recently published prospective randomized trial compared BES to DES in the treatment of pancreatic SOD (pSOD). Eighty-nine patients underwent successful ERCP with SOM for the indication of IRAP. pSOD was found in 69 patients (77.5%). Patients were randomized after SOM to receive a BES alone (n = 33) or a DES (n = 36). The rate of RAP was similar for the pSOD patients in both treatment arms (48.5% BES vs 47.2% DES; P = .20) over a median of 78 months (interquartile range, 23–108 months). No significant differences were seen between BES and DES, but the study was only powered for detection of a 50% absolute risk reduction, so is likely underpowered. There was a parallel cohort including 20 patients with IRAP and normal pancreatic SOM randomized to sham (n = 9) or BES (n = 11); in these groups, the rate of RAP was very low and not different between the 2 groups (11% vs 27%), although this comparison had even lower power. Post-ERCP pancreatitis occurred in 13 of 89 (14.6%) patients and was not significantly different between the BES and DES groups; however, again, this is likely underpowered. The findings of this study suggest the benefit of DES over BES may be lower than previously thought in reducing episodes or RAP, and that those patients with normal pancreatic SOM have a good prognosis and do not likely benefit from (empiric) endoscopic therapy.[77] The lack of a control group in the pSOD cohort, however, does not provide answers as to whether endoscopic sphincterotomy (of either type) reduces RAP compared with no therapy. Regarding sphincterotomy technique, both needle-knife and pull-type pancreatic sphincterotomies seem safe, although one study found slightly higher risk in the needle-knife group.[79]

In summary, ERCP with SOM is an important diagnostic test for the evaluation of IRAP and detects elevated basal SO pressures in 15% to 72% of patients.[10,64,66–69] Diagnosing SOD in IRAP and ablative treatment of the SO, based on nonrandomized data, seems effective in reducing the risk of RAP, but the role of DES over BES in these patients is not clear, and the effect of this therapy on the risk of subsequent chronic pancreatitis is not known.[80] Larger prospective, ideally randomized, studies with longer term follow-up are needed to further the understanding of the associations between SOD, RAP, and chronic pancreatitis.

MISCELLANEOUS CAUSES OF RECURRENT ACUTE PANCREATITIS
Anomalous Pancreaticobiliary Junction

Anomalous Pancreaticobiliary Junction (APBJ) is a congenital anomaly associated with a long common channel shared by the terminal pancreas and bile duct. It is defined as a common channel greater than 15 mm as measured from the duodenal wall to the separation of the respective ducts. APBJ is associated with choledochal cysts and can lead to both biliary and pancreatic disease. Acute, chronic, and recurrent pancreatitis have all been described in patients with APBJ. The mechanism for how pancreatitis develops is not completely understood. One theory is that intraductal pressures in the pancreas rise as a result of refluxing bile which may also lead to activation of pancreatic enzymes. Radiolucent protein plugs have also been described which may lead to transient ductal obstruction. Takuma et al[81] reviewed 381 patients with acute and recurrent acute pancreatitis and found APBJ in 26%. Longer common channel segments (>21 mm), common channels >5 mm in diameter, filling defects, and other ductal anomalies were associated with a higher incidence of pancreatitis in 16 of 58 patients with APBJ.[82] The Indianapolis group performed endoscopic sphincterotomy ± choledochal cyst excision in 15 patients with APBJ associated acute pancreatitis resulting in a decrease in symptoms and frequence of pancreatitis in 13 patients.[83] Given the strong association of choledochal cyst and the risk of gallbladder and or cholangiocarcinoma, prophylactic surgical removal of the gallbladder and/or cysts remains the primary consideration in these patients. It is unclear whether prophylactic endoscopic therapy prevents acute pancreatitis or progression to chronic pancreatitis.

Duodenal Duplication Cysts

Duodenal Duplication Cysts (DDC) are the rarest form of congenital gastrointestinal duplication cysts and are a rare cause of acute and recurrent forms of pancreatitis. They may be difficult to distinguish from type III choledochal cysts, but confirmation can be made with a cholangiogram, although EUS and MRI offer effective, less invasive diagnostic tests. DDC are fluid filled with normal duodenal mucosa on the inner and outer sides with intervening muscularis mucosae on histology. This double sided mucosa is easily demonstrated with EUS. They appear as a bulging mass in the duodenal lumen and often involve the major papilla. Endoscopic marsupialization of the luminal side of the cyst causes decompression via drainage of the fluid contents. Antaki et al followed up 8 patients with DDC, 7 with acute or recurrent acute pancreatitis and all treated with marsupialization of the cyst. There were no recurrent symptoms in any patients with a median follow up of 7.3 years (5 months to 13 years).[84]

SUMMARIES OF APPROACH AND DIAGNOSTIC ALGORITHM
Summary of Imaging and Initial Evaluation

If the initial evaluation with a thorough history (including alcohol and smoking patterns and medication review), examination, and laboratory testing (triglycerides, calcium) is abnormal and the gallbladder is still present, then good-quality abdominal ultrasonography should be performed to look for cholelithiasis or sludge. An EUS and/or magnetic resonance imaging (MRI)/MRCP should then be performed to outline anatomy, identify PD, uncover occult cholelithiasis or chronic pancreatitis (especially obstructive pancreatopathy), and identify tumors (solid or cystic). These noninvasive pancreatobiliary imaging studies detect gallbladder sludge/stones, chronic pancreatitis, pancreatic mass lesions, or abnormal pancreatic ductal anatomy, such as divisum, in 57% of cases; pSOD cannot be detected with these tests. The performance of EUS and MRI seems comparable for diagnosing most of these abnormalities; however, several studies have demonstrated improved detection of subtle gallbladder stones/sludge, minimal-change chronic pancreatitis, and small pancreatic/ampullary tumors with EUS[85]; as such, the authors' group prefers EUS in patients with gallbladder in situ, chronic pain, and older age or unexplained weight loss, respectively. Regarding the first indication, Yusoff and colleagues[16] found stones or sludge in 17% of patients with RAP with a gallbladder, whereas the diagnostic yield for biliary disease was much lower in patients with prior cholecystectomy, and almost zero in the RAP postcholecystectomy group. There are conflicting studies regarding the performance of the 2 in diagnosing PD, but both MRCP (with and without secretin) and EUS had a high PPV in the FRAMES study (Romagnuolo et al, Unpublished data, 2013).[86,87] **Fig. 1** shows the authors' suggested approach to the management of IRAP.

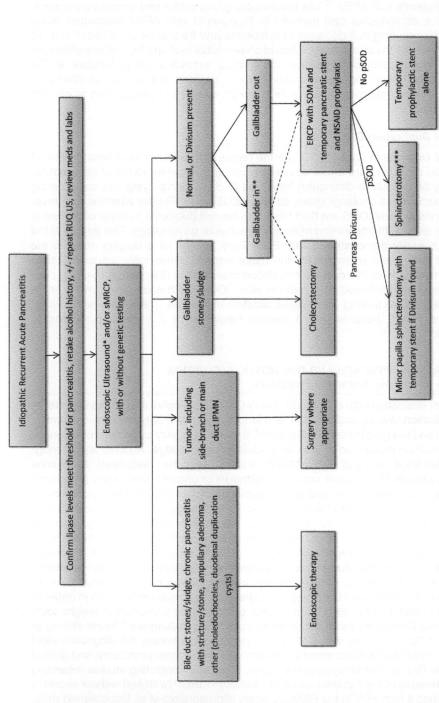

Fig. 1. Management of idiopathic RAP. *Preferred if gallbladder in situ, weight loss, or age greater than 60 years. **If normal, especially including EUS of the gallbladder, ERCP with manometry is justifiable, although some clinicians prefer empiric cholecystectomy, reserving manometry for postchole-cystectomy patients. There are no good data to support empiric cholecystectomy. ***One underpowered study suggested biliary and dual sphincter-otomy were equivalent; however, experts still think this is controversial. IPMN, intraductal papillary mucinous neoplasm; NSAID, nonsteroidal anti-inflammatory drug; RUQ, right upper quadrant; sMRCP, secretin magnetic resonance cholangiopancreatography; US, ultrasound.

Summary of Steps After Imaging

IRAP with normal findings on EUS or MRI should be considered for genetic testing and be considered for referral for ERCP with SOM to evaluate for pSOD. BES/DES with temporary pancreatic stenting and rectal indomethacin prophylaxis should be performed; the decision of which sphincter to treat at this time must be left to the discretion of the clinician because the data are sparse and underpowered.[77] Hepatobiliary iminodiacetic acid scan (HIDA), secretin EUS (sEUS), and secretin magnetic resonance cholangiopancreatography (sMRCP) are unfortunately not good at predicting pSOD.[87–89] As discussed above, empiric biliary sphincterotomy is not indicated and is high risk, and not likely helpful when pSOM is normal.[77] Bile collection for crystals via ERCP takes on the risks of an ERCP and is likely of extremely low yield in postcholecystectomy subjects, and bile collection via EUS FNA of the gallbladder has been shown to be also high risk; the data do not support either of these maneuvers.[90]

Although often deferred by patients, genetic testing is an appropriate consideration at any point during the evaluation of IRAP because perhaps 50% of patients will have mutations in SPINK1, PRSS1, or CFTR genes; however, there are no gene-guided therapeutic options in these patients unless a coexisting obstructive abnormality such as PD is found.[91] The tests remain expensive and only partially covered by insurance; although there are legal protections from discrimination based on these test results, there may be stigma related to harboring a genetic predisposition to disease, and genetic counseling is recommended for positive results, especially PRSS1 because of the high penetrance and cancer risk. Trials are underway with drugs that may improve CFTR function and could be used in the future. Studies have shown an increased prevalence of PD in patients with CFTR mutations without phenotypic cystic fibrosis supporting the theory of gene mutations as cofactors in pancreatitis. Overall, SPINK-1 appears to be the most common mutation in sporadic IRAP. In familial or hereditary pancreatitis, PRSS1 mutations are the most commonly found abnormalities in an autosomal-dominant inheritance pattern and is associated with an increased lifetime risk of pancreatic cancer of 40%.[7] There are no guidelines on screening tests or intervals for pancreatic cancer in these individuals. Although rarely autoimmune pancreatitis can present as AP without a mass or other autoimmune features, this phenotype is uncommon, and not likely worth routine IgG4 in all these patients; selective testing may be considered.

Approach to Refractory or Recurrent Disease

Some patients continue to have RAP despite the above-mentioned factors. If genetic testing has not been performed, it should now be reconsidered. If a cluster of RAP occurs months after endoscopic therapy, restenosis should be considered. After pancreatic sphincterotomy, this is known to occur in 20% to 30% of patients[44,77]; pancreatic restenosis or residual pSOD is found in about two-thirds of such patients.[77] Biliary restenosis is rare (<5%); most often, pSOD is the only finding, if any, in the post-BES patients who have ongoing symptoms. However, one should understand that many PD and SOD patients also likely have a genetic predisposition, so a single recurrent attack that happens in the future is not completely unexpected and does not necessarily require extensive investigation. Clusters of attacks, however, usually lead to repeat manometry. Manometric restenosis can be treated with further sphincterotomy, often with a traction technique with a miniature sphincterotome; if there is no more room to cut, a small dilating balloon matched to the duct size (eg, 4 mm diameter) can be used to perform balloon sphincteroplasty. Patients who recurrently restenose sometimes require multiple plastic stents for short periods, and/or consideration of surgical sphincteroplasty. Finally, those with unstable metabolic abnormalities (refractory hypertriglyceridemia, for example) may continue to have attacks, and there is little role for endoscopic therapy here.

For those with frequent RAP without signs of SOD, PD, or restenosis, with or without a metabolic or genetic abnormality, there are few options. Empiric sphincter therapy is not recommended, nor is long-term stenting. Total pancreatectomy with islet cell autotransplantation is indicated for patients with intractable pain or very frequent attacks.[92] Chronic pancreatitis patients with these symptoms, but for pure RAP without proven chronic pancreatitis, it is more controversial. Nonetheless, in patients without other options, with poor quality of life due to these recurrent attacks, total pancreatectomy with islet cell autotransplantation may be a consideration.

In summary, endoscopy plays an important role in both the diagnosis and the initial management of RAP, as well as the investigation of refractory disease, but it has known limitations and risks. Sound selective use of these therapies, complemented with other lines of investigation such as genetic testing, can dramatically improve frequency of attacks and associated quality of life. Whether endoscopic therapy can reduce progression to chronic pancreatitis, or reduce the risk of malignancy, is debatable and remains to be proven.

REFERENCES

1. Lankisch PG, Breuer N, Bruns A, et al. Natural history of acute pancreatitis: a long-term population-based study. Am J Gastroenterol 2009;104:2797–805 [quiz: 2806].
2. Nojgaard C, Becker U, Matzen P, et al. Progression from acute to chronic pancreatitis: prognostic factors, mortality, and natural course. Pancreas 2011; 40:1195–200.
3. Takeyama Y. Long-term prognosis of acute pancreatitis in Japan. Clin Gastroenterol Hepatol 2009;7:S15–7.
4. Romagnuolo J, Guda N, Freeman M, et al. Preferred designs, outcomes, and analysis strategies for treatment trials in idiopathic recurrent acute pancreatitis. Gastrointest Endosc 2008;68:966–74.
5. Pelli H, Lappalainen-Lehto R, Piironen A, et al. Risk factors for recurrent acute alcohol-associated pancreatitis: a prospective analysis. Scand J Gastroenterol 2008;43:614–21.
6. Pelli H, Sand J, Laippala P, et al. Long-term follow-up after the first episode of acute alcoholic pancreatitis: time course and risk factors for recurrence. Scand J Gastroenterol 2000;35:552–5.
7. Guda N, Romagnuolo J, Freeman M. Recurrent and relapsing pancreatitis. Curr Gastroenterol Rep 2011;13:140–9.
8. Yadav D, Hawes R, Brand R, et al. Alcohol consumption, cigarette smoking, and the risk of recurrent acute and chronic pancreatitis. Arch Intern Med 2009; 169(11):1035–45.
9. Steinberg W, Tenner S. Acute pancreatitis. N Engl J Med 1994;330:1198–210.
10. Thomson SR, Hendry WS, McFarlane GA, et al. Epidemiology and outcome of acute pancreatitis. Br J Surg 1987;74:398–401.
11. Venu RP, Geenen JE, Hogan W, et al. Idiopathic recurrent pancreatitis. An approach to diagnosis and treatment. Dig Dis Sci 1989;34:56–60.
12. Soergel KH. Acute pancreatitis. In: Sleisenger MH, Fordtran JS, editors. Gastrointestinal disease. 5th edition. Philadelphia: WB Saunders; 1993. p. 1628–51.

13. Lee SP, Nicholls JF, Park HZ. Biliary sludge as a cause of acute pancreatitis. N Engl J Med 1992;326:589–93.
14. Ros E, Navarro S, Bru C, et al. Occult microlithiasis in "idiopathic" acute pancreatitis: prevention of relapses by cholecystectomy or ursodeoxycholic acid therapy. Gastroenterology 1991;101:1701–9.
15. Fischer M, Hassan A, Sipe B, et al. Endoscopic retrograde cholangiopancreatography and manometry findings in 1,241 idiopathic pancreatitis patients. Pancreatology 2010;10(4):444–52.
16. Yusoff IF, Raymond G, Sahai AV. A prospective comparison of the yield of EUS in primary vs. recurrent idiopathic acute pancreatitis. Gastrointest Endosc 2004; 60:673–8.
17. Somogyi L, Martin S, Venkateson T, et al. Recurrent acute pancreatitis: an algorithmic approach to the identification and elimination of inciting factors. Gastroenterology 2001;120:708–17.
18. Frey C. Gallstone pancreatitis. Surg Clin North Am 1981;61:922–38.
19. Kelly T, Swaney P. Gallstone pancreatitis. The second time around. Surgery 1987;92:571–5.
20. Kelly T. Gallstone pancreatitis: the timing of surgery. Surgery 1980;88: 345–50.
21. Paloyan D, Simonowitz D, Skinner D. The timing of biliary tract operations in patients with pancreatitis associated with gallstones. Surg Gynecol Obstet 1975;141:737–9.
22. Wilson P, Neoptolemos J. Gallstone-associated acute pancreatitis. In: Howard J, Idezuki Y, Ihse I, et al, editors. Surgical diseases of the pancreas. 3rd edition. Baltimore (MD): Williams & Wilkins; 1998. p. 240–5.
23. Vazques-Iglesias L, Gonzalez-Conde B, Lopez-Rose L, et al. Endoscopic sphincterotomy for prevention of the recurrence of acute biliary pancreatitis in patients with gallbladder in situ: Long-term follow-up of 88 patients. Surg Endosc 2004;18:1442–6.
24. Uomo G, Manes G, Laccetti M, et al. Endoscopic sphincterotomy and recurrence of acute pancreatitis in gallstone patients considered unfit for surgery. Pancreas 1997;14:28–31.
25. Billi P, Barakat B, D'Imperio N, et al. Relapses of biliary acute pancreatitis in patients with previous attack of biliary pancreatitis and gallbladder in situ. Dig Liver Dis 2003;35:653–5.
26. Kaw M, Al-Antably Y, Kaw P. Management of gallstone pancreatitis: cholecystectomy or ERCP and endoscopic sphincterotomy. Gastrointest Endosc 2002; 56:61–5.
27. Alempijevic T, Stimec B, Kovacevic N. Anatomical features of the minor duodenal papilla in pancreas divisum. Surg Radiol Anat 2006;28:620–4.
28. Kin T, Shapiro A, Lakey J. Pancreas divisum: a study of the cadaveric donor pancreas for islet isolation. Pancreas 2005;30:325–7.
29. Borak G, Romagnuolo J, Alsolaiman M, et al. Long-term clinical outcomes after endoscopic minor papilla therapy in symptomatic patients with pancreas divisum. Pancreas 2009;38(8):903–6.
30. Fogel E, Sherman S, Kalayci C, et al. Manometry and native minor papillae and post minor papilla therapy: experience at a tertiary referral center. Gastrointest Endosc 1999;49:187A.
31. Lans J, Geenan J, Johansen J, et al. Endoscopic therapy in patients with pancreas divisum and acute pancreatitis: a prospective, randomized, controlled clinical trial. Gastrointest Endosc 1992;38:430–4.

32. Kozarek R, Ball T, Patterson D, et al. Endoscopic approach to pancreas divisum. Dig Dis Sci 1995;40:1974–81.

33. Lehman G, Sherman S, Nisi R, et al. Pancreas divisum: results of minor papilla sphincterotomy. Gastrointest Endosc 1993;39:1–8.

34. Bernard J, Sahel J, Giovannini M, et al. Pancreas divisum is a probable cause of acute pancreatitis: a report of 137 cases. Pancreas 1990;5:248–54.

35. Cotton P. Congenital anomaly of pancreas divisum as cause of obstructive pain and pancreatitis. Gut 1980;21:105–14.

36. Richter J, Schapiro R, Mulley A, et al. Association of pancreas divisum and pancreatitis and its treatment by sphincteroplasty of the accessory papilla. Gastroenterology 1981;81:1104–10.

37. Delhaye M, Engelholm L, Cremer M. Pancreas divisum: congenital anatomic variant or anomaly? Contribution of endoscopic retrograde dorsal pancreatography. Gastroenterology 1985;89:951–8.

38. Brenner P, Duncombe V, Ham J. Pancreatitis and pancreas divisum: aetiological and surgical considerations. Aust N Z J Surg 1990;60:899–903.

39. Morgan D, Logan K, Baron T, et al. Pancreas divisum: implications for diagnostic and therapeutic pancreatography. AJR Am J Roentgenol 1999;173:193–8.

40. Gelrud A, Sheth S, Banarjee S, et al. Analysis of cystic fibrosis gene product (CFTR) function in patients with pancreas divisum and recurrent acute pancreatitis. Am J Gastroenterol 2004;99:1557–62.

41. Bertin C, Pelletier A, Vullierme M, et al. Pancreas divisum is not a cause of pancreatitis by itself but acts as a partner of genetic mutations. Am J Gastroenterol 2012;107:311–7.

42. Choudari C, Imperiale T, Sherman S, et al. Risk of pancreatitis with mutation of the cystic fibrosis gene. Am J Gastroenterol 2004;99:1358–63.

43. Garg PK, Khajuria R, Kabra M, et al. Association of SPINK1 gene mutation and CFTR gene polymorphisms in patients with pancreas divisum presenting with idiopathic pancreatitis. J Clin Gastroenterol 2009;43(9):848–52.

44. Attwell A, Borak G, Hawes R, et al. Endoscopic pancreatic sphincterotomy for pancreas divisum by using a needle-knife or standard pull-type technique: safety and reintervention rates. Gastrointest Endosc 2006;64:705–11.

45. Morgan KA, Romagnuolo J, Adams DB. Transduodenal sphincteroplasty in the management of sphincter of Oddi dysfunction and pancreas divisum in the modern era. J Am Coll Surg 2008;206:908–17.

46. Satterfield S, McCarthy J, Geenen J, et al. Clinical experience in 82 patients with pancreas divisum: preliminary results of manometry and endoscopic therapy. Pancreas 1988;3:248–53.

47. McCarthy J, Geenen J, Hogan W. Preliminary experience with endoscopic stent placement in benign pancreatic diseases. Gastrointest Endosc 1988;34:16–8.

48. Coleman S, Eisen G, Troughton A, et al. Endoscopic treatment in pancreas divisum. Am J Gastroenterol 1994;89:1152–5.

49. Jacob L, Geenen J, Catalano M, et al. Clinical presentation and short-term outcome of endoscopic therapy of patients with symptomatic incomplete pancreas divisum. Gastrointest Endosc 1999;49:53–7.

50. Ertan A. Long-term results after endoscopic pancreatic stent placement without pancreatic papillotomyin acute recurrent pancreatitis due to pancreas divisum. Gastrointest Endosc 2000;52:9–14.

51. Heyries L, Barthet M, Delvasto C, et al. Long-term results of endoscopic management of pancreas divisum with recurrent acute pancreatitis. Gastrointest Endosc 2002;55:376–81.

52. Linder J, Bukeirat F, Geenen J, et al. Long-term response to pancreatic duct stent placement in symptomatic patients with pancreas divisum. Gastrointest Endosc 2003;57:208A.
53. Bierig L, Chen Y, Shah R. Patient outcomes following minor papilla endotherapy (MPE) for pancreas divisum (PD). Gastrointest Endosc 2006;63:313A.
54. Kwan V, Loh S, Walsh P, et al. Minor papilla sphincterotomy for pancreatitis due to pancreas divisum. ANZ J Surg 2008;78:257–61.
55. Romagnuolo J, Durkalski V, Fogel EL, et al. Prospective study of imaging predictive value and agreement in diagnosing pancreas divisum: the FRAMES (Frequency of Recurrent Acute Pancreatitis After Minor Papilla Endoscopic Sphincterotomy) study [abstract]. Gastrointestinal Endoscopy 2013;77(Suppl 5).
56. Devereaux B, Fein S, Purich E, et al. A new synthetic porcine secretin for facilitation of cannulation of the dorsal pancreatic duct at ERCP in patients with pancreas divisum: a multicenter, randomized, double-blind comparative study. Gastrointest Endosc 2003;57(6):643–747.
57. Park S, de Bellis M, McHenry L, et al. Use of methylene blue to identify the minor papilla or its orifice in patients with pancreas divisum. Gastrointest Endosc 2003;57(3):358–63.
58. Elta G. Sphincter of Oddi dysfunction and bile duct mircolithiasis in acute idiopathic pancreatitis. World J Gastroenterol 2008;14:1023–6.
59. Fazel A, Geenen J, Moezardalan K, et al. Intrapancreatic ductal pressure in sphincter of Oddi dysfunction. Pancreas 2005;30:359–62.
60. Coyle W, Pineau B, Tarnasky P, et al. Evaluation of unexplained acute and acute recurrent pancreatitis using endoscopic retrograde cholangiopancreatography, sphincter of Oddi manometry, and endoscopic ultrasound. Endoscopy 2002;34: 617–23.
61. Fogel E, Toth T, Lehman G, et al. Does endoscopic therapy favorably affect the outcome of patients who have recurrent acute pancreatitis and pancreas divisum? Pancreas 2007;34(1):21–45.
62. Guda NM, Freeman ML. True culprit or guilt by association? Is sphincter of Oddi manometry the cause of post-ERCP pancreatitis in patients with suspected sphincter of Oddi dysfunction, or is it the patients' susceptibility? Rev Gastroenterol Disord 2004;4(4):211–3.
63. Hogan W, Geenen J, Dodds W. Dysmotility disturbances of the biliary tract: classification, diagnosis and treatment. Semin Liver Dis 1987;7(4): 302–10.
64. Choudari C, Fogel E, Sherman S, et al. Idiopathic pancreatitis: yield of ERCP correlated with patient age. Am J Gastroenterol 1998;93:1654A.
65. Toouli J, Francesco V, Saccone G, et al. Division of sphincter of Oddi for treatment of dysfunction associated with recurrent pancreatitis. Br J Surg 1996;83: 1205–10.
66. Guelrud M, Mendoz S, Viera L. Idiopathic recurrent pancreatitis and hypercontractilesphincter of Oddi. Treatment with endoscopic sphincterotomy and pancreatic duct dilation. Gastroenterology 1986;90:1443.
67. Gregg JA. Function and dysfunction of the sphincter of Oddi. In: Jacobson IM, editor. ERCP: diagnostic and therapeutic applications. New York: Elsevier; 1989. p. 137–70.
68. Sherman S, Jamidar P, Reber H, et al. Idiopathic acute pancreatitis (IAP): endoscopic diagnosis and therapy. Am J Gastroenterol 1993;88:1541A.
69. Kaw M, Brodmerkel G. ERCP, biliary crystal analysis, and sphincter of Oddi manometry in idiopathic pancreatitis. Gastrointest Endosc 2002;55:157–62.

70. Sherman S, Hawes R, Madura J, et al. Comparison of intraoperative and endo-scopic manometry of the sphincter of Oddi. Surg Gynecol Obstet 1992;175:410–8.
71. Madura J, Madura J 2nd, Sherman S, et al. Surgical sphincteroplasty in 446 patients. Arch Surg 2005;140:504–11.
72. Lans J, Parikh N, Geenen J, et al. Applications of sphincter of Oddi manometry in routine clinical investigations. Endoscopy 1991;23:139–43.
73. Guelrud M, Plaz J, Mendosa S, et al. Endoscopic treatment in Type II pancreatic sphincter dysfunction. Gastrointest Endosc 1995;41:A398.
74. Okolo P, Pasricha P, Kalloo A. what are the long-term results of endoscopic pancreatic sphincterotomy. Gastrointest Endosc 2000;52:15–9.
75. Park S, Watkins J, Foegl E, et al. Long-term outcome of endoscopic dual sphinc-terotomy in patients with manometry-documented sphincter of Oddi dysfunction and normal pancreatogram. Gastrointest Endosc 2003;57:483–91.
76. Wehrmann T, Schmitt T, Arndt A, et al. Endoscopic botulinum toxin injection for treatment of idiopathic recurrent pancreatitis due to sphincter of Oddi dysfunc-tion. Aliment Pharmacol Ther 2000;14:1469–77.
77. Cote G, Imperiale T, Schmidt S, et al. Similar efficacies of biliary, with or without pancreatic, sphincterotomy in treatment of idiopathic recurrent acute pancrea-titis. Gastroenterology 2012;143(6):1502–9.
78. Eversman D, Fogel E, Rusche M, et al. Frequency of abnormal pancreatic and biliary sphincter manometry compared with clinical suspicion of sphincter of Oddi dysfunction. Gastrointest Endosc 1999;50:637–41.
79. Varadalajulu S, Wilcox M. Randomized trial comparing needle-knife and pull-sphincterotome techniques for pancreatic sphincterotomy in high-risk patients. Gastrointest Endosc 2006;64:716–22.
80. Layer P, Yamamoto H, Kalthoff L, et al. The different courses of early- and late-onset idiopathic and alcoholic chronic pancreatitis. Gastroenterology 1994;107:1481–7.
81. Takuma K, Kamisawa T, Hara S, et al. Etiology of recurrent acute pancreatitis, with special emphasis on pancreaticobiliary malformation. Advanced in Medical Sciences 2012;57(2):244–50.
82. Jeong J, Whang J, Ryu J, et al. Risk factors for pancreatitis in patients with anomalous union of pancreatobiliary duct. Hepatogastroenterology 2004;5(58):1187–90.
83. Ramanujan S, Sherman S, Lehman G. Endoscopic therapy in anomalous pan-creatobiliary duct junction. Gastrointest Endosc 1999;50:623–7.
84. Antaki F, Tringali A, Deviere J, et al. A case series of symptomatic intraluminal duodenal duplication cysts: presentation, endoscopic therapy, and long-term outcome. Gastrointest Endo 2008;67(1):163–8.
85. Ortega A, Gomez-Rodriguez R, Romero M, et al. Prospective comparison of endoscopic ultrasonography and magnetic resonance cholangiopancreatogra-phy in the etiological diagnosis of "idiopathic" acute pancreatitis. Pancreas 2011;40:289–94.
86. Lai R, Freeman M, Cass O, et al. Accurate diagnosis of pancreas divisum by linear-array endoscopic ultrasonography. Endoscopy 2004;36:705–9.
87. Carnes M, Romagnuolo J, Cotton P. Miss rate of pancreas divisum by magnetic resonance cholangiopancreatography in clinical practice. Pancreas 2008;37:151–3.
88. Catalano M, Lahoti S, Alcocer E, et al. Dynamic imaging of the pancreas using real-time endoscopic ultrasonography with secretin stimulation. Gastrointest Endosc 1998;48(6):580–7.

89. Aisen A, Sherman S, Jennings S, et al. Comparison of secretin-stimulated magnetic resonance pancreatography and manometry results in patients with suspected sphincter of Oddi dysfunction. Acad Radiol 2008;15(5): 601–9.
90. Jacobson B, Waxman I, Parmar K, et al. Endoscopic ultrasound-guided gallbladder bile aspiration in idiopathic pancreatitis carries a significant risk of bile peritonitis. Pancreatology 2002;2(1):26–9.
91. Joergensen M, Brusgaard K, Gylling D, et al. Incidence, prevalence, etiology, and prognosis of first-time chronic pancreatitis in young patients: a nationwide cohort study. Dig Dis Sci 2010;55:2988–98.
92. Sutherland DE, Radosevich DM, Bellin MD, et al. Total pancreatectomy and islet autotransplantation for chronic pancreatitis. J Am Coll Surg 2012;214(4):409–24 [discussion: 424–6].

Endoscopic Therapy for Chronic Pancreatitis

Jean-Marc Dumonceau, MD, PhD

KEYWORDS

- Chronic pancreatitis • Pain • Guideline • Treatment
- Endoscopic retrograde cholangio-pancreatography
- Extracorporeal shockwave lithotripsy • Endoscopic ultrasonography
- Celiac plexus block

KEY POINTS

- Endoscopic therapy is the first-line interventional therapy for painful chronic pancreatitis (CP) with an obstacle on the main pancreatic duct (MPD) and no locoregional complication.
- Calcified stones that obstruct the MPD are first treated by extracorporeal shockwave lithotripsy (ie, before or in place of ERCP).
- Dominant MPD strictures are treated with a single, large, plastic stent that should be exchanged within 1 year even in asymptomatic patients.
- In the case of unsatisfactory clinical response at 6–8 weeks, the patient's case should be discussed in a multidisciplinary team.
- Treatment of pancreatic pseudocysts should be performed by endoscopy. Compared with surgery, results are better at short term and similar at long term.

INTRODUCTION

In chronic pancreatitis (CP), endoscopic therapy aims to provide pain relief and to treat local complications. Pain may be caused by multiple factors, including neuropathy, increased intraductal and parenchymal pancreatic pressure, pancreatic ischemia, and acute inflammation during a flare. Complications such as pseudocysts, strictures of the common bile duct (CBD), and pancreatic cancer may also cause pancreatic-type pain.

In the case of uncomplicated CP, most nonsurgical therapeutic interventions aim at relieving outflow obstruction of the main pancreatic duct (MPD). In a large

Disclosure: The author has no competing interest relevant to this article.
Division of Gastroenterology and Hepatology, Geneva University Hospitals, Rue Gabrielle Perret Gentil 4, Geneva 1211, Switzerland
E-mail addresses: dumonceau123@yahoo.com; jmdumonceau@hotmail.com

Gastrointest Endoscopy Clin N Am 23 (2013) 821–832
http://dx.doi.org/10.1016/j.giec.2013.06.004
1052-5157/13/$ – see front matter © 2013 Elsevier Inc. All rights reserved.

multicenter study of endoscopic treatment of CP, MPD obstruction was caused by strictures (47% of the patients), stones (18%), or a combination of both (32%).[1] Depending on the type of MPD obstruction, extracorporeal shockwave lithotripsy (ESWL), endoscopic retrograde cholangio-pancreatography (ERCP), or a combination of both may be used to restore MPD outflow. CP-related complications amenable to endoscopic treatment consist of pseudocysts and CBD strictures; in the multicenter study cited above, they were treated in 17% and 23% of patients, respectively.

The recommendations presented here are based on a Guideline that has recently been issued by the European Society of Gastrointestinal Endoscopy (ESGE).[2] Importantly, they do not apply to patients with CP that is mild in severity at pancreatography as assessed by the Cambridge classification.[3]

PLANNING TREATMENT
Differential Diagnosis and Local Disease Assessment

Before deciding on which treatment to apply, it is necessary to confirm the diagnosis of CP, to rule out the presence of a pancreatic cancer reasonably, and to assess the local anatomy.

The differential diagnosis of CP mostly includes intraductal papillary mucinous neoplasm (IPMN) and autoimmune pancreatitis:

- Approximately 10% of patients with IPMN are first inappropriately diagnosed with CP.[4] Demographic and imaging data may help in making the correct diagnosis:
  - Patients with IPMN are more often women, are older, drink less alcohol, and smoke fewer cigarettes than those with CP[4];
  - An MPD dilation without downstream stone or stricture evidenced at magnetic resonance cholangiopancreatography (MRCP) or endoscopic ultrasonography (EUS) is highly suggestive of IPMN;
  - Consensus guidelines for the management of IPMN have recently been updated.[5]
- The diagnosis of autoimmune pancreatitis requires a combination of imaging, histopathology, serology (IgG_4), evaluation of other organ involvement, and response to steroids.[6]

CP is one of the factors that increase the risk of pancreatic cancer.[7] It is not a main cause of pancreatic cancer except in patients with the rare autosomal-dominant hereditary form of pancreatitis. Nevertheless, pancreatic cancer may be overlooked, in particular, at the time of the initial diagnosis of CP. Special attentiveness for pancreatic cancer should be paid in patients greater than 50 years, of female gender, of white race, those presenting with jaundice or exocrine insufficiency, as well as in the absence of pancreatic calcifications.[8,9]

Assessment of the local anatomy is usually performed by a combination of computed tomographic (CT) scan without contrast medium injection (CT scan is the most sensitive examination for the detection of pancreatic calcifications and it allows broad assessment of the pancreatic parenchyma) and of MRCP (for assessing the pancreatic ducts, including MPD strictures and relevant anatomic variants such as pancreas divisum). Magnetic resonance and EUS may be superior to CT scan for the workup of pancreatic fluid collections because these techniques depict solid necrotic debris inside collections that may impede its effective drainage.[10,11]

Choice of Treatment

Surgical and endoscopic interventions for the treatment of pain in CP have been compared in 2 randomized controlled trials (RCT).[12,13] Criticisms of the nonsurgical treatment performed in these studies aside, these RCTs showed that surgery provides pain relief in more patients than endoscopic treatment but that complete pain relief is infrequent after surgical as well as endoscopic treatment. Hence, the ESGE recommended endoscopic therapy as the first-line therapy for painful uncomplicated CP because

- Surgery is not a "definitive" treatment of CP (except in the case of total pancreatectomy, with its long-term complications); pain eventually relapses following surgery in most patients.[12,13] Total pancreatectomy with islet autotransplantation is an emerging option for definitive therapy, particularly in younger patients with aggressive hereditary pancreatitis such as that associated with mutations of the cationic trypsinogen gene (PRSS-1).[14,15]
- Death is not exceptional after surgery, even in its least risky form (ie, MPD drainage; mortality, 0%–4%).[16] Complications are extremely common after pancreatic resection for CP (20%–50%).[17] In contrast, morbidity and mortality of nonsurgical interventions for CP are in the range of 3% to 9% and 0% to 0.5%, respectively,[1,18,19] which is likely related to the relative protection against post-ERCP pancreatitis conferred by CP.[20,21]
- Most patients present a satisfactory long-term outcome after nonsurgical treatment for CP. For example, in a selection of independent series (Table 1), 59% to 79% of patients had no further pancreatic intervention during long-term (4–14 years) follow-up after nonsurgical intervention for CP.

Therefore, in centers with both endoscopic and surgical expertise, a nonsurgical intervention is often proposed as a first-step procedure for the treatment of painful uncomplicated CP. Some factors that may help in the choice between the surgical and nonsurgical options are as follows:

- The location of obstructive calcifications in the head of the pancreas, a short disease duration, and a low frequency of pain attacks before a nonsurgical intervention predict a good clinical outcome.[22]
- Conversely, if the lesions targeted by nonsurgical interventions are located in the pancreatic tail *exclusively*, pancreatic tail resection may be favored as a possible

Table 1
Long-term outcome after nonsurgical treatment of CP

First Author, Year	N	Follow-Up (mo)	Surgery (%)	Ongoing Endoscopic Treatment (%)	No Further Intervention (%)
Binmoeller et al,[45] 1995	93	58	26	13	61
Rösch et al,[1] 2002	1018	58	24	16	60
Delhaye et al,[25] 2004	56	173	21	18	61
Tadenuma et al,[27] 2005	70	75	1	20	79
Inui et al,[33] 2005	555	44	4	—	—
Farnbacher et al,[26] 2006	98	46	23	18	59

Adapted from Dumonceau JM, Delhaye M, Tringali A, et al. Endoscopic treatment of chronic pancreatitis: European Society of Gastrointestinal Endoscopy (ESGE) Clinical Guideline. Endoscopy 2012;44(8):784–800; with permission.

first-intent option. Nevertheless, it should be noted that patients with MPD obstruction located in both the head and the tail of the pancreas may have a favorable clinical outcome after relieving the MPD obstacle located in the head of the pancreas only.

- In the unusual cases where a pancreatic cancer cannot be reasonably excluded based on a detailed pretherapeutic workup,[23] pancreatic resection may be performed as a diagnostic and therapeutic procedure (intraoperative needle aspiration is not adequate to exclude the presence of a cancer).
- The absence of MPD stricture predicts a good long-term outcome.
- Discontinuation of alcohol and tobacco during follow-up predicts a good outcome; help should be offered to the patients to succeed in this difficult task, independently of the treatment elected, and preferably before beginning treatment.[24–27]

If nonsurgical treatment is elected, the clinical response should be evaluated at 6 to 8 weeks; if it seems unsatisfactory, the patient's case should be discussed in a multidisciplinary team with endoscopists, surgeons, and radiologists and surgical options should be considered, in particular in patients with a predicted poor outcome following endoscopic therapy.

MANAGEMENT OF PANCREATIC STONES

Stones targeted by nonsurgical interventions for the treatment of PC are those that obstruct or are susceptible to obstruct the MPD. A significant exception to this general rule includes large stones that are located in a secondary duct and impede the communication between a pseudocyst and the MPD. Complete MPD stone clearance at initial ERCP predicts a good clinical outcome.[22]

Infrequently, stones obstructing the MPD are not calcified. Such noncalcified stones are usually easy to extract at ERCP using a Dormia basket and/or a balloon following pancreatic sphincterotomy. Much more frequently, stones obstructing the MPD are calcified; such calcified stones can be cleared using ESWL alone, ERCP alone, a combination of ESWL plus ERCP, or medications. ESWL has become the core, first-line, therapy (except for stones smaller than 4 mm that are difficult to target at ESWL) because of the following:

- Endoscopic attempts at stone extraction using Dormia baskets without prior stone fragmentation have yielded unsatisfactory results in terms of both success rates (approximately 10%) and morbidity rates (3 times higher than those reported for biliary stones).[28,29]
- Advanced intraductal lithotripsy techniques such as laser or electrohydraulic lithotripsy are not readily available in many endoscopy units; their use has been reported in small case series only and they have provided low success rates compared with ESWL.[30] These techniques may be useful in the case of failed ESWL.
- Medications able to dissolve pancreatic stones are not approved for that use by health organizations. They have never been tested in comparative trials; treatment duration is long, and side effects may be significant.[31,32]

On the contrary, ESWL is largely available because of its widespread use to treat urological stones and it has consistently been reported to be highly effective to fragment calcified MPD stones. MPD stones are successfully fragmented in approximately 90% of the cases.[19,22] The material and the techniques of ESWL used to fragment MPD stones are critical to ensure such high success rates and less favorable results have been reported, particularly in low case-volume centers.[33] A meta-analysis of 17 studies (total of 491 patients) showed that ESWL is useful to clear MPD stones and to decrease pain.[34]

Performance of ESWL before endoscopic attempt at stone removal is independently associated with the success of MPD stone clearance.[24] In practice, ESWL is always performed before ERCP to extract calcified MPD stones of significant size to avoid failure of stone extraction. After ESWL, successful MPD stone clearance is more likely for stones that are solitary or confined to the head of the pancreas.[24,35]

ESWL may also be used alone to treat painful uncomplicated CP. Initial uncontrolled studies showed that stone fragments are spontaneously eliminated in the stools, through the intact pancreatic sphincter, in approximately 75% of patients subjected to ESWL alone; 78% of patients had long-term pain relief.[33,36] Then, an RCT showed that, compared with ESWL combined with ERCP, ESWL alone provided a similar decrease in the MPD diameter and in the number of yearly pain attacks.[37] The only significant differences between ESWL alone or combined with ERCP were a longer hospital stay and a higher treatment cost in the combination group (ESWL plus ERCP). Therefore, ESWL alone may be the preferred first-line intervention to treat painful uncomplicated CP, in particular, if no MPD stricture is evidenced at MRCP and if the center has expertise with pancreatic ESWL. Otherwise, endoscopic extraction of stone fragments is performed immediately after satisfactory stone fragmentation has been obtained.

Morbidity related to ESWL alone or combined with ERCP was reviewed based on 4 large (>100 patients) series: significant complications were reported in 104 of 1801 patients, including one death (morbidity and mortality: 5.8% and 0.05%, respectively).[19,27,33,38] Complications related to the treatment of CP by ESWL alone were reported in 3 series that involved 165 patients[27,36,37]; the morbidity rate was 6.0%. For both ESWL alone or combined with ERCP, complications consisted of pancreatitis in most cases. Contraindications to ESWL are rarely encountered in patients with CP.

MANAGEMENT OF MPD STRICTURES

Temporary stent placement for a duration of at least 1 year has become the standard of care for the endoscopic treatment of dominant MPD strictures because repeated balloon dilation without stenting or MPD stenting for a short duration has been shown to be ineffective.[39] The principles and technique of temporary MPD stricture dilation using stents is similar to those applied for benign biliary strictures.[40] Technical points specific to MPD strictures are as follows:

- Pancreatic sphincterotomy always precedes stent insertion, contrary to what is performed for biliary stenting, carrying a 10% risk of post-ERCP pancreatitis but the flare is usually mild.[18,20] Biliary sphincterotomy is associated with pancreatic sphincterotomy in specific cases only (ie, to facilitate catheterization of the MPD or to prevent cholangitis in patients who are at risk of this complication, including those with a bilirubin level ≥ 3 mg/dL, a diameter of the CBD ≥ 12 mm, or alkaline phosphatases >2 times the upper limit of normal values).[41]
- Stricture dilation is performed before stenting in most cases because of the resilience of CP-related MPD strictures; bougies/balloons are used or, in most difficult cases, the Soehendra's stent retriever.[42]

The ESGE recommended treating dominant MPD stricture by inserting a single 10-French plastic stent, with stent exchange planned within 1 year even in asymptomatic patients to prevent complications related to long-standing pancreatic stent occlusion.[2] Simultaneous placement of multiple, side-by-side, pancreatic stents is being applied more and more extensively, either at first treatment attempt or in patients with MPD strictures persisting after 12 months of single plastic stenting. At this time, all available options (eg, endoscopic placement of multiple simultaneous MPD stents, surgery) should be discussed in a multidisciplinary team.

The insertion of plastic stents in the MPD is technically successful in greater than 90% of attempted cases; it is followed by immediate and long-term pain relief in approximately 80% and 50% of the patients, respectively (**Table 2**).[39,43–45] Simultaneous insertion of multiple, side-by-side, MPD stents has been investigated in a single series of 19 patients, with encouraging results.[46] This strategy might be particularly useful in patients (1) with MPD strictures persisting after 12 months of single plastic stenting and (2) with a pancreas divisum because this anatomy is associated with a more frequent relapse of MPD stricture and of pain after stent removal compared with a fused pancreas.[43]

Placement of a fully covered self-expandable metal stent (SEMS) into the MPD for 2 to 3 months is another option that is currently under investigation.[47–49] Potential complications include spontaneous SEMS migration and the development of de novo focal MPD strictures. This, together with the very short follow-up available up to now, currently limits the use of fully covered SEMS to clinical research.

ROLE OF EUS IN THE TREATMENT OF UNCOMPLICATED CP
EUS-guided Access and Drainage of the MPD

Various techniques of EUS-guided access and drainage (ESGAD) have been described[50–52]; this section is reviewed in more detail in another article of the present issue of the *Gastrointestinal Endoscopy Clinics of North America*. In short, ESGAD consists of puncturing the MPD through the gastric or duodenal wall under EUS guidance with a large needle and to proceed with either standard, transpapillary, drainage (rendezvous technique) or with transmural drainage. Potential indications for ESGAD of the MPD include patients with a symptomatic MPD obstruction and failed conventional MPD decompression. Initial results are relatively promising: in small series, immediate pain relief has followed successful ESGAD in 50% to 100% of patients.

Table 2
Selected series of treatment with plastic stents for MPD strictures in CP

First Author, Year	N	Stents (F)	Follow-up (mo)	Early Pain Relief (%)	Sustained Pain Relief (%)	Patients Operated on (%)
Cremer et al,[72] 1991	75	10	37	94	NA	15
Ponchon et al,[39] 1995	23	10	14	74	52	15
Smits et al,[73] 1995	49	10	34	82	82	6
Binmoeller et al,[45] 1995	93	5-7-10	58	74	65	26
Morgan et al,[74] 2003	25	5-7-8.5	NA	65	NA	NA
Vitale et al,[44] 2004	89	5-7-10	43	83	68	12
Eleftheriadis et al,[43] 2005	100	8.5-10	69	70	62	4
Ishihara et al,[75] 2006	20	10	21	95	90	NA
Weber et al,[76] 2007	17	7-8.5-10-11.5	24	89	83	NA

Abbreviation: NA, not available.

Adapted from Dumonceau JM, Delhaye M, Tringali A, et al. Endoscopic treatment of chronic pancreatitis: European Society of Gastrointestinal Endoscopy (ESGE) Clinical Guideline. Endoscopy 2012;44(8):784–800; with permission.

However patients seem to deteriorate as time elapses.[53] Furthermore, ESGAD is technically challenging and severe complications have been reported. For these reasons, the ESGE recommended that ESGAD of the MPD be performed only in carefully selected patients referred to tertiary centers with appropriate equipment and expertise.[2]

EUS-guided Celiac Plexus Block

Celiac plexus block (CPB) consists of injecting corticoids (usually mixed with a local anesthetic) into celiac plexus nerves to disrupt the signaling of painful stimuli through pancreatic nerves. It differs from celiac plexus neurolysis (CPN), whose goal is to ablate the nerve fibers by injecting alcohol. The use of CPN is classically restricted to patients with pain related to unresectable cancer because alcohol injection may cause fibrosis that would make pancreatic surgery more difficult. Both interventions have long been performed through the percutaneous route before being performed under EUS guidance. Based on an RCT,[54] CPB under EUS guidance is thought to be more effective than percutaneous CPB.

The ESGE recommended considering EUS-guided CPB only as a second-line treatment for pain in CP[2] based on the facts that

- If present, pain relief is short-lived. For example, in a prospective series of 90 patients, the proportion of patients with pain relief decreased from 55% immediately after EUS-guided CPB to 10% at 24 weeks.[55]
- Complications are frequent after EUS-guided CPB; they include transient diarrhea, hypotension, and pain exacerbation. Less frequently, severe infection may occur.[56]
- The efficacy of CPB to relieve pain in CP has been questioned: the single RCT that has compared EUS-guided injection of a local anesthetic either alone or mixed with corticoids into the celiac plexus found no difference in pain relief between allocation groups.[57]
- Procedure-related death has been reported with CPN.[58]

CP-RELATED LOCOREGIONAL COMPLICATIONS
Pseudocysts

Endoscopic drainage is recommended as the first-line therapy for uncomplicated chronic pancreatic pseudocysts (PPC) that are within endoscopic reach.[2] Treatment of PPC is indicated in the presence of symptoms (abdominal pain, gastric outlet obstruction, early satiety, weight loss, or jaundice), of infection, or if the PPC enlarges.[59] Some authors also recommend treating PPC in asymptomatic patients to prevent complications (eg, if a major vessel is compressed) because spontaneous resolution of PPC is rare in patients with established CP.[60]

Endoscopic and surgical treatments of PPC were compared in a large review of historical series: procedure-related morbidity and recurrence rate of PPC at long term were similar with both approaches but procedure-related mortality was lower with the endoscopic method (0.2% vs 2.5%).[61] More recently, an RCT directly compared endoscopic and surgical treatments of uncomplicated PPC in a small group of patients[62]; it found that endoscopic treatment was significantly better than surgery in terms of cost, length of hospital stay, and quality of life up to 3 months after procedure. At a median follow-up of 18 months, clinical outcomes and quality of life were similar for both allocation groups.

At endoscopy, PPC may be treated by inserting a drain into the PPC either through the papilla (transpapillary drainage) or through the gastroduodenal wall (transmural drainage):

- Transpapillary PPC drainage is feasible only if a communication is evidenced between the PPC and the MPD (this represents approximately half of the cases), and it is used only for relatively small collections (generally ≤50 mm). Transpapillary drainage provides similar long-term success and is associated with significantly fewer complications than transmural drainage.[63–65] Therefore, it is recommended to attempt transpapillary drainage first for small collections communicating with the MPD and located in the head or the body of the pancreas.[2]
- Transmural PPC drainage may be performed with or without EUS guidance; drainage without EUS guidance is possible only if the PPC bulges into the digestive lumen, which is the case in approximately half of the cases.[63] This requirement accounts for the higher technical success rates that were reported in 2 RCTs when endoscopic drainage was performed with EUS guidance versus without EUS guidance.[66,67] However, in the cases where the 2 approaches were technically feasible (per-protocol analysis), they provided similar results in terms of morbidity and clinical outcome. If the transmural approach is chosen, it is recommended to insert at least 2 double-pigtail plastic stents[68]; these should not be retrieved before cyst resolution as determined by cross-sectional imaging and not before at least 2 months of stenting.[69] In patients with disconnected pancreatic duct, leaving stents in place indefinitely is associated with significantly fewer recurrences of the fluid collections.[70]

Biliary Strictures

This section is reviewed in more detail in another article of the present issue of the *Gastrointestinal Endoscopy Clinics of North America*. In short, treatment of CP-related biliary strictures is recommended in the case of symptoms, secondary biliary cirrhosis, biliary stones, progression of biliary stricture, or asymptomatic elevation of serum alkaline phosphatase (>2 or 3 times the upper limit of normal values) and/ or of serum bilirubin for longer than 1 month.[2] The choice between endoscopic and surgical treatment should rely on local expertise, local or systemic patient comorbidities (eg, portal cavernoma, cirrhosis), and expected patient's compliance with repeat endoscopic procedures. If endoscopic therapy is elected, temporary (1-year) placement of multiple, side-by-side, plastic biliary stents is recommended.[2,71]

REFERENCES

1. Rösch T, Daniel S, Scholz M, et al. Endoscopic treatment of chronic pancreatitis: a multicenter study of 1000 patients with long-term follow-up. Endoscopy 2002; 34(10):765–71.
2. Dumonceau JM, Delhaye M, Tringali A, et al. Endoscopic treatment of chronic pancreatitis: European Society of Gastrointestinal Endoscopy (ESGE) clinical guideline. Endoscopy 2012;44(8):784–800.
3. Sarner M, Cotton PB. Classification of pancreatitis. Gut 1984;25(7):756–9.
4. Talamini G, Zamboni G, Salvia R, et al. Intraductal papillary mucinous neoplasms and chronic pancreatitis. Pancreatology 2006;6(6):626–34.
5. Tanaka M, Fernandez-del Castillo C, Adsay V, et al. International consensus guidelines 2012 for the management of IPMN and MCN of the pancreas. Pancreatology 2012;12(3):183–97.

6. Shimosegawa T, Chari ST, Frulloni L, et al. International consensus diagnostic criteria for autoimmune pancreatitis: guidelines of the International Association of Pancreatology. Pancreas 2011;40(3):352–8.

7. Raimondi S, Maisonneuve P, Lowenfels AB. Epidemiology of pancreatic cancer: an overview. Nat Rev Gastroenterol Hepatol 2009;6(12):699–708.

8. Varadarajulu S, Tamhane A, Eloubeidi MA. Yield of EUS-guided FNA of pancreatic masses in the presence or the absence of chronic pancreatitis. Gastrointest Endosc 2005;62(5):728–36 [quiz: 751, 753].

9. Arvanitakis M, Van Laethem JL, Parma J, et al. Predictive factors for pancreatic cancer in patients with chronic pancreatitis in association with K-ras gene mutation. Endoscopy 2004;36(6):535–42.

10. Morgan DE, Baron TH, Smith JK, et al. Pancreatic fluid collections prior to intervention: evaluation with MR imaging compared with CT and US. Radiology 1997; 203(3):773–8.

11. Pamuklar E, Semelka RC. MR imaging of the pancreas. Magn Reson Imaging Clin N Am 2005;13(2):313–30.

12. Cahen DL, Gouma DJ, Nio Y, et al. Endoscopic versus surgical drainage of the pancreatic duct in chronic pancreatitis. N Engl J Med 2007;356(7):676–84.

13. Díte P, Ruzicka M, Zboril V, et al. A prospective, randomized trial comparing endoscopic and surgical therapy for chronic pancreatitis. Endoscopy 2003; 35(7):553–8.

14. Bellin MD, Freeman ML, Schwarzenberg SJ, et al. Quality of life improves for pediatric patients after total pancreatectomy and islet autotransplant for chronic pancreatitis. Clin Gastroenterol Hepatol 2011;9(9):793–9.

15. Sutherland DE, Radosevich DM, Bellin MD, et al. Total pancreatectomy and islet autotransplantation for chronic pancreatitis. J Am Coll Surg 2012;214(4):409–24 [discussion: 424–6].

16. Isaji S. Has the Partington procedure for chronic pancreatitis become a thing of the past? A review of the evidence. J Hepatobiliary Pancreat Sci 2010;17(6): 763–9.

17. Diener MK, Rahbari NN, Fischer L, et al. Duodenum-preserving pancreatic head resection versus pancreatoduodenectomy for surgical treatment of chronic pancreatitis: a systematic review and meta-analysis. Ann Surg 2008;247(6): 950–61.

18. Hookey LC, RioTinto R, Delhaye M, et al. Risk factors for pancreatitis after pancreatic sphincterotomy: a review of 572 cases. Endoscopy 2006;38(7):670–6.

19. Tandan M, Reddy DN, Santosh D, et al. Extracorporeal shock wave lithotripsy and endotherapy for pancreatic calculi-a large single center experience. Indian J Gastroenterol 2010;29(4):143–8.

20. Dumonceau JM, Andriulli A, Deviere J, et al. European Society of Gastrointestinal Endoscopy (ESGE) Guideline: prophylaxis of post-ERCP pancreatitis. Endoscopy 2010;42(6):503–15.

21. Freeman ML, DiSario JA, Nelson DB, et al. Risk factors for post-ERCP pancreatitis: a prospective, multicenter study. Gastrointest Endosc 2001;54(4):425–34.

22. Nguyen-Tang T, Dumonceau JM. Endoscopic treatment in chronic pancreatitis, timing, duration and type of intervention. Best Pract Res Clin Gastroenterol 2010;24(3):281–98.

23. Dumonceau JM, Polkowski M, Larghi A, et al. Indications, results, and clinical impact of endoscopic ultrasound (EUS)-guided sampling in gastroenterology: European Society of Gastrointestinal Endoscopy (ESGE) clinical guideline. Endoscopy 2011;43(10):897–912.

24. Dumonceau JM, Devière J, Le Moine O, et al. Endoscopic pancreatic drainage in chronic pancreatitis associated with ductal stones: long-term results. Gastrointest Endosc 1996;43(6):547–55.

25. Delhaye M, Arvanitakis M, Verset G, et al. Long-term clinical outcome after endoscopic pancreatic ductal drainage for patients with painful chronic pancreatitis. Clin Gastroenterol Hepatol 2004;2(12):1096–106.

26. Farnbacher MJ, Mühldorfer S, Wehler M, et al. Interventional endoscopic therapy in chronic pancreatitis including temporary stenting: a definitive treatment? Scand J Gastroenterol 2006;41(1):111–7.

27. Tadenuma H, Ishihara T, Yamaguchi T, et al. Long-term results of extracorporeal shockwave lithotripsy and endoscopic therapy for pancreatic stones. Clin Gastroenterol Hepatol 2005;3(11):1128–35.

28. Farnbacher MJ, Schoen C, Rabenstein T, et al. Pancreatic duct stones in chronic pancreatitis: criteria for treatment intensity and success. Gastrointest Endosc 2002;56(4):501–6.

29. Thomas M, Howell DA, Carr-Locke D, et al. Mechanical lithotripsy of pancreatic and biliary stones: complications and available treatment options collected from expert centers. Am J Gastroenterol 2007;102(9):1896–902.

30. Fishman DS, Tarnasky PR, Patel SN, et al. Management of pancreaticobiliary disease using a new intra-ductal endoscope: the Texas experience. World J Gastroenterol 2009;15(11):1353.

31. Noda A, Okuyama M, Murayama H, et al. Dissolution of pancreatic stones by oral trimethadione in patients with chronic calcific pancreatitis. J Gastroenterol Hepatol 1994;9(5):478–85.

32. Sarles H, Verine H, Lohse J, et al. Dissolution of pancreatic calculi during prolonged oral administration of citrate. Nouv Presse Med 1979;8(21):1767–8 [in French].

33. Inui K, Tazuma S, Yamaguchi T, et al. Treatment of pancreatic stones with extracorporeal shock wave lithotripsy: results of a multicenter survey. Pancreas 2005; 30(1):26–30.

34. Guda NM, Partington S, Freeman ML. Extracorporeal shock wave lithotripsy in the management of chronic calcific pancreatitis: a meta-analysis. JOP 2005;6(1):6–12.

35. Adamek HE, Jakobs R, Buttmann A, et al. Long term follow up of patients with chronic pancreatitis and pancreatic stones treated with extracorporeal shock wave lithotripsy. Gut 1999;45(3):402–5.

36. Ohara H, Hoshino M, Hayakawa T, et al. Single application extracorporeal shock wave lithotripsy is the first choice for patients with pancreatic duct stones. Am J Gastroenterol 1996;91(7):1388–94.

37. Dumonceau JM, Costamagna G, Tringali A, et al. Treatment for painful calcified chronic pancreatitis: extracorporeal shock wave lithotripsy versus endoscopic treatment: a randomised controlled trial. Gut 2007;56(4):545–52.

38. Delhaye M, Vandermeeren A, Baize M, et al. Extracorporeal shock-wave lithotripsy of pancreatic calculi. Gastroenterology 1992;102(2):610–20.

39. Ponchon T, Bory RM, Hedelius F, et al. Endoscopic stenting for pain relief in chronic pancreatitis: results of a standardized protocol. Gastrointest Endosc 1995;42(5):452–6.

40. Dumonceau JM, Heresbach D, Devière J, et al. Biliary stents: models and methods for endoscopic stenting. Endoscopy 2011;43(7):617–26.

41. Kim MH, Myung SJ, Kim YS, et al. Routine biliary sphincterotomy may not be indispensable for endoscopic pancreatic sphincterotomy. Endoscopy 1998; 30(8):697–701.

42. Ziebert JJ, DiSario JA. Dilation of refractory pancreatic duct strictures: the turn of the screw. Gastrointest Endosc 1999;49(5):632–5.

43. Eleftherladis N, Dinu F, Delhaye M, et al. Long-term outcome after pancreatic stenting in severe chronic pancreatitis. Endoscopy 2005;37(3):223–30.

44. Vitale GC, Cothron K, Vitale EA, et al. Role of pancreatic duct stenting in the treatment of chronic pancreatitis. Surg Endosc 2004;18(10):1431–4.

45. Binmoeller KF, Jue P, Seifert H, et al. Endoscopic pancreatic stent drainage in chronic pancreatitis and a dominant stricture: long-term results. Endoscopy 1995;27(9):638–44.

46. Costamagna G, Bulajic M, Tringali A, et al. Multiple stenting of refractory pancreatic duct strictures in severe chronic pancreatitis: long-term results. Endoscopy 2006;38(3):254–9.

47. Park DH, Kim MH, Moon SH, et al. Feasibility and safety of placement of a newly designed, fully covered self-expandable metal stent for refractory benign pancreatic ductal strictures: a pilot study (with video). Gastrointest Endosc 2008;68(6):1182–9.

48. Sauer B, Talreja J, Ellen K, et al. Temporary placement of a fully covered self-expandable metal stent in the pancreatic duct for management of symptomatic refractory chronic pancreatitis: preliminary data (with videos). Gastrointest Endosc 2008;68(6):1173–8.

49. Moon SH, Kim MH, Park DH, et al. Modified fully covered self-expandable metal stents with antimigration features for benign pancreatic-duct strictures in advanced chronic pancreatitis, with a focus on the safety profile and reducing migration. Gastrointest Endosc 2010;72(1):86–91.

50. Shami VM, Kahaleh M. Endoscopic ultrasonography (EUS)-guided access and therapy of pancreatico-biliary disorders: EUS-guided cholangio and pancreatic drainage. Gastrointest Endosc Clin N Am 2007;17(3):581–93, vii–viii.

51. Kahaleh M, Hernandez AJ, Tokar J, et al. EUS-guided pancreaticogastrostomy: analysis of its efficacy to drain inaccessible pancreatic ducts. Gastrointest Endosc 2007;65(2):224–30.

52. Barkay O, Sherman S, McHenry L, et al. Therapeutic EUS-assisted endoscopic retrograde pancreatography after failed pancreatic duct cannulation at ERCP. Gastrointest Endosc 2010;71(7):1166–73.

53. Tessier G, Bories E, Arvanitakis M, et al. EUS-guided pancreatogastrostomy and pancreatobulbostomy for the treatment of pain in patients with pancreatic ductal dilatation inaccessible for transpapillary endoscopic therapy. Gastrointest Endosc 2007;65(2):233–41.

54. Santosh D, Lakhtakia S, Gupta R, et al. Clinical trial: a randomized trial comparing fluoroscopy guided percutaneous technique vs. endoscopic ultrasound guided technique of coeliac plexus block for treatment of pain in chronic pancreatitis. Aliment Pharmacol Ther 2009;29(9):979–84.

55. Gress F, Schmitt C, Sherman S, et al. Endoscopic ultrasound-guided celiac plexus block for managing abdominal pain associated with chronic pancreatitis: a prospective single center experience. Am J Gastroenterol 2001;96(2):409–16.

56. Kaufman M, Singh G, Das S, et al. Efficacy of endoscopic ultrasound-guided celiac plexus block and celiac plexus neurolysis for managing abdominal pain associated with chronic pancreatitis and pancreatic cancer. J Clin Gastroenterol 2010;44(2):127–34.

57. Stevens T, Costanzo A, Lopez R, et al. Adding triamcinolone to endoscopic ultrasound-guided celiac plexus blockade does not reduce pain in patients with chronic pancreatitis. Clin Gastroenterol Hepatol 2012;10(2):186–191.e1.

58. Gimeno-García AZ, Elwassief A, Paquin SC, et al. Fatal complication after endoscopic ultrasound-guided celiac plexus neurolysis. Endoscopy 2012;44(Suppl 2 UCTN):E267.

59. Jacobson BC, Baron TH, Adler DG, et al. ASGE guideline: the role of endoscopy in the diagnosis and the management of cystic lesions and inflammatory fluid collections of the pancreas. Gastrointest Endosc 2005;61(3):363-70.

60. Lerch MM, Stier A, Wahnschaffe U, et al. Pancreatic pseudocysts: observation, endoscopic drainage, or resection? Dtsch Arztebl Int 2009;106(38):614-21.

61. Rosso E, Alexakis N, Ghaneh P, et al. Pancreatic pseudocyst in chronic pancreatitis: endoscopic and surgical treatment. Dig Surg 2003;20(5):397-406.

62. Varadarajulu S, Bang JY, Sutton BS, et al. Equal efficacy of endoscopic and surgical cystogastrostomy for pancreatic pseudocyst drainage in a randomized trial. Gastroenterology 2013 May 31. [Epub ahead of print].

63. Barthet M, Lamblin G, Gasmi M, et al. Clinical usefulness of a treatment algorithm for pancreatic pseudocysts. Gastrointest Endosc 2008;67(2):245-52.

64. Binmoeller KF, Seifert H, Walter A, et al. Transpapillary and transmural drainage of pancreatic pseudocysts. Gastrointest Endosc 1995;42(3):219-24.

65. Hookey LC, Debroux S, Delhaye M, et al. Endoscopic drainage of pancreatic-fluid collections in 116 patients: a comparison of etiologies, drainage techniques, and outcomes. Gastrointest Endosc 2006;63(4):635-43.

66. Varadarajulu S, Christein JD, Tamhane A, et al. Prospective randomized trial comparing EUS and EGD for transmural drainage of pancreatic pseudocysts (with videos). Gastrointest Endosc 2008;68(6):1102-11.

67. Park DH, Lee SS, Moon SH, et al. Endoscopic ultrasound-guided versus conventional transmural drainage for pancreatic pseudocysts: a prospective randomized trial. Endoscopy 2009;41(10):842-8.

68. Cahen D, Rauws E, Fockens P, et al. Endoscopic drainage of pancreatic pseudocysts: long-term outcome and procedural factors associated with safe and successful treatment. Endoscopy 2005;37(10):977-83.

69. Arvanitakis M, Delhaye M, Bali MA, et al. Pancreatic-fluid collections: a randomized controlled trial regarding stent removal after endoscopic transmural drainage. Gastrointest Endosc 2007;65(4):609-19.

70. Devière J, Antaki F. Disconnected pancreatic tail syndrome: a plea for multidisciplinarity. Gastrointest Endosc 2008;67(4):680-2.

71. Dumonceau JM, Tringali A, Blero D, et al. Biliary stenting: indications, choice of stents and results: European Society of Gastrointestinal Endoscopy (ESGE) clinical guideline. Endoscopy 2012;44(3):277-98.

72. Cremer M, Devière J, Delhaye M, et al. Stenting in severe chronic pancreatitis: results of medium-term follow-up in seventy-six patients. Endoscopy 1991; 23(3):171-6.

73. Smits ME, Badiga SM, Rauws EA, et al. Long-term results of pancreatic stents in chronic pancreatitis. Gastrointest Endosc 1995;42(5):461-7.

74. Morgan DE, Smith JK, Hawkins K, et al. Endoscopic stent therapy in advanced chronic pancreatitis: relationships between ductal changes, clinical response, and stent patency. Am J Gastroenterol 2003;98(4):821-6.

75. Ishihara T, Yamaguchi T, Seza K, et al. Efficacy of s-type stents for the treatment of the main pancreatic duct stricture in patients with chronic pancreatitis. Scand J Gastroenterol 2006;41(6):744-50.

76. Weber A, Schneider J, Neu B, et al. Endoscopic stent therapy for patients with chronic pancreatitis: results from a prospective follow-up study. Pancreas 2007; 34(3):287-94.

ERCP for Biliary Strictures Associated with Chronic Pancreatitis

Pietro Familiari, MD, PhD, Ivo Boškoski, MD, PhD, Vincenzo Bove, MD,
Guido Costamagna, MD*

KEYWORDS

- Chronic pancreatitis • Benign biliary strictures • ERCP • Plastic stent
- Self-expandable metal stent • Dilation • Surgery • Pancreatic cancer

KEY POINTS

- The vast majority of chronic pancreatitis (CP)-related biliary strictures occur as a consequence of progressive fibrosis of pancreatic parenchyma and should be considered as permanent. CP-related biliary strictures are more resistant to endoscopic dilation than other benign biliary strictures.
- Surgical drainage is considered the gold standard for the definitive treatment of CP-related biliary strictures.
- Endoscopic biliary stenting is initially recommended in patients who present with jaundice, especially occurring after an acute exacerbation of pancreatitis, because this may resolve with the resolution of the acute inflammation.
- Endoscopic stenting may be indicated in patients unfit for surgery or in those who refuse surgery.
- Removable, fully covered self-expandable metal stents (FCSEMSs) seem to be a promising alternative for common bile duct strictures related to CP.

INTRODUCTION

A stricture of the intrapancreatic common bile duct (CBD) will develop in approximately 3% to 46% of patients with CP[1–8] and can seriously compromise the clinical course of the disease. Biliary strictures usually complicate a long-lasting disease, as a result of severe fibrosis of the pancreatic head parenchyma, which compresses and narrows the distal CBD. However, CP-related CBD strictures may also be seen in patients with a recently diagnosed disease.

Digestive Endoscopy Unit, Gemelli University Hospital, Università Cattolica del Sacro Cuore, Rome 00167, Italy
* Corresponding author. Digestive Endoscopy Unit, Gemelli University Hospital, 8 Largo Gemelli, Rome 00167, Italy.
E-mail address: gcostamagna@rm.unicatt.it

Gastrointest Endoscopy Clin N Am 23 (2013) 833–845
http://dx.doi.org/10.1016/j.giec.2013.06.007
1052-5157/13/$ – see front matter © 2013 Elsevier Inc. All rights reserved.

The real incidence of CP-related biliary strictures is unknown. Many patients remain asymptomatic for years before the stricture will cause increasing cholestasis, jaundice, or cholangitis, and this may contribute to underestimate their incidence. Furthermore, many patients with CP have a history of alcohol addiction, being less compliant to medical care and follow-up.

The management of CP-related biliary strictures is still controversial. Traditionally, a surgical bypass, choledochoduodenostomy, choledochojejunostomy, or hepaticojejunostomy, was the only treatment option. Despite the benefits of a definitive solution, because of the morbidity and mortality associated with surgery, alternative drainage techniques have been investigated, especially endoscopic biliary stent placement. Both treatments, endoscopic and surgical, have, as usual, advantages and disadvantages.

Despite some CP-related biliary strictures resolving with time, the vast majority of clinically significant strictures should be considered as permanent. These strictures are usually more resistant to endoscopic dilation than other benign biliary strictures, especially those occurring after biliary surgery or orthotopic liver transplantation.[9,10] Furthermore, patients with CP have a risk of pancreatic cancer substantially higher than the general population.[11] Cancer usually occurs many years after the clinical onset of CP. Therefore, in certain circumstances, surgery might also be recommended to rule out cancer.[12,13]

Many patients potentially curable with surgery are not good candidates because of their compromised general status, adverse local conditions (ie, postoperative adhesions, portal vein thrombosis with portal hypertension, consequences of severe necrotizing pancreatitis, and so on) or refusal of surgery. Endoscopic drainage offers a chance to this selected group of patients or may be considered as a bridge to surgery.

The pathogenesis of CP-related biliary strictures, the diagnostic workup, the indication to endoscopic treatment, the results of endotherapy, and the future developments in this field are discussed in this review.

PATHOGENESIS

Different mechanisms contribute to the development of biliary strictures in patients with CP. The strictures usually involve the distal third of the CBD, which passes through the pancreatic head before it reaches the papilla of Vater and the duodenum. The intrapancreatic portion of the CBD varies in length from 1.5 to 6 cm, and this accounts for the variability of stricture length seen in clinical practice.[14]

The vast majority of biliary strictures associated with CP occur as a consequence of progressive fibrosis of the pancreatic parenchyma due to recurrent acute or chronic inflammation, which may eventually result in permanent periductal fibrosis. Parenchymal fibrosis in CP is a slow, irreversible process, and these strictures usually occur late in the natural history of the disease. The strictures occurring in patients with calcified pancreatic stones are particularly fibrotic and thus resistant to dilation.[15–17] CBD strictures can also develop earlier in the course of the disease and be the result of an acute pancreatic inflammation as an exacerbation of the chronic illness: the edema of the pancreatic head compresses the CBD, usually between one to few days after the acute bout. These strictures may resolve spontaneously, few days or weeks after the clinical onset, or, in more severe cases, be persistent and require biliary drainage.

Biliary strictures can also be caused by the extrinsic compression of the CBD from a pancreatic retention cyst, a pseudocyst, or a walled-off pancreatic necrosis.[18] These strictures are usually reversible and are managed by draining the pancreatic fluid collection. However, 2 or more mechanisms may contribute to the development of the biliary stricture; as a consequence, the drainage of the collection might be sufficient to make the jaundice disappear, but subclinical cholestasis may persist and eventually require drainage.[19] Furthermore, the stricture can also be caused by a pancreatic cancer, which can additionally complicate the course of the CP. This danger should always be carefully investigated and excluded when the patient is seen for the first time or in case of a long-lasting disease.

CLINICAL PRESENTATION AND DIAGNOSIS

Biliary strictures have a broad spectrum of presentation, varying from mildly elevated levels in liver function tests to severe jaundice in case of complete biliary obstruction. Acute cholangitis is uncommon in patients with an intact papilla but may become the predominant symptom in case of prior biliary sphincterotomy.

The "incidental finding" of a CP-related biliary stricture accounts for up to 17% of cases.[20]

Abdominal pain is usually considered the predominant symptom in most patients, but it is doubtful that a biliary stricture per se might be a major contributing factor to pain development.[19] Pain is more likely to be caused by a bout of acute pancreatitis or a stricture of the pancreatic duct than by a biliary stricture.

Jaundice may be present in 30% to 50% of patients at the diagnosis.[20,21] Transient jaundice is typically seen in patients with exacerbation of the chronic illness, as a result of the edema and acute inflammation of the pancreatic head. In these cases, jaundice will usually recede spontaneously with the resolution of the acute process. Alteration of liver function test results and biochemical markers of cholestasis, including alkaline phosphatase and gamma-glutamyl transferase, may be persistent for some weeks after the normalization of bilirubin levels.

Acute cholangitis may be life threatening and thus becomes a clear indication to an emergency biliary drainage, but it rarely represents the leading symptom at diagnosis.

Jaundice and elevation of alkaline phosphatase level greater than 2-fold lasting for more than 1 month has been advocated as a precise marker of biliary stricture. However, biochemical findings should always be confirmed by radiological imaging, especially before endoscopic drainage.

The demonstration of a dilated CBD at transabdominal ultrasound examination, associated with elevation of levels of biochemical markers of cholestasis, is usually sufficient for the diagnosis. However, a computed tomographic (CT) scan is usually required, especially at the first episode of jaundice, to better clarify the nature of the pancreatic disease, accurately delineate the parenchymal and ductal changes, demonstrate the severity and localization of calcifications, exclude fluid collections, and, importantly, demonstrate suspicious masses. Furthermore, CT scan is fundamental to plan the subsequent treatment of patients. The decision whether to operate or not a patient is also based on the CT scan findings: portal vein thrombosis, a large peripancreatic mass, liver metastases, and cirrhosis are commonly considered contraindications to surgical biliary bypass.

The differentiation between pancreatic cancer and CP is particularly difficult. CT scan offers good visualization of the pancreatic parenchyma, but in the absence of distant metastases, fibrotic and inflammatory masses associated with CP or groove pancreatitis cannot be discriminated with certainty from neoplasms. Cross-sectional imaging by magnetic resonance can provide a better anatomic detail but again often does not permit a definite diagnosis of malignancy. At cholangiography, including magnetic resonance cholangiopancreatography (MRCP), benign biliary strictures appear smooth, tapering and regular, whereas malignant ones are irregular, tightened, and abrupt. However, cholangiographic features are unreliable because of a wide variability of the cholangiographic appearances of the stricture. Endoscopic retrograde cholangiopancreatography (ERCP) is still more accurate than MRCP in delineating the main pancreatic duct and side branches morphology and CBD stricture and may assist in the differential diagnosis (**Fig. 1**).

Neoplastic biochemical markers are of help for the discrimination between malignant and benign strictures. Markedly increased levels of CA 19-9 (>1000 U/mL) are strongly associated with pancreatic cancer,[22] but this is not a common finding. Unfortunately, moderately increased levels of CA-19.9 are frequently seen also in patients with benign biliary strictures as a result of elevated biliary pressure that causes leakage of CA 19-9 into serum.[23]

Nowadays, a cytologic or histologic confirmation is often advocated to definitely rule out the presence of malignancy. Brush cytology and endobiliary biopsies can be obtained during ERCP, but the sensitivity of the sampling is low for pancreatic cancer and not routinely recommended. Endoscopic ultrasound-guided fine-needle aspiration is becoming the predominant technique to obtain cytologic and histologic sampling from pancreatic masses because of its high safety profile and diagnostic accuracy.[24]

When the suspicion of malignancy is strong, every effort should be made to convince the more reluctant patient to undergo surgery, or at least, the diagnostic test and histologic sampling should be repeated and repeated at short time intervals.

INDICATIONS FOR ENDOSCOPIC DRAINAGE AND PROCEDURAL ASPECTS

Cholangitis is per se a life-threatening complication and an obvious indication for drainage. However, jaundice and subclinical persistent cholestasis usually require drainage too, as they may lead to secondary biliary cirrhosis. Biliary cirrhosis in patients with CBD stenosis secondary to CP has been observed in about 7% of patients,[25] but reports are old and contradictory. Alcohol addiction and "unorthodox" behaviors are common in patients with CP and may be per se the cause of liver cirrhosis. However, Hammel and colleagues[26] found regression of liver fibrosis in patients with CP-related biliary stricture after biliary drainage. Therefore, every biliary stricture that persists for more than 1 month and is associated with increased levels

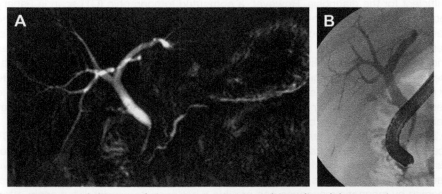

Fig. 1. Patient with history of chronic pancreatitis and jaundice. (*A*) Magnetic resonance cholangiopancreatography showing a tapered, smooth, and regular stricture of the distal common bile duct. (*B*) Endoscopic retrograde cholangiopancreatography confirming MRCP findings.

of biochemical markers of cholestasis should be drained by either surgery or endoscopy.[1,27]

Biliary decompression is also clearly indicated when frequent relapses of biliary obstruction occur, to minimize the risk of secondary biliary cirrhosis and cholangitis. Asymptomatic patients or those with slightly elevated levels of biochemical markers of cholestasis should be treated conservatively with close monitoring of liver functions test results at regular intervals. A conservative approach is also initially recommended for patients who present with jaundice, especially occurring after an acute exacerbation of pancreatitis, because this may resolve with the resolution of the acute inflammation. However, most biliary strictures associated with CP are permanent, and these patients are usually young, with a long life expectancy.

Every biliary stent, whether plastic or metallic, will inevitably occlude over time, leading to recurrent jaundice or cholangitis. Endoscopic bile duct stricture dilation with stent placement has become standard of care for most postoperative biliary strictures. However, CP-related strictures are much more resistant to endoscopic dilation than postoperative strictures, and when successfully dilated, strictures frequently recur, months or years after the end of the stenting period.

Endoscopic biliary stent placement is therefore not recommended as a definitive treatment of CP-related biliary strictures. Surgical drainage is still considered as the gold standard, by either a biliary bypass (ie, hepaticojejunostomy or choledocoduodenostomy) or more complex operations, in patients with pain due to concomitant pancreatic duct obstruction (duodenopancreatectomy or duodenal preserving pancreatectomy, as the Frey or the Beger procedure). However, due to its morbidity and mortality, surgery should be carefully balanced in patients with potentially reversible strictures, which might regress spontaneously or after a short stenting period. Some other patients are not good surgical candidates, because of comorbidities, postoperative adhesions, portal biliopathy, or other anatomic situations that can make surgery more difficult or impossible. Furthermore, some patients with CP refuse surgery and prefer repeated endoscopies to a definitive operation with a potentially complicated postoperative course.

Endoscopic biliary stenting has a high technical success rate and provides short-term resolution of jaundice and cholangitis, but because of the long-term recurrences, it should be proposed as a first-line therapy in a selected group of patients, including (1) symptomatic patients, with jaundice or cholangitis and with a potentially reversible biliary stricture; (2) patients unfit for surgery; (3) patients unwilling to undergo surgery; (4) as a temporary measure, in patients with severe jaundice or in those with acute cholangitis in case of delayed definitive surgery.

Procedural Aspects

From a procedural point of view, biliary stent placement for CP-related CBD strictures does not substantially differ from that for palliation of malignant biliary strictures. After CBD cannulation and cholangiography, a biliary sphincterotomy is performed. Biliary sphincterotomy facilitates stent insertion and future repeat access to the biliary tree and enables placement of single/multiple stents in the course of the treatment. Despite the fibrosis of the pancreatic parenchyma, CP-related biliary strictures are easily traversed with a guidewire and a guiding catheter. Balloon dilation before single stent placement is seldom necessary, and placement of a plastic Amsterdam-type 10F or 11.5F stent over the guiding catheter is usually not technically demanding.

The patency of a large-bore (10–11.5F) biliary plastic stent is 3–4 months, on average. To avoid cholangitis, ERCP is repeated after 3 months, and the stent is removed. The stricture is reevaluated and biopsies or biliary brushing repeated if necessary. The stricture is considered sufficiently dilated when the stricture-waist has disappeared, the ERCP catheter passes through the stricture without resistance, and the contrast agent injected into the bile ducts rapidly flows into the duodenum.

If the stricture persists after 3 months, stenting has to be repeated. The length of treatment should be individualized, according to the patient's fitness and willingness to undergo surgery. To maximize the dilation of the stricture, some authors recommend the placement of multiple plastic stents, side by side, similarly to that for other benign biliary strictures. Nevertheless, if stricture resolution is not observed after a 1-year treatment, a successful outcome is unlikely and surgery should be again considered (**Fig. 2**).[28]

Recently, SEMSs have been used for the treatment of CP-related biliary strictures.[29–31]

Permanent placement of uncovered SEMSs has to be avoided because of the inevitable hyperplastic reaction of the CBD mucosa, which eventually occludes the stent after 6 to 24 months. Temporary placement of SEMSs, usually fully covered and equipped with an extraction lasso to make them easily removable, may offer an alternative to dilation with plastic stents.

Placement of a FCSEMS for a CP biliary stricture is not per se technically demanding. After sphincterotomy, a guidewire is pushed into the bile ducts, through the stricture. The SEMS delivery system is advanced over the wire, and the SEMS deployed across the stricture under fluoroscopic and endoscopic controls.

OUTCOMES OF ENDOSCOPIC TREATMENT
Plastic Stents

A single plastic stent is placed to resolve chronic cholestasis and its complications as first-line treatment and as "bridge" to surgery or to definitive diagnosis.

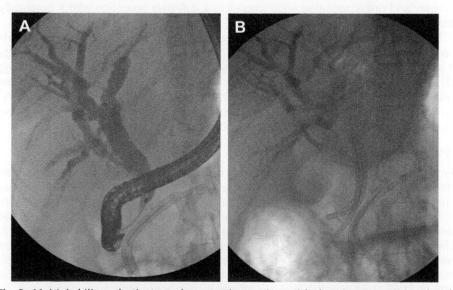

Fig. 2. Multiple biliary plastic stent placement in a patient with chronic pancreatitis–related biliary stricture. (*A*) ERCP shows a tight, smooth, and tapered stricture of the distal common bile duct. Two 10F pancreatic stents have been placed for a main pancreatic duct stricture. (*B*) Placement of 3 biliary plastic stents to dilate the stricture.

Single plastic stent placement in CP-related CBD strictures has given disappointing long-term results (**Table 1**). Poor outcomes are mostly due to the fact that CBD strictures related to CP are more resistant to endoscopic treatment compared with strictures of the CBD related to other benign causes.[9,10] Furthermore, the presence of pancreatic head calcifications has been found to be associated with even poorer outcomes.[32,33] For instance, Kahl and colleagues[32] in 2003 found that the presence of calcifications in the pancreatic head was associated with a 17-fold increased risk of treatment failure.

As for benign biliary strictures due to other nature, endoscopic placement of multiple plastic stents for strictures due to CP requires frequent reinterventions (usually 4 per year). This approach has shown promising results (**Table 2**). The rationale is that multiple stents gradually dilate the stricture resulting in a progressive tissue remodeling (**Fig. 2**).

Draganov and colleagues[34] performed multiple plastic stenting in 9 patients with CP-related CBD strictures. Stricture resolution was found in 44% of the patients. Multiple plastic stenting was also performed by Catalano and colleagues[35] in 12 patients with CP-related CBD stricture. In 92% of the patients, there was a resolution of the CBD stricture during a mean follow-up of 3.9 years. In 2004, Pozsar and colleagues[36] performed multistenting with plastic stents in 29 patients with CP-related CBD strictures. There was a complete resolution in 60% after a mean follow-up period of 1 year.

According to these results, a temporary simultaneous placement of multiple plastic stents seems to be a suitable approach in patients with CP-related CBD strictures. Although stricture recurrences in these patients are not rare, recurrences can be successfully re-treated by ERCP.

Patients undergoing planned plastic multistenting should be evaluated for compliance before the procedure. Noncompliance of these patients has been found to be associated with high rate of septic complications, which are even fatal, particularly in alcoholics.[37]

Self-Expandable Metal Stents

The concept of placing a single metal stent to cure CP-related CBD strictures is based on the characteristics of these stents. SEMSs are larger in diameter, allowing better

Table 1
Studies on treatment of common bile duct strictures related to chronic pancreatitis with endoscopic placement of single biliary plastic stents

Author and Reference, Year	No. of Patients	Long-term Success (%)	Mean Stenting Duration (mo)	Stent Dysfunction for Any Cause (%)	Follow-Up Post Stent Removal (mo)
Deviere et al,[43] 1990	25	12	NA	72	14
Barthet et al,[44] 1994	19	10	10	NA	18
Smits et al,[45] 1996	58	28	10	64	49
Farnbacher et al,[46] 2000	31	32	10	52	28
Vitale et al,[47] 2000	25	80	13	20	32
Eickoff et al,[48] 2001	39	31	9	43	58
Kahl et al,[32] 2003	61	26	12	34	40
Catalano et al,[35] 2004	34	24	21	41	50
Bartoli et al,[49] 2005	9	44	9	22	16

Abbreviation: NA, not available.

Table 2
Studies on treatment of common bile duct strictures related to chronic pancreatitis with endoscopic placement of multiple biliary plastic stents

Author and Reference, Year	No. of Patients	Long-term Success (%)	Mean Stenting Duration (mo)	Stent Dysfunction for Any Cause (%)	Follow-Up Post Stent Removal (mo)
Draganov et al,[34] 2002	9	44	14	NA	48
Catalano et al,[35] 2004	12	92	14	8	47
Pozsar et al,[36] 2004	29	60	21	NA	12

Abbreviation: NA, not available.

biliary drainage and longer patency, allowing only 2 ERCP sessions, one for stent placement and one for stent removal (**Fig. 3**).

In the past, uncovered SEMSs were used to treat all types of strictures of the CBD, including CP-related strictures.[38] At present, placement of uncovered SEMSs is

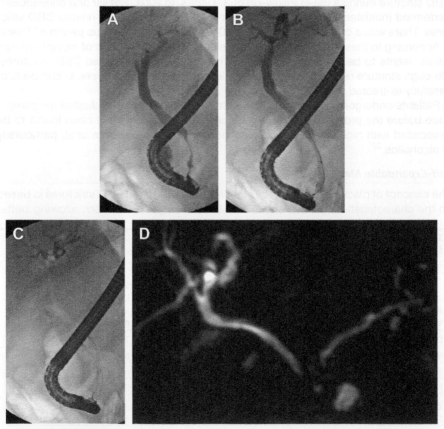

Fig. 3. Fully covered SEMS placement. (*A*) ERCP shows a stricture of the distal common bile duct. (*B*) Placement of a fully covered, removable, biliary SEMS. (*C*) Complete biliary drainage and pneumobilia after SEMS placement. (*D*) MRCP shows complete SEMS migration 4 months after the placement. The patient is asymptomatic, with a good dilation of the biliary stricture.

strongly discouraged, because their removal may be impossible because of tissue hyperplasia through the meshes of the stents.[35,39,40]

Covered SEMSs are designed to prevent tissue ingrowth. However, loss of the integrity of the stent covering may sometimes preclude removability of partially and FCSEMSs.[33]

In 1993, Deviere and colleagues[39] published a report on permanent uncovered SEMS placement in patients with CP-related CBD stricture. The overall stent patency rate was 90% in 20 patients after a mean follow-up of 33 months. At cholangioscopy, the metal mesh was rapidly covered by hyperplasia, which occluded the stent only in 2 patients, who required further treatment.

Partially covered metal stents were used by Cantù and colleagues[41] in 14 patients with CP-related CBD strictures but with no intention to remove the stents. At 18 months, all the stents remained patent; however, after a mean period of 22 months, 50% of the patients developed stent dysfunction, caused by tissue ingrowth and stent migration.

FCSEMSs were used by Kahaleh and colleagues[9] in 79 patients with benign biliary strictures due to different causes: 32 were due to CP. Of these patients, only 22 were evaluable: the stricture resolved in 77% at a median follow-up of 12 months after removal. In this study, distal migration of the fully covered stent was the most common problem.

Temporary placement of partially covered SEMSs was performed by Behm and colleagues[29] in 20 patients, obtaining a stricture resolution in 90% of the patients 6 months after stent removal. However, removal of the stents was possible only in 18 patients. Complications were bleeding in one patient and pancreatitis in another patient.

FCSEMSs should prevent the risk of tissue ingrowth that can occur in partially covered stents, making them difficult or impossible to extract. However, the risk of migration of these stents is higher (Fig. 3, Table 3).

To prevent migration of FCSEMSs, some investigators proposed the use of stents with anchoring flaps. FCSEMSs with either an anchoring flap or a flared end at the proximal end were tried by Park and colleagues[31] in 43 patients with benign biliary strictures due to different causes: in this cohort, 11 patients had strictures related to CP. In these series, 6 months after placement, 100% of the stents with anchoring flaps were in situ, whereas 33% of the stents with proximal flared end migrated. All stents in situ were removed in both groups.

Mahajan and colleagues[10] used FCSEMSs in 44 patients with benign biliary strictures due to different causes: in 19 patients, the strictures were due to CP. The

Table 3
Studies on treatment of common bile duct strictures due to chronic pancreatitis with partially and fully covered removable SEMS

Author and Reference, Year	No. of Patients	Stent Design	Median Time to SEMS Removal (mo)	Stricture Resolution Rate at SEMS Removal (%)	Migration Rate (%)	Median Follow-Up Post Stent Removal (mo)
Cahen et al,[30] 2008	6	FCSEMS	5.5	67	33	20.5
Behm et al,[29] 2009	20	PCSEMS	5	80	5	22
Perri et al,[33] 2012	7	UE-FCSEMS	6	43	100	24
	10	FE-FCSEMS		90	40	

Abbreviations: FE, flared ends; PC, partially covered; UE, unflared ends.

stricture resolved in 58% after a median follow-up time of 3.8 months; stent migration was found only in one patient. Complications in these patients were pancreatitis in one and bleeding in another.

In a case series, Cahen and colleagues[30] placed an FCSEMS, with a distal lasso to pull the stents, in 6 patients with CP-related CBD strictures. Stricture resolution was found in 37% of patients after a median time of 5.5 months. Proximal migration was observed in 2 cases; in both stent removal failed.

Perri and colleagues[33] analyzed the resolution rate of CP-related CBD strictures after temporary insertion of unflared-ends and flared-ends FCSEMS in 17 patients. The authors found migration in 100% of the unflared-ends stents, compared with 40% of the flared-ends stents. The stents were removed after 6 months. After a median follow-up of 24 months, stricture resolution was found in 43% of patients with unflared-ends stents and in 90% of patients with flared-ends stents. Five patients had cholangitis during the course of the study.

Table 3 shows the results of studies on partially and fully covered SEMSs.

In selected patients, covered SEMSs seem to be a promising alternative for CBD strictures related to CP.[40] Even in these cases, stricture recurrences can be successfully re-treated by ERCP.

Biodegradable Stents

Biodegradable stents might theoretically solve the problems of metallic stents and replace metal stents for the treatment of benign biliary strictures of different causes.

Yamamoto and colleagues[42] performed an experimental study with biodegradable stents in normal canine bile ducts with the intention to clarify the advantages in terms of mucosal reaction and biodegradation after placement. The stent placed in 3 dogs was a balloon-expandable Z stent consisting of poly-L-lactic acid with platinum markers. Follow-up was done at 1, 3, 6, and 9 months. The bile duct lumen was examined macroscopically and histologically. Stent degradation was also examined by electron microscopy. None of the stent migrated, and stent obstruction was absent. There was moderate epithelial hyperplasia. Degradation of stents was evident macroscopically and on electron microscopy. Even if placed in normal bile ducts, these encouraging results suggest that biodegradable stents could have a future for the treatment of benign biliary strictures, including CBD strictures due to CP. Further studies are needed to evaluate the application of these stents for tight strictures of the CBD as those induced by CP.

SUMMARY

CP-related CBD strictures are more difficult to treat endoscopically compared with benign biliary strictures because of their nature, particularly in patients with calcific CP.

Before any attempt at treatment, malignancy must be excluded.

Single plastic stents can be used for immediate symptom relief and as "bridge to surgery and/or bridge to decision," but are not suitable for definitive treatment of CP-related CBD strictures because of long-term poor results.

Temporary simultaneous placement of multiple plastic stents has a high technical success rate and provides good long-term results. This treatment requires a mean of approximately 4 ERCPs during a 1-year period. Stricture recurrences are not rare and can be successfully re-treated endoscopically.

The use of uncovered metal stents should be avoided because they cannot be removed.

Temporary placement of covered SEMSs is still under investigation, and further trials are needed to confirm their suitability for CP-related CBD strictures.

Physicians should always be aware that "forgetting" patients with a stent or their lack of compliance can lead to severe and even fatal septic complications.

Biodegradable stents that do not have impact on the mucosa of the CBD and have enough axial and radial forces might be the future alternative, solving also the problem of noncompliance.

REFERENCES

1. Afroudakis A, Kaplowitz N. Liver histopathology in chronic common bile duct stenosis due to chronic alcoholic pancreatitis. Hepatology 1981;1:65–72.
2. Huizinga WK, Thomson SR, Spitaels JM, et al. Chronic pancreatitis with biliary obstruction. Ann R Coll Surg Engl 1992;74:119–23.
3. Petrozza JA, Dutta SK. The variable appearance of distal common bile duct stenosis in chronic pancreatitis. J Clin Gastroenterol 1985;7:447–50.
4. Sand JA, Nordback IH. Management of cholestasis in patients with chronic pancreatitis: evaluation of a treatment protocol. Eur J Surg 1995;161:587–92.
5. Stabile BE, Calabria R, Wilson SE, et al. Stricture of the common bile duct from chronic pancreatitis. Surg Gynecol Obstet 1987;165:121–6.
6. Wislooff F, Jakobsen J, Osnes M. Stenosis of the common bile duct in chronic pancreatitis. Br J Surg 1982;69:52–4.
7. Yadegar J, Williams RA, Passaro E Jr, et al. Common duct stricture from chronic pancreatitis. Arch Surg 1980;115:582–6.
8. Aranha GV, Prinz RA, Freeark RJ, et al. The spectrum of biliary tract obstruction from chronic pancreatitis. Arch Surg 1984;119:595–600.
9. Kahaleh M, Behm B, Clarke BW, et al. Temporary placement of covered self-expandable metal stents in benign biliary strictures: a new paradigm? (with video). Gastrointest Endosc 2008;67:446–54.
10. Mahajan A, Ho H, Sauer B, et al. Temporary placement of fully covered self-expandable metal stents in benign biliary strictures: midterm evaluation (with video). Gastrointest Endosc 2009;70:303–9.
11. Lowenfels AB, Maisonneuve P, Cavallini G, et al. Pancreatitis and the risk of pancreatic cancer. International Pancreatitis Study Group. N Engl J Med 1993; 328:1433–7.
12. Nealon WH, Urrutia F. Long-term follow-up after bilioenteric anastomosis for benign bile duct stricture. Ann Surg 1996;223:639–45.
13. Adler DG, Lichtenstein D, Baron TH, et al. The role of endoscopy in patients with chronic pancreatitis. Gastrointest Endosc 2006;63:933–7.
14. Eckhauser FE, Knol JA, Strodel WE, et al. Common bile duct strictures associated with chronic pancreatitis. Am Surg 1983;49:350–8.
15. Kasugai T, Kuno N, Kizu M. Endoscopic pancreatocholangiography with special reference to manometric method. Med J Aust 1973;2:717–25.
16. Kasugai T, Kuno N, Kobayashi S, et al. Endoscopic pancreatocholangiography. I. The normal endoscopic pancreatocholangiogram. Gastroenterology 1972;63: 217–26.
17. Smanio T. Varying relations of the common bile duct with the posterior face of the pancreatic head in Negroes and white persons. J Int Coll Surg 1954;22: 150–73.
18. Delhaye M, Arvanitakis M, Bali M, et al. Endoscopic therapy for chronic pancreatitis. Scand J Surg 2005;94:143–53.

19. Abdallah AA, Krige JE, Bornman PC. Biliary tract obstruction in chronic pancreatitis. HPB (Oxford) 2007;9:421–8.
20. Kalvaria I, Bornman PC, Marks IN, et al. The spectrum and natural history of common bile duct stenosis in chronic alcohol-induced pancreatitis. Ann Surg 1989; 210:608–13.
21. Sarles H, Sahel J. Cholestasis and lesions of the biliary tract in chronic pancreatitis. Gut 1978;19:851–7.
22. Steinberg W. The clinical utility of the CA 19-9 tumor-associated antigen. Am J Gastroenterol 1990;85:350–5.
23. Minghini A, Weireter LJ Jr, Perry RR. Specificity of elevated CA 19-9 levels in chronic pancreatitis. Surgery 1998;124:103–5.
24. Lewis JJ, Kowalski TE. Endoscopic ultrasound and fine needle aspiration in pancreatic cancer. Cancer J 2012;18:523–9.
25. Frey CF, Suzuki M, Isaji S. Treatment of chronic pancreatitis complicated by obstruction of the common bile duct or duodenum. World J Surg 1990;14: 59–69.
26. Hammel P, Couvelard A, O'Toole D, et al. Regression of liver fibrosis after biliary drainage in patients with chronic pancreatitis and stenosis of the common bile duct. N Engl J Med 2001;344:418–23.
27. Warshaw AL, Schapiro RH, Ferrucci JT Jr, et al. Persistent obstructive jaundice, cholangitis, and biliary cirrhosis due to common bile duct stenosis in chronic pancreatitis. Gastroenterology 1976;70:562–7.
28. Cahen DL, van Berkel AM, Oskam D, et al. Long-term results of endoscopic drainage of common bile duct strictures in chronic pancreatitis. Eur J Gastroenterol Hepatol 2005;17:103–8.
29. Behm B, Brock A, Clarke BW, et al. Partially covered self-expandable metallic stents for benign biliary strictures due to chronic pancreatitis. Endoscopy 2009; 41:547–51.
30. Cahen DL, Rauws EA, Gouma DJ, et al. Removable fully covered self-expandable metal stents in the treatment of common bile duct strictures due to chronic pancreatitis: a case series. Endoscopy 2008;40:697–700.
31. Park DH, Lee SS, Lee TH, et al. Anchoring flap versus flared end, fully covered self-expandable metal stents to prevent migration in patients with benign biliary strictures: a multicenter, prospective, comparative pilot study (with videos). Gastrointest Endosc 2011;73:64–70.
32. Kahl S, Zimmermann S, Genz I, et al. Risk factors for failure of endoscopic stenting of biliary strictures in chronic pancreatitis: a prospective follow-up study. Am J Gastroenterol 2003;98:2448–53.
33. Perri V, Boskoski I, Tringali A, et al. Fully covered self-expandable metal stents in biliary strictures caused by chronic pancreatitis not responding to plastic stenting: a prospective study with 2 years of follow-up. Gastrointest Endosc 2012; 75:1271–7.
34. Draganov P, Hoffman B, Marsh W, et al. Long-term outcome in patients with benign biliary strictures treated endoscopically with multiple stents. Gastrointest Endosc 2002;55:680–6.
35. Catalano MF, Linder JD, George S, et al. Treatment of symptomatic distal common bile duct stenosis secondary to chronic pancreatitis: comparison of single vs. multiple simultaneous stents. Gastrointest Endosc 2004;60:945–52.
36. Pozsar J, Sahin P, Laszlo F, et al. Medium-term results of endoscopic treatment of common bile duct strictures in chronic calcifying pancreatitis with increasing numbers of stents. J Clin Gastroenterol 2004;38:118–23.

37. Kiehne K, Folsch UR, Nitsche R. High complication rate of bile duct stents in patients with chronic alcoholic pancreatitis due to noncompliance. Endoscopy 2000;32:377–80.
38. Dumonceau JM, Deviere J, Delhaye M, et al. Plastic and metal stents for postoperative benign bile duct strictures: the best and the worst. Gastrointest Endosc 1998;47:8–17.
39. Deviere J, Cremer M, Baize M, et al. Management of common bile duct stricture caused by chronic pancreatitis with metal mesh self-expandable stents. Gut 1994;35:122–6.
40. Dumonceau JM, Tringali A, Blero D, et al. Biliary stenting: indications, choice of stents and results: European Society of Gastrointestinal Endoscopy (ESGE) clinical guideline. Endoscopy 2012;44:277–98.
41. Cantù P, Hookey LC, Morales A, et al. The treatment of patients with symptomatic common bile duct stenosis secondary to chronic pancreatitis using partially covered metal stents: a pilot study. Endoscopy 2005;37:735–9.
42. Yamamoto K, Yoshioka T, Furuichi K, et al. Experimental study of poly-L-lactic acid biodegradable stents in normal canine bile ducts. Cardiovasc Intervent Radiol 2011;34:601–8.
43. Deviere J, Devaere S, Baize M, et al. Endoscopic biliary drainage in chronic pancreatitis. Gastrointest Endosc 1990;36:96–100.
44. Barthet M, Bernard JP, Duval JL, et al. Biliary stenting in benign biliary stenosis complicating chronic calcifying pancreatitis. Endoscopy 1994;26:569–72.
45. Smits ME, Rauws EA, van Gulik TM, et al. Long-term results of endoscopic stenting and surgical drainage for biliary stricture due to chronic pancreatitis. Br J Surg 1996;83:764–8.
46. Farnbacher MJ, Rabenstein T, Ell C, et al. Is endoscopic drainage of common bile duct stenoses in chronic pancreatitis up-to-date? Am J Gastroenterol 2000;95:1466–71.
47. Vitale GC, Reed DN Jr, Nguyen CT, et al. Endoscopic treatment of distal bile duct stricture from chronic pancreatitis. Surg Endosc 2000;14:227–31.
48. Eickhoff A, Jakobs R, Leonhardt A, et al. Endoscopic stenting for common bile duct stenoses in chronic pancreatitis: results and impact on long-term outcome. Eur J Gastroenterol Hepatol 2001;13:1161–7.
49. Bartoli E, Delcenserie R, Yzet T, et al. Endoscopic treatment of chronic pancreatitis. Gastroenterol Clin Biol 2005;29:515–21.

Endoscopic Ultrasonography–Guided Drainage of the Pancreatic Duct

Jessica Widmer, DO, Reem Z. Sharaiha, MD, MSc,
Michel Kahaleh, MD*

KEYWORDS

- Endoscopic ultrasonography • Endoscopic retrograde cholangiopancreatography
- Pancreatic access • Pancreatic drainage • Pancreaticogastrostomy

KEY POINTS

- Endoscopic ultrasonography–guided techniques for drainage of the pancreatic duct continue to evolve as less invasive alternatives to surgery.
- Drainage of the pancreatic duct can be transluminal or transpapillary, with or without the rendezvous technique.
- This method is technically challenging and requires advanced expertise.
- Complications can be severe.
- Dedicated devices are needed to improve the safety profile and efficacy.

INTRODUCTION

Endoscopic retrograde pancreatography (ERP) is the conventional method for evaluating and treating obstruction of the pancreatic duct caused by strictures, stones, or congenital anomalies such as pancreatic divisum. Even in expert hands, ERP is not technically possible in approximately 3% to 10% of patients, owing to surgically altered anatomy, tight strictures, complete ductal obstruction, or a disrupted duct.[1] Surgery and/or interventional radiology alternatives have been posited, with their known respective morbidity.[2–7] Over the last 2 decades there has been continuing development in endoscopic ultrasonography (EUS) with therapeutic techniques, such as celiac plexus block and EUS-guided pseudocyst or abscess drainage, replacing surgical or radiologic interventions. EUS-guided pancreatic drainage was the next

---

Division of Gastroenterology & Hepatology, Department of Medicine, Weill Cornell Medical College, 1305 York Avenue, 4th Floor, New York, NY 10021, USA
* Corresponding author.
E-mail address: mkahaleh@gmail.com

Gastrointest Endoscopy Clin N Am 23 (2013) 847–861
http://dx.doi.org/10.1016/j.giec.2013.06.011
1052-5157/13/$ – see front matter © 2013 Elsevier Inc. All rights reserved.

step on this continuum. EUS-guided pancreatic drainage methods include antero-grade or retrograde pancreatography with drainage and the rendezvous procedure.

BACKGROUND

Obstruction of the main pancreatic duct caused by strictures, stones, or anatomic anomalies is typically treated by ERP, interventional radiology, or surgical drainage.[2–8] It is thought that the obstruction to the flow of pancreatic juices causes high pressures in the pancreatic duct, which lead to pain.[9] Pharmacologic pain management and celiac plexus block are often used in an attempt to relieve pain, but do not address the obstruction.[10,11] In symptomatic patients with obstruction of the pancreatic duct and retention of pancreatic juice within the pancreatic duct, ERP with drainage is considered the primary therapy.[12–15] Indications for drainage of the pancreatic duct include chronic pancreatitis, groove pancreatitis, post-Whipple strictures, disrupted pancreatic duct after acute pancreatitis or trauma, pancreatic fistula and ascites, and endoscopic snare ampullectomy when prophylactic stent insertion has failed.[16–21]

Before performing pancreatic decompression, a tumor should be excluded as a possible cause of pancreatic obstruction, and adequate sampling of the pancreatic stricture should be performed.[22] Decompression of the duct using ERP leads to complete or partial relief in 60% to 80% of patients.[23,24] In 5% to 10% of these patients, the pancreatic duct cannot be drained via ERP.[1] Reasons for failure include postinflammatory changes of the periampullary region, pancreatic divisum with a stenotic minor papillary orifice, surgically altered anatomy, and gastric outlet or duodenal obstruction.[22,25,26] Patients who fail ERP may require interventional radiology, surgery, or enteral feeding until the acute flare is resolved.[27]

Surgical interventions permit both ductal decompression and pancreatic resection, if indicated. The type of surgery is typically determined by the anatomy of the pancreatic duct. In patients with a dilated main pancreatic duct, a lateral pancreaticojejunostomy is performed.[26,28] Resection of the diseased portion of the pancreas is indicated when there is focal disease, particularly in the absence of pancreatic ductal dilatation. In these cases a Whipple procedure, a duodenum-preserving resection of the pancreatic head, or distal pancreatectomy is performed.[28] Total pancreatectomy with auto-islet cell transplantation has been recommended for patients with chronic pancreatitis with adequate endocrine reserve, and seems to be the most appropriate option for patients failing endoscopic treatment.[29]

However, surgical interventions have limitations. Lateral pancreaticojejunostomy has a high complication rate (range, 6%–30%) and mortality rate (range, 0%–2%). Up to 20% of patients develop recurrent pain from inadequate drainage.[30–35] Pain may occur after pancreatic resection owing to the development of anastomotic strictures, which occur in approximately 5% of patients undergoing a Whipple procedure.[23,30,31] Steatorrhea occurs in 30% to 40% of patients undergoing drainage procedures and in up to 60% of patients requiring pancreatic resections.[36–38] Diabetes can occur after pancreatic resection as a consequence of surgery or progression of the disease state.[39]

In patients with a high operative risk or those who decline surgical intervention, EUS-guided pancreatic drainage is a promising alternative diagnostic and therapeutic option.[25] With the evolution of the linear-array echoendoscopy, and the ability to direct a needle within the field of intervention, the biliary and pancreatic ducts become reasonable targets for EUS when not accessible by conventional endoscopic retrograde cholangiopancreatography (ERCP). The method of EUS-guided pancreatography was first described by Harada and colleagues[40] in 1995 as a case report of a patient requiring removal of a pancreatic duct stone following pancreaticoduodenectomy.

Since then, interventional endosonography has been described as a platform for access to and drainage of the pancreatic duct either by rendezvous or transmural drainage. The rendezvous technique combines EUS with ERP by puncturing the dilated pancreatic duct under EUS guidance with insertion of a guide wire into the duct, then exiting the papilla.[25] Data show that rendezvous is often unsuccessful, and patients may require transluminal drainage with either pancreaticogastrostomy or pancreaticoduodenostomy.

METHODS
Procedure Considerations

Only experienced endoscopists trained in EUS and ERCP should attempt this procedure. If ERP initially fails, the patient should be referred to a tertiary care center with expertise in ERCP. Before considering EUS-guided drainage, various methods to obtain pancreatic access should be attempted including standard cannulation techniques, hydrophilic guide wires, or needle knife precut sphincterotomy of the major and/or minor papilla. Dedicated pancreaticobiliary surgeons should be available in the event of complications.

Patient Selection and Evaluation

Specific informed consent for EUS-guided pancreatic drainage should be obtained from all patients after a detailed discussion of the indications, risks, benefits, and alternatives to the procedure. Cross-sectional imaging should be reviewed and eventually repeated, if inadequate, before the procedure, to use as a roadmap. All procedures should be performed under general anesthesia with fluoroscopic guidance. Carbon dioxide is exclusively used for insufflation. Antibiotics are administered as a prophylactic measure.

Materials and Instruments

A therapeutic channel linear-array echoendoscope with a large working channel (3.8 mm) is needed to allow the use of a broad variety of accessories and to allow for the insertion of large-caliber stents (10F).

If the goal of the procedure is to perform ductography, it may be advantageous to use a smaller-gauge needle to determine whether contrast freely flows across the stricture, a finding suggesting absence of critical stenosis and precluding therapeutic intervention.[19] For interventional cases, a 19-gauge fine-needle aspiration (FNA) needle should be used, offering the ability to manipulate a larger 0.025-in (0.635 mm) or 0.035-in (0.889 mm) guide wire, which may facilitate crossing strictures and promote passage of other accessories. 0.035-in wires have maximal stiffness but may be subject to shearing at the tip of the 19-gauge needle. The authors do not recommend using a 0.018-in (0.457 mm) guide wire because such wires are floppy and can make interventions challenging.[19] For difficult stenoses or angles, a hydrophilic wire or an angled wire may facilitate traversal of narrowed or tortuous segments.[19]

TECHNIQUE

The technique may vary as regards EUS duct access for rendezvous as opposed to a transenteric approach to stent placement. After endosonographic examination of the pancreas, the main pancreatic duct (MPD) is localized using an echoendoscope below the esophagogastric junction (**Fig. 1**). To provide a larger area to target and enable

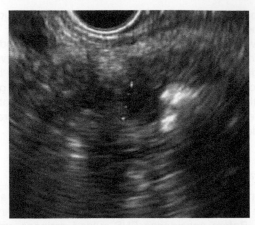

Fig. 1. Endoscopic ultrasound of dilated main pancreatic duct targeted for the drainage.

antegrade passage of the guide wire, it is ideal to orient the echoendoscope parallel to the long axis of the MPD (**Fig. 2**).[26] The tip of the scope is positioned in either the stomach or the duodenal bulb, depending on which position provides the least distance between the gastrointestinal (GI) tract and the MPD, which technique is selected (retrograde or antegrade) (**Fig. 3**) with the fewest vessels between the scope and the pancreatic duct, and the location with maximal scope stability.

Under both fluoroscopic and endosonographic guidance, the MPD is then punctured with either a 19- or 22-gauge FNA needle or the inner needle of a cystoenterostome. The stylet is removed. Pancreatic fluid is then aspirated to confirm location. Contrast is injected, mapping the pancreatic duct. Volume and concentration of contrast injection should be limited in an attempt to reduce the risk of inadvertent parenchyma or vascular injection and to help maintain visualization of targeted areas.[19]

A guide wire is advanced through the FNA needle into the pancreatic duct (**Figs. 4 and 5**). The needle is then removed, leaving the guide wire in place. If the goal is

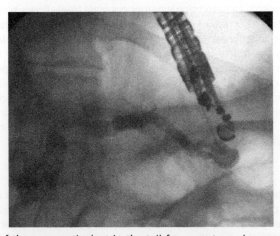

Fig. 2. Puncture of the pancreatic duct in the tail for an antegrade approach.

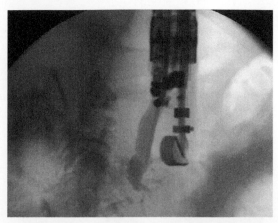

Fig. 3. Puncture of the pancreatic duct above an anastomotic stricture for a retrograde approach.

rendezvous access via a luminal endoscopic route and the wire can be passed through the stricture or anastomosis into the bowel lumen, no further tract dilation is necessary. If transenteric stent placement is planned, a bougie dilator (SBDC-7 or -6, Wilson Cook), a 4- or 6-mm balloon dilator (Boston Scientific) (**Figs. 6** and **7**), or administration of electrocautery using a diathermic sheath is used to enlarge the newly created fistula.[16,17,22,28]

Selection of Access Site (Choice of Approach)

Pancreaticogastrostomy is most frequently described in the current literature, likely attributable to accessibility to the pancreatic duct from the stomach, even in patients with surgically altered anatomy. Pancreaticoduodenostomy is a more recently described technique used by Tessier and colleagues,[16] who prefer the transbulbar and retrograde approach because the "long" scope position allows a better view of the MPD and better stability during the procedure, and facilitates stent placement.

Selection of Drainage Route

Transpapillary pancreatic drainage (rendezvous and antegrade)

The preference is always to advance the guide wire in an antegrade fashion into the duodenum or the jejunum, whenever possible, in patients with surgically altered

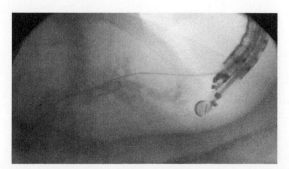

Fig. 4. Advancement of the guide wire in an antegrade fashion in the main pancreatic duct.

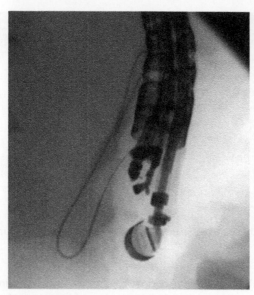

Fig. 5. Advancement of the guide wire in a retrograde fashion in the main pancreatic duct.

anatomy.[28] A rendezvous procedure is possible when the endoscope can be advanced to the papillary orifice or the surgical anastomosis for retrieval of the guide wire looped into the small bowel.[26,28,41]

ERP can then be performed using a standard duodenoscope. In patients with surgically altered anatomy, ERP is performed with a pediatric colonoscope or an enteroscope.[42] Cannulation of the pancreatic duct can be achieved alongside the guide wire or by retrieving the guide wire into the working channel of the endoscope for subsequent therapeutic intervention.[28] The wire is grasped with a snare or a biopsy forceps and is withdrawn into the working channel for retrograde introduction of a sphincterotome over the wire.[18] Subsequently, conventional transpapillary drainage can be performed.

Antegrade or retrograde drainage
If rendezvous ERCP is not possible, 2 options exist: (1) stent placement across the papilla or anastomosis for "downstream" drainage, or (2) stent placement above the

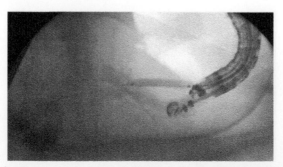

Fig. 6. Dilation of the fistula created before placement of the transgastric stent (antegrade).

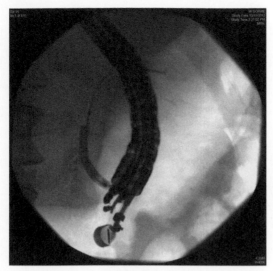

Fig. 7. Dilation of the fistula created before placement of the transgastric stent (retrograde).

stricture and across the puncture tract for "upstream" drainage. Downstream drainage is typically preferred, though not always possible (**Figs. 8–10**).[43]

Transmural drainage (pancreaticogastrostomy and pancreaticoduodenostomy)
Once pancreatic duct access has been obtained and a guide wire is coiled within the duct, the newly created fistula is dilated with bougie or balloon catheters. Typically 7F

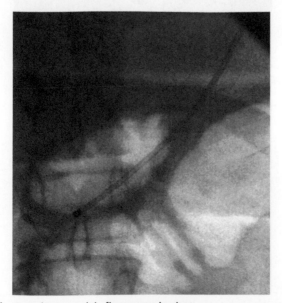

Fig. 8. Transgastric stent (antegrade), fluoroscopic view.

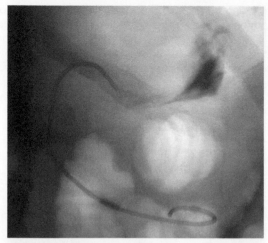

Fig. 9. Transgastric stent (retrograde), fluoroscopic view.

plastic stents with or without pigtails are then advanced across the fistula. The stents should be long, with flanges or pigtails, to avoid intrapancreatic migration.[44]

EVOLUTION AND EXPERIENCE WITH EUS-GUIDED DRAINAGE TECHNIQUES

The goal of EUS-guided pancreatic access is to puncture in a plane parallel to the long axis of the duct with the needle tip directed to toward the point of obstruction. This

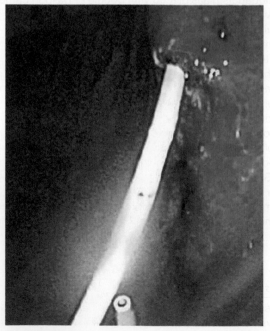

Fig. 10. Transgastic stent, endoscopic view.

approach limits buckling of the guide wire and allows a greater force to be exerted against the obstruction with the guide wire.[42] Often, the guide wire may be inadvertently advanced into a ductal side branch if the endoscope is nearly perpendicular to the desired duct. By changing the needle angle of entry or by using a different wire such as a glide wire or angle-tipped wire, access to the desired areas is typically attained.[19] The risk of wire shearing, which occurs when retracting the wire back into the needle at an acute angle, can be minimized by avoiding the acute angle while advancing the needle, or by using a smaller-caliber guide wire such as 0.025-in (0.635 mm) or 0.021-in (0.533 mm). When resistance is felt, the wire and the needle can be withdrawn simultaneously.[19] Ultimately, if antegrade guide-wire placement fails after EUS-guided pancreatography and a transenteric fistula has been created, transgastric stenting should be performed to decompress the pancreatic duct, thus reducing the risk of a leak.[18,22,42]

There can also be difficulty in passing a catheter or balloon across the gastric or duodenal wall, anastomosis, or other area of obstruction. Initial dilatation with the needle sheath can aid passage.[19] A needle-knife can be used to facilitate stent insertion if an inadequate fistula has been formed.

FOLLOW-UP

Patients are routinely hospitalized for observation and continued intravenous fluids and antibiotics following the procedure. Patients are given nothing by mouth for at least 24 to 48 hours to allow adequate healing of the puncture site. Pain medications and antiemetics are given as needed.

Follow-up recommendations are variable, and no standard of care has been established as yet. Typically, cross-sectional imaging is repeated within a month of the procedure and every 6 months thereafter. Secretin-enhanced magnetic resonance imaging/cholangiopancreatography is helpful in demonstrating a decompressed pancreatic duct with contrast emptying into the small bowel or transmurally, suggesting a patent fistula.[17]

Endoscopic treatment is repeated if necessary. Stent revisions are performed approximately 2 to 3 months after the index procedure. In the interim, if stent dysfunction occurs, exchange can be performed if the patient is symptomatic or the MPD is dilated on imaging studies.[16,25,44] A high rate of stent obstruction may be due to the smaller caliber of the drainage stents used. A high migration rate may be related to the limited intraductal length of the stents and the intragastric location, which may be subject to strong expulsive contractions.[16,44] Serial dilatations and repeated stent exchanges are often required until stents can be removed.[42]

There are reports of patients with the subsequent presentation with pancreatic cancer after EUS-guided drainage of the pancreatic duct.[22,44] Patients with chronic pancreatitis with a tight duct stricture that may require drainage are at high risk of cancer development. Therefore detailed multidisciplinary evaluation should be performed before the procedure, and close surveillance during the follow-up period is paramount.[22,44]

DISCUSSION
Technical Success and Outcomes

Technical success of EUS-guided pancreatic drainage is described in the literature as 25% to 100%, with complications developing in 15% to 50% of patients (**Table 1**).[45] Clinical success is probably lower, with series suggesting pain relief in only 50% to

Table 1
Results from published series on pancreatic drainage by EUS-guided pancreatography

Authors,[Ref.] Year	Patients (n)	Technical Success		Ductography	Drainage				Complications		Follow-Up Interventions
					Transpapillary		Transmural				
		n	%		RV	Non-RV	PGS	PDS	n	%	
Harada et al,[40] 1995	1	1	100	1	—	—	—	—	0	0	
Gress et al,[48] 1996	1	1	100	1	—	—	—	—	0	0	
Francois et al,[17] 2002	4	4	100	—	—	—	4	—	0	0	1 endoscopy
Bataille and Deprez,[49] 2002	1	1	100	—	1	—	—	—	0	0	
Mallery et al,[42] 2004	4	1	25	—	4	—	—	—	1 fever	25	1 endoscopy 1 surgery
Tessier et al,[16] 2007	36	33	92	—	—	—	26	7	1 hematoma 1 severe pancreatitis with pseudocyst 3 other	13	20 endoscopy 3 surgery
Kahaleh et al,[22] 2007	13	10	77	—	—	—	10	—	1 bleeding 1 perforation	15	8 endoscopy
Papachristou et al,[50] 2007	2	2	100	—	—	—	—	—	0	0	
Will et al,[25] 2007	13	9	69	—	4	—	5	—	4 pain 1 bleeding 1 perforation 1 pseudocyst	54	3 endoscopy 4 surgery

Study								
Keenan et al,[20] 2007	1	1	100	—	—	1	0	—	0
Saftiou et al,[51] 2007	1	1	100	—	—	1	0	—	0
Das et al,[47] 2010	1	1	100	—	—	1	100	1 peripancreatic fluid collection	1 endoscopy
Kinney et al,[21] 2009	9	4	44	—	—	9	11	1 fever	—
Brauer et al,[18] 2009	8	7	87	3	—	3	0	—	1 surgery
Barkay et al,[46] 2010	21	10	48	—	6	4	10	2	—
Ergun et al,[44] 2011	20	18	90	16	—	5	10	1 bleeding 1 perigastric collection	9 endoscopy
Shah et al,[43] 2012	25	19	88	8	—	14	16	1 pneumoperitoneum 2 mild pancreatitis 1 severe pancreatitis	3 surgery 2 endoscopy
Mori et al,[52] 2012	1	1	100	—	—	1	0	—	None
Vila et al,[45] 2012	19	—	—	5	—	14	—	1 pseudocyst	—

Abbreviations: PDS, pancreaticoduodenostomy; PGS, pancreaticogastrostomy; RV, rendezvous.

70% of patients.[16,26,28] Approximately 20% to 25% of patients develop recurrence of symptoms after endoscopic therapy, requiring multiple interventions or surgery.[26]

Ductography is typically successful. The key to successful EUS-guided pancreatic drainage with the rendezvous technique is the passage of the guide wire through the stenotic anastomosis or the papilla. Two major reasons for failure of passage of the guide wire include a tight stricture, and a suboptimal angle of the tip of the guide wire toward the pancreatic tail rather than the small bowel.[46] Technical failures with stenting may be due to difficulty in orienting the echoendoscope along the axis of the MPD, particularly if it has not been dilated, or to an inability to dilate the transmural tract because of fibrosis.[26]

Complications

Complications include bleeding, fever, perforation, hematoma requiring endoscopic drainage, and pancreatitis with pseudocyst formation requiring endoscopic drainage.[16,22,42,47] Complications are typically higher for pancreaticogastrostomy than for simple rendezvous, and are summarized in **Table 1**.

Role in Clinical Practice: Physician Experience and Training

The endoscopist performing EUS-guided pancreatic drainage must have a broad skill set with extensive dedicated training in both EUS and ERCP. In advanced endoscopy training programs, fellows are typically introduced to techniques during the first half of the year and obtain more hands-on experience in the second half of the year. Because of the delayed exposure and procedure complexity with a limited number of procedures, most trainees will not have sufficient experience to independently perform these techniques.[19] It is recommended to first develop skills in EUS-guided procedures such as celiac plexus block and pseudocyst drainage. As the field continues to evolve there is as yet no standardization for credentialing this procedure, although some experts suggest that at least 10 to 20 cases are necessary to become proficient.

Future Considerations

As a result of the complexity of these procedures, new techniques and equipment are needed. Most technical failures are related to unsuccessful manipulation of the guide wire, whereas most of the complications are related to the management of the transmural fistula. To improve technical success and limit complications, adequate devices facilitating access and drainage are required.[19,28,45]

There are limited data regarding technical details, safety, outcomes, and skills required to perform the procedures.[45] A dedicated prospective registry is therefore needed to capture these data. The creation of an international consortium on EUS-guided procedures during Digestive Disease Week in Chicago in 2011 was a first step toward this crucial aim. Finally, standardization of billing for these procedures is necessary to compensate for the complicated nature of this technique and the long procedural time.

SUMMARY

EUS-guided pancreatic drainage is an evolving procedure that can be offered to those patients who are high-risk surgical candidates and in whom the pancreatic duct cannot be accessed at ERP.[26] This procedure is a minimally invasive alternative option to surgery and interventional radiology. However, because of its complexity and its potential for fulminant complications, it is recommended that these procedures are only performed by highly skilled endoscopists. Additional data are needed to define risks and long-term outcomes more accurately via a dedicated prospective registry.

REFERENCES

1. Fink AS, Perez de Ayala V, Chapman M, et al. Radiologic pitfalls in endoscopic retrograde pancreatography. Pancreas 1986;1(2):180–7.
2. Cahen DL, Gouma DJ, Nio Y, et al. Endoscopic versus surgical drainage of the pancreatic duct in chronic pancreatitis. N Engl J Med 2007;356(7):676–84.
3. Schnelldorfer T, Adams DB. Outcome after lateral pancreaticojejunostomy in patients with chronic pancreatitis associated with pancreas divisum. Am Surg 2003;69(12):1041–4 [discussion: 1045–6].
4. Byrne RL, Gompertz RH, Venables CW. Surgery for chronic pancreatitis: a review of 12 years experience. Ann R Coll Surg Engl 1997;79(6):405–9.
5. Kalady MF, Broome AH, Meyers WC, et al. Immediate and long-term outcomes after lateral pancreaticojejunostomy for chronic pancreatitis. Am Surg 2001; 67(5):478–83.
6. Bradley EL 3rd. Long-term results of pancreatojejunostomy in patients with chronic pancreatitis. Am J Surg 1987;153(2):207–13.
7. Thuluvath PJ, Imperio D, Nair S, et al. Chronic pancreatitis. Long-term pain relief with or without surgery, cancer risk, and mortality. J Clin Gastroenterol 2003; 36(2):159–65.
8. Bradley EL 3rd. A fifteen year experience with open drainage for infected pancreatic necrosis. Surg Gynecol Obstet 1993;177(3):215–22.
9. Ebbehoj N, Borly L, Bulow J, et al. Evaluation of pancreatic tissue fluid pressure and pain in chronic pancreatitis. A longitudinal study. Scand J Gastroenterol 1990;25(5):462–6.
10. Wilder-Smith CH, Hill L, Osler W, et al. Effect of tramadol and morphine on pain and gastrointestinal motor function in patients with chronic pancreatitis. Dig Dis Sci 1999;44(6):1107–16.
11. Gress F, Schmitt C, Sherman S, et al. Endoscopic ultrasound-guided celiac plexus block for managing abdominal pain associated with chronic pancreatitis: a prospective single center experience. Am J Gastroenterol 2001;96(2): 409–16.
12. Cremer M, Deviere J, Delhaye M, et al. Stenting in severe chronic pancreatitis: results of medium-term follow-up in seventy-six patients. Endoscopy 1991;23(3): 171–6.
13. Costamagna G, Bulajic M, Tringali A, et al. Multiple stenting of refractory pancreatic duct strictures in severe chronic pancreatitis: long-term results. Endoscopy 2006;38(3):254–9.
14. Dumonceau JM, Deviere J, Le Moine O, et al. Endoscopic pancreatic drainage in chronic pancreatitis associated with ductal stones: long-term results. Gastrointest Endosc 1996;43(6):547–55.
15. Cremer M, Deviere J, Delhaye M, et al. Non-surgical management of severe chronic pancreatitis. Scand J Gastroenterol Suppl 1990;175:77–84.
16. Tessier G, Bories E, Arvanitakis M, et al. EUS-guided pancreatogastrostomy and pancreatobulbostomy for the treatment of pain in patients with pancreatic ductal dilatation inaccessible for transpapillary endoscopic therapy. Gastrointest Endosc 2007;65(2):233–41.
17. Francois E, Kahaleh M, Giovannini M, et al. EUS-guided pancreaticogastrostomy. Gastrointest Endosc 2002;56(1):128–33.

18. Brauer BC, Chen YK, Fukami N, et al. Single-operator EUS-guided cholangiopancreatography for difficult pancreaticobiliary access (with video). Gastrointest Endosc 2009;70(3):471–9.
19. Levy MJ. EUS-guided drainage of biliary and pancreatic ductal systems. In: Hawes RH, Fockens P, Varadarajulu S, editors. Endosonography: expert consult. 2nd edition. Philadelphia: Elsevier Saunders; 2010. p. 264–74.
20. Keenan J, Mallery JS, Freeman ML. EUS rendezvous for pancreatic stent placement during endoscopic snare ampullectomy. Gastrointest Endosc 2007;66(4): 850–3.
21. Kinney TP, Li R, Gupta K, et al. Therapeutic pancreatic endoscopy after Whipple resection requires rendezvous access. Endoscopy 2009;41:898–901.
22. Kahaleh M, Hernandez AJ, Tokar J, et al. EUS-guided pancreaticogastrostomy: analysis of its efficacy to drain inaccessible pancreatic ducts. Gastrointest Endosc 2007;65(2):224–30.
23. Rosch T, Daniel S, Scholz M, et al. Endoscopic treatment of chronic pancreatitis: a multicenter study of 1000 patients with long-term follow-up. Endoscopy 2002; 34(10):765–71.
24. Delhaye M, Arvanitakis M, Verset G, et al. Long-term clinical outcome after endoscopic pancreatic ductal drainage for patients with painful chronic pancreatitis. Clin Gastroenterol Hepatol 2004;2(12):1096–106.
25. Will U, Fueldner F, Thieme AK, et al. Transgastric pancreatography and EUS-guided drainage of the pancreatic duct. J Hepatobiliary Pancreat Surg 2007; 14(4):377–82.
26. Gines A, Varadarajulu S, Napoleon B. EUS 2008 Working Group document: evaluation of EUS-guided pancreatic-duct drainage (with video). Gastrointest Endosc 2009;69(Suppl 2):S43–8.
27. Makola D, Krenitsky J, Parrish CR. Enteral feeding in acute and chronic pancreatitis. Gastrointest Endosc Clin N Am 2007;17(4):747–64.
28. Varadarajulu S, Trevino JM. Review of EUS-guided pancreatic duct drainage (with video). Gastrointest Endosc 2009;69(Suppl 2):S200–2.
29. Sutherland DE, Radosevich DM, Bellin MD, et al. Total pancreatectomy and islet autotransplantation for chronic pancreatitis. J Am Coll Surg 2012;214: 409–24.
30. Reid-Lombardo KM, Ramos-De la Medina A, Thomsen K, et al. Long-term anastomotic complications after pancreaticoduodenectomy for benign diseases. J Gastrointest Surg 2007;11(12):1704–11.
31. Adams DB, Ford MC, Anderson MC. Outcome after lateral pancreaticojejunostomy for chronic pancreatitis. Ann Surg 1994;219(5):481–7 [discussion: 487–9].
32. Prinz RA, Greenlee HB. Pancreatic duct drainage in 100 patients with chronic pancreatitis. Ann Surg 1981;194(3):313–20.
33. Nealon WH, Thompson JC. Progressive loss of pancreatic function in chronic pancreatitis is delayed by main pancreatic duct decompression. A longitudinal prospective analysis of the modified Puestow procedure. Ann Surg 1993;217(5): 458–66 [discussion: 466–8].
34. Blondet JJ, Carlson AM, Kobayashi T, et al. The role of total pancreatectomy and islet autotransplantation for chronic pancreatitis. Surg Clin North Am 2007;87(6): 1477–501, x.
35. Markowitz JS, Rattner DW, Warshaw AL. Failure of symptomatic relief after pancreaticojejunal decompression for chronic pancreatitis. Strategies for salvage. Arch Surg 1994;129(4):374–9 [discussion: 379–80].

36. Jimenez RE, Fernandez-del Castillo C, Rattner DW, et al. Outcome of pancreaticoduodenectomy with pylorus preservation or with antrectomy in the treatment of chronic pancreatitis. Ann Surg 2000;231(3):293–300.
37. Sakorafas GH, Farnell MB, Farley DR, et al. Long-term results after surgery for chronic pancreatitis. Int J Pancreatol 2000;27(2):131–42.
38. Izbicki JR, Bloechle C, Broering DC, et al. Extended drainage versus resection in surgery for chronic pancreatitis: a prospective randomized trial comparing the longitudinal pancreaticojejunostomy combined with local pancreatic head excision with the pylorus-preserving pancreatoduodenectomy. Ann Surg 1998; 228(6):771–9.
39. Hsu JT, Yeh CN, Hwang TL, et al. Outcome of pancreaticoduodenectomy for chronic pancreatitis. J Formos Med Assoc 2005;104(11):811–5.
40. Harada N, Kouzu T, Arima M, et al. Endoscopic ultrasound-guided pancreatography: a case report. Endoscopy 1995;27(8):612–5.
41. Kikuyama M, Itoi T, Ota Y, et al. Therapeutic endoscopy for stenotic pancreatodigestive tract anastomosis after pancreatoduodenectomy (with videos). Gastrointest Endosc 2011;73(2):376–82.
42. Mallery S, Matlock J, Freeman ML. EUS-guided rendezvous drainage of obstructed biliary and pancreatic ducts: report of 6 cases. Gastrointest Endosc 2004;59(1):100–7.
43. Shah JN, Marson F, Weilert F, et al. Single-operator, single-session EUS-guided anterograde cholangiopancreatography in failed ERCP or inaccessible papilla. Gastrointest Endosc 2012;75(1):56–64.
44. Ergun M, Aouattah T, Gillain C, et al. Endoscopic ultrasound-guided transluminal drainage of pancreatic duct obstruction: long-term outcome. Endoscopy 2011;43(6):518–25.
45. Vila JJ, Perez-Miranda M, Vazquez-Sequeiros E, et al. Initial experience with EUS-guided cholangiopancreatography for biliary and pancreatic duct drainage: a Spanish national survey. Gastrointest Endosc 2012;76(6):1133–41.
46. Barkay O, Sherman S, McHenry L, et al. Therapeutic EUS-assisted endoscopic retrograde pancreatography after failed pancreatic duct cannulation at ERCP. Gastrointest Endosc 2010;71(7):1166–73.
47. Das K, Kitano M, Komaki T, et al. Pancreatic ductal drainage by endoscopic ultrasound-assisted rendezvous technique for pain caused by ductal stricture with chronic pancreatitis. Dig Endosc 2010;22(3):217–9.
48. Gress F, Ikenberry S, Sherman S, et al. Endoscopic ultrasound-directed pancreatography. Gastrointest Endosc 1996;44(6):736–9.
49. Bataille L, Deprez P. A new application for therapeutic EUS: main pancreatic duct drainage with a "pancreatic rendezvous technique". Gastrointest Endosc 2002;55(6):740–3.
50. Papachristou GI, Gleeson FC, Petersen BT, et al. Pancreatic endoscopic ultrasound-assisted rendezvous procedure to facilitate drainage of nondilated pancreatic ducts. Endoscopy 2007;39(suppl 1):E324–5.
51. Saftoiu A, Dumitrescu D, Stoica M, et al. EUS-assisted rendezvous stenting of the pancreatic duct for chronic calcifying pancreatitis with multiple pseudocysts. Pancreatology 2007;7(1):74–9.
52. Mori N, Imazu H, Futagawa Y, et al. EUS-guided rendezvous drainage for pancreatic duct obstruction from stenosis of pancreatojejunal anastomosis after pancreatoduodenostomy. Surg Laparosc Endosc Percutan Tech 2012;22(4): e236–8.

Endoscopic Therapy for Pancreatic Duct Leaks and Disruptions

Shyam Varadarajulu, MD[a],*, Surinder S. Rana, MD, DM[b],
Deepak K. Bhasin, MD, DM[b]

KEYWORDS

- Pseudocyst • Acute pancreatitis • Chronic pancreatitis • Computed tomography
- Stent • Pancreatic sphincterotomy • Endoscopic ultrasound

KEY POINTS

- Pancreatic duct (PD) disruption can lead to pseudocysts, pancreatic ascites/pleural effusion, and external pancreatic fistulas.
- Endoscopic transpapillary drainage is a safe and effective treatment modality for treating PD disruptions.
- The best results following endoscopic transpapillary drainage are obtained if the PD disruption is partial and is bridged by the endoprosthesis.
- Pseudocyst occurring as a consequence of PD disruptions can also be treated with endoscopic transmural drainage, with or without endoscopic ultrasound (EUS) guidance.
- For patients with disconnected pancreatic duct syndrome (DPDS) and an associated peripancreatic fluid collection, placement of permanent indwelling transmural stents is effective for drainage of the upstream gland.
- For patients with DPDS and an external fistula, in the absence of an associated peripancreatic fluid collection, the "outside-in" transluminal puncture technique or EUS-guided PD stent placement may be considered for drainage of the upstream gland.

Pancreatic duct (PD) disruption with leakage of pancreatic juice is a complication resulting from episodes of acute or chronic pancreatitis, pancreatic malignancy, or abdominal trauma, or following abdominal surgery.[1–6] The PD disruption may involve the main PD or one of its side branches. The clinical consequences of PD disruption depend on several factors including the etiology, site and extent of disruption, rate of secretion of pancreatic juice, location of the leak relative to anatomic tissue planes, ability of the systemic inflammatory response in containing the leak, and the presence of downstream obstruction of the PD by strictures/calculi.[1,5] A normal PD with a small leak of pancreatic juice from one of the side branches may resolve spontaneously,

a Center for Interventional Endoscopy, Florida Hospital, 601 East Rollins Street, Orlando, FL 32803, USA; b Department of Gastroenterology, Post Graduate Institute of Medical Education and Research (PGIMER), Sector 12, Chandigarh 160012, India
* Corresponding author.
E-mail address: svaradarajulu@yahoo.com

Gastrointest Endoscopy Clin N Am 23 (2013) 863–892
http://dx.doi.org/10.1016/j.giec.2013.06.008
1052-5157/13/$ – see front matter © 2013 Elsevier Inc. All rights reserved.

whereas a persistent leak from a major main PD disruption may be complicated by pseudocyst formation, internal fistula formation causing ascites or pleural effusion, or external pancreatic fistulas (EPFs).

Following PD disruption, the pancreatic secretions leak from the ductal defect and collect in the peripancreatic area. This pancreatic fluid collection (PFC) evolves and, depending on the path the pancreatic juice takes, leads to formation of a pseudocyst, internal pancreatic fistula (IPF), or EPF.[7] If the pancreatic juice remains confined to the retroperitoneum, mediastinum, or lesser sac, it subsequently becomes enclosed by a well-formed nonepithelialized wall and evolves into a pseudocyst over a 4- to 6-week period. If the pancreatic secretions track into internal spaces like peritoneal or pleural cavities, an IPF is created. An anterior PD rupture leads to leakage of the pancreatic juice into the peritoneal cavity with development of pancreatic ascites, whereas a posterior PD disruption directs the pancreatic juice superiorly into the mediastinum through the aortic or esophageal hiatus and into the pleural cavity, resulting in pleural effusion.[8] The IPFs can occasionally communicate with other spaces such as the pericardium or organs such as bronchus, stomach, and small or large bowel.[7,8] The pancreatic juice can also find its way externally to the skin surface, and an EPF develops as a consequence. This process may occur spontaneously but usually follows a surgical or radiologic intervention of the PFC.[7,9]

PANCREATIC DUCTAL DISRUPTION IN ACUTE NECROTIZING PANCREATITIS

In contrast to other causes of PD disruption, there are limited data on the incidence and consequences of PD disruption in acute necrotizing pancreatitis (ANP). Neoptolemos and colleagues[4] retrospectively evaluated the integrity of the PD in 105 patients with acute pancreatitis using endoscopic retrograde pancreatography (ERP). Patients were divided into 2 groups. In the first group, patients (n = 89) had clinically mild pancreatitis or severe disease (<25% necrosis on contrast-enhanced computed tomography [CECT]) but did not require surgery for local complications. In the second group (n = 16), patients had clinically severe pancreatitis and underwent surgery for local complications and/or had necrosis of 25% or more. There was no PD disruption in the first group, but 7 of 16 (44%) patients in the second group had PD disruption. The investigators concluded that ANP was associated with ductal disruption and that patients with ductal disruption needed surgery more often. In 75 consecutive patients with ANP and suspected biliary etiology who underwent endoscopic retrograde cholangiopancreatography (ERCP) within 7 days of admission, Uomo and colleagues[10] observed that main PD was satisfactorily visualized in 59 of 75 (84.3%) patients, and PD disruption was noted in 18 patients (31%).[10] Most patients with PD disruption (13/18; 72%) were managed nonsurgically. Lau and colleagues[11] retrospectively studied 144 patients (82 males; average age 55 years) with severe pancreatitis for the presence of PD disruption and its impact on the length of hospital stay, mortality, and need for surgery. PD disruption was present in 37% of patients and was significantly associated with necrosis ($P = .0006$), prolonged hospital stay (≥ 20 days; $P = .007$), percutaneous drain placement ($P<.0001$), and a short-term PD stent ($P<.0001$). However, the PD leak was not significantly associated with the mortality or need for surgical necrosectomy.

Despite the limited data, it is important to remember that PD disruption in ANP is different from other causes of PD disruption because it is accompanied by variable degree of pancreatic and peripancreatic necrosis, which has important therapeutic implications. The PFCs occurring in this setting contain both solid and liquid debris and are termed walled-off pancreatic necrosis (WOPN).[12] These collections are different from pseudocysts, which contain only liquid. Moreover, most PD disruptions occurring in the setting of ANP are complete disruptions that lead to disconnected pancreatic duct syndrome (DPDS), an entity discussed later in this review.[13–15]

MANAGEMENT OF PANCREATIC DUCT LEAKS AND DISRUPTIONS

As PD leaks are not common, the current scientific evidence regarding the clinical management of PD leaks and disruptions is limited to case reports and case series. There are no randomized controlled trials that have evaluated the relative efficacy of medical, endoscopic, radiologic, or surgical treatment modalities. The management of PD disruptions involves stabilization of the patient, identification of the PD anatomy, the type of disruption, and definitive management of the PD disruption.[5–9] Careful attention to maintenance of hydration, nutrition, and electrolyte balance through the management of the disease process is of prime importance for successful clinical outcomes.

Diagnosis and Characterization of PD Disruption

The diagnosis and characterization of the PD disruption is a necessary first step for selection of an appropriate management strategy. ERP has been noted to have the highest accuracy in diagnosing PD disruption through visualization of detailed images of the PD as well as the ability to identify precisely the location (head, neck, body, or tail of pancreas) and extent of the disruption.[1,2,16,17] On ERP, PD disruption is defined as extravasation of contrast medium from the ductal system,[1,16] and can be further defined as partial (opacification of the proximal PD upstream to the site of disruption) or complete (no visualization of the PD upstream to the leak).[1,2,16,17] ERP can also provide information about the presence of stricture or calculi in the downstream portion of the duct. However, ERP is invasive, requires expertise, and the rates of cannulation of the PD are operator dependent, with failed cannulation or inadequate pancreatography observed in up to 10% of patients.[18–20] Furthermore, ERP can be associated with serious adverse effects such as postprocedure pancreatitis and the risk of infection of sterile PFCs.[18–20] To overcome these limitations of ERP, there has been an increasing number of attempts to detect and characterize the PD disruption using noninvasive cross-sectional imaging modalities. Recent advances in imaging, such as thin multislice helical CECT and magnetic resonance imaging (MRI), may help in noninvasively detecting PD disruptions.

CECT has been shown to be a useful technique for imaging pancreatic parenchyma and for identification and localization of PFCs. The location of the fluid collections seen on CECT can be suggestive of the site of PD disruption (**Fig. 1**).[8] Newer computed tomography (CT) technology with thinner collimation as well as use of multirow detector CT (MDCT) with postprocessing techniques such as multiplanar reformations has led to improved visualization of the PD.[21] Anderson and Soto[22] used the portal venous phase on a 64-row MDCT scan in 11 patients with pancreatic cystic lesions, and noted that it could correctly identify the ductal communication with the PFC in all 9 patients who had communicating PFC noted on standard of reference examination. O'Toole and colleagues[23] used helical CT in 16 patients with PD disruption and observed accurate delineation of the site of PD disruption in 50% patients, and the accuracy improved to 94% when CT was combined with magnetic resonance cholangiopancreatography (MRCP). MRCP, when used alone as the imaging method of choice, accurately identified the anatomy of PD disruption only in 67% of the patients. Similarly, Wong and colleagues[24] evaluated the clinical utility of multiphasic CT in 9 patients with PD disruption, and found the overall accuracy of multiphasic CT to be 97.9% (in parenchymal phase), 100.0% (in portal venous phase), and 96.8% (in equilibrium

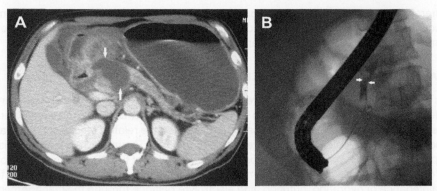

Fig. 1. (A) Contrast-enhanced computed tomography (CECT) showing a fluid collection adjacent to proximal body of pancreas (*arrows*), suggesting possible pancreatic duct (PD) disruption. (B) Endoscopic retrograde pancreatography (ERP) confirming complete PD disruption (*arrows*) at same level.

phase). These studies have demonstrated that MDCT is a promising noninvasive imaging method for the diagnosis of PD disruptions. However, there is a need for multicenter studies with a larger sample size to validate these results and also help develop an optimal CT-based protocol.

MRCP can noninvasively evaluate the pancreatic parenchyma and also delineate the PD morphology. Its usefulness in various benign, malignant, and congenital anomalies of the pancreas with excellent visualization of the PD has been well reported.[18] MRCP has also been shown to be useful for detecting PD disruptions.[25,26] A recent study using MRCP in 31 patients with suspected PD disruptions reported that it could correctly identify intact PD in all 8 (100%) patients and localize the PD disruption in 21 of 23 (91%) patients with ductal disruption.[25] One of the limitations of MRCP is the absence of visualization of ductal filling and extravasation in real time, as seen on ERCP, thus giving rise to the possibility of missed diagnosis of PD injury in nondilated ducts.[27] To overcome this limitation, dynamic secretin-stimulated MRCP was studied in 17 patients with suspected PD disruption.[28] After secretin administration, changes in the duodenal and jejunal fluid content were evaluated as well as the size or signal intensity of PFC recorded. In healthy individuals with no PD disruption, secretin administration increases the duodenal and jejunal fluid content, with less than 1 mm transient increase in PD diameter. Any increase in fluid outside these anatomic regions is suggestive of PD disruption. Dynamic MRCP was able to identify PD disruption in 10 of 17 (59%) patients, and the investigators concluded that this is a safe and noninvasive technique, providing the requisite information about PD integrity and anatomy, thus facilitating appropriate management. An additional advantage of MRCP over ERP is its ability to characterize the PD upstream of the site of complete disruption, an area that is not visualized on ERP (**Fig. 2**).[25] Though helpful in diagnosis, one of the most important limitations of MRCP is the inability to intervene therapeutically at the time of diagnosis.

Definitive Management of PD Disruption

After the PD anatomy and site of PD disruption have been confirmed, a definitive management plan focusing on healing of the ductal disruptions is required. The traditional options for management of PD disruption include conservative medical therapy or surgery.[29,30] The conservative management includes adequate drainage of pancreatic secretions for prevention or control of sepsis, aggressive treatment if the patient

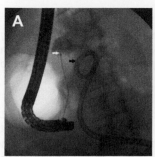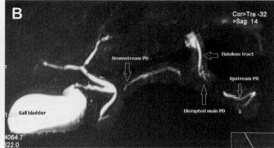

Fig. 2. (*A*) ERP in a patient with an external pancreatic fistula: complete PD disruption with contrast extravasation (*white arrow*). PD upstream to disruption not visualized. Percutaneous catheter is noted (*black arrow*). (*B*) magnetic resonance cholangiopancreatography in the same patient demonstrating upstream PD, disrupted PD, and a fistulous tract from upstream duct.

becomes septic, optimal nutritional support through the recovery process, correction of electrolyte imbalance, and decreased pancreatic exocrine secretions for pancreatic rest with administration of total parenteral nutrition (TPN), jejunal nutrition, or with use of drugs such as anticholinergic agents, carbonic anhydrase inhibitors, glucagon, calcitonin, somatostatin, or octreotide.[7,9] This treatment approach is based on the rationale that reduction of the pancreatic secretion would decrease the flow of the pancreatic juice through the PD disruption and thus expedite its healing. This conservative approach of prolonged pancreatic rest may be sufficient to heal the ductal disruption, but occurs at the cost of prolonged hospitalization with a concomitant increase in the cost of treatment, and an increased risk of hospital-acquired infections. Moreover, the conservative therapy fails in a significant proportion of patients with large disruptions or ductal obstruction downstream of the disruption. The other major alternative is surgical management, which is not without the associated risks of significant morbidity and mortality.[29,30]

The last 2 decades have seen considerable advancement in therapeutic pancreatic endoscopy, and over the years endoscopic drainage has been used, with encouraging results, to treat PD disruptions and the resultant consequences of pancreatic pseudocyst, pancreatic fistulas, and pancreatic ascites/pleural effusion. The various options for endoscopic drainage include[31]:

1. Transmural drainage. This technique involves creating a communication between the pseudocyst and the gastroduodenal lumen (cystogastrostomy or cystoduodenostomy). This internal drainage of pancreatic juice collapses the cavity of the pseudocyst and facilitates resolution of the PD disruption (see later discussion).
2. Transpapillary drainage. This method of drainage involves placement of an endoprosthesis in the PD through the papilla. The transpapillary stent or nasopancreatic drain (NPD) promotes healing of duct disruptions by blockage of the leaking duct by bridging the disruption, and also, by traversing the pancreatic sphincter and thus converting the high-pressure PD system to a low-pressure system with preferential flow of the pancreatic juice through the stent.[32] This route can also be used when there is PD disruption with no associated PFC, as in patients with pancreatic ascites, pleural effusion, and EPF.
3. Endoscopic pancreaticoduodenostomy or pancreaticogastrostomy. This recent approach can be used for reconnecting a completely disconnected PD to the gastrointestinal (GI) tract lumen.

PSEUDOCYSTS

Pseudocysts developing as a consequence of PD disruption may be drained through the transpapillary or transmural route, or a combination of the 2 routes.[1,33–67] The endoscopic management of WOPN involves more aggressive endoscopic therapy and is not discussed in this review.

Transmural Drainage

The transmural drainage of pseudocysts is achieved by placing 1 or more stents through the endoscopically created communication between the pseudocyst and the gastroduodenal lumen. The technical details of the procedure are not discussed here, but in brief it involves the following steps: site localization, cyst puncture, guide-wire insertion, tract dilation, and placement of stents. These steps can be done with or without endoscopic ultrasound (EUS) guidance.[40,41] EUS offers the advantage of excellent visualization of pancreas and peripancreatic areas, and provides real-time guidance to advance the needle safely into the pseudocyst cavity without inadvertent puncture of any intervening blood vessels (**Fig. 3**). Therefore, EUS-guided drainage should be considered in patients with nonbulging fluid collections, patients at high risk of bleeding complications, prior failed transmural attempt

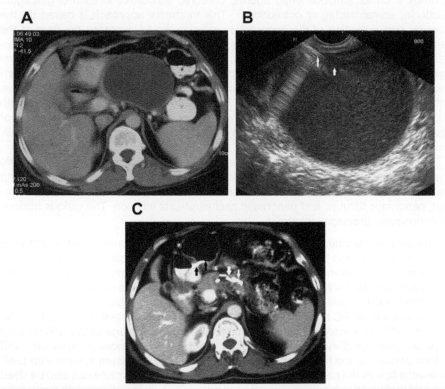

Fig. 3. (A) CECT: pseudocyst of pancreas. (B) Endoscopic ultrasound (EUS)-guided drainage using a 19-gauge needle for puncture (arrows). (C) Computed tomography (CT) demonstrating resolution of pseudocyst. Transmural stents were left indefinitely (gastric end shown by black arrows and the cyst end by white arrows), as ERP had demonstrated complete disruption of PD.

without EUS guidance, and collections inaccessible by standard endoscopic techniques (eg, pseudocysts located at the tail end of the pancreas).[39–41] Observational case studies have demonstrated that transmural drainage of pancreatic pseudocysts is safe and effective (**Table 1**). A nonrandomized, retrospective, matched case-controlled study by Varadarajulu and colleagues[44] compared patients undergoing surgical (n = 10) versus EUS-guided transmural cystogastrostomy (n = 20). There were no significant differences in the rates of treatment success (100% vs 95%, $P = .36$), procedural complications (none in either cohort), or need for reinterventions (10% vs 0%, $P = .13$) between the surgery and EUS-guided cystogastrostomy groups. However, the mean length of postprocedure hospital stay was significantly shorter in the EUS group (2.65 vs 6.5 days, $P = .008$), as was the average direct cost per case ($9077 vs $14,815, $P = .01$).

Transmural drainage causes internal diversion of the pancreatic juice leading to the collapse of the pseudocyst cavity, and it is presumed that this will cause healing of the PD disruption. However, there is a paucity of studies that have directly looked at PD disruption and its healing following endoscopic transmural drainage. Satisfactory clinical outcomes in the majority of patients would be suggestive of resolution of PD disruption, or alternatively might reflect persistent patency of the transmural tract that is preventing recurrence of the PFC.[45] In a randomized controlled study, Arvanitakis and colleagues[46] compared the clinical outcomes of leaving transmural stents in place indefinitely following drainage with removal of stents after resolution of the PFC. Five of 13 patients in the stent-retrieval group had recurrence of the same PFC, whereas in the group with indwelling stents there was no recurrence noted in any patients. Most patients with recurrence had PD disruption, suggesting that following transmural drainage the PD disruption may not heal. The investigators suggested that long-term transmural stent placement should be considered in patients with complete PD disruption or a communicating PFC in the setting of chronic pancreatitis.

Cahen and colleagues[47] evaluated the role of endoscopic therapy in 92 patients with pseudocysts, and on multivariate analyses showed that leaving stents for longer than 6 weeks was associated with a more favorable outcome ($P = .01$). An alternative to long-term indwelling transmural stents would be the combined use of transpapillary and transmural drainage. With this technique, the transpapillary stent assists in the continued healing of the ductal disruption and further lowers the risk of PFC recurrence after removal of the stents.[45] However, data on the role of combined drainage are limited and inconsistent. Hookey and colleagues[34] performed endoscopic drainage of PFC in 116 patients and documented no significant difference in the success rates between patients who underwent transmural drainage alone (90%) in comparison with those who had combined transmural and transpapillary drainage (82.9%). On the contrary, there was a trend toward higher recurrence rates in patients with combined drainage than in those who underwent transmural stenting alone (26.8% vs 8.3%, $P = .015$). The investigators hypothesized that transmural drainage may allow the cystenterostomy fistula to remain patent for a longer time, even in the event of stent blockage, and that the addition of transpapillary drainage may hinder this process.

In a retrospective study of PFC drainage, Trevino and colleagues[48] reported that treatment was significantly more successful in patients who underwent combined drainage than in those who underwent transmural drainage alone (97.5% vs 80%; crude risk ratio [RR] = 1.22; 95% confidence interval [CI]: 1.06–1.26; $P = .01$); the significance of these findings was demonstrated on multivariable analysis (adjusted RR = 1.14; 95% CI: 1.01–1.29; $P = .036$), even after adjusting for cause of pancreatitis, type and location of PFC, luminal compression at endoscopy, enteral nutrition, white blood cell count, and number of endoscopic interventions.

Table 1
Selected studies on endoscopic transmural drainage alone of pancreatic pseudocysts (studies in which results of endoscopic transmural drainage alone are given separately)

Authors,[Ref.] Year	No. of Patients	EUS Guidance	Success	Complications of Procedure	Recurrence
Kozarek et al,[50] 1985	4	No	2/4 (50%)	Infection: 1 Bleeding: 1	Nil
Cremer et al,[54] 1989	33	No	Technical: 32/33 (97%) Clinical: 26/32 (82%)	Bleeding: 1 Infection: 1	4/32 (12%)
Smits et al,[55] 1995	17	No	10/17 (59%)	Bleeding: 2 Perforation: 2 Apnea: 1	—[a]
Binmoeller et al,[52] 1995	24	No	Technical: 20/24 (83%) Clinical: 19/20 (95%)	Bleeding: 2 Gallbladder perforation: 1	6/19 (32%)
Sharma et al,[56] 2002	33	No	33/33 (100%)	Bleeding: 1 Infection: 3 (stent block) Perforation: 1	—[a]
Sanchez Cortes et al,[60] 2002	33 patients 34 attempts	Yes	Technical: 32/33 (97%) Clinical: 31/32 (97%)	Bleeding: 2 Pneumoperito- neum: 1	1/32 (3%)
Cahen et al,[47] 2005	54	No	36/54 (67%)	39%	—[a]
Krüger et al,[53] 2006	35	Yes	Technical: 33/35 (94%) Clinical: 29/33 (88%)	None	4/29 (14%)
Antillon et al,[58] 2006	33	Yes	Technical: 31/33 (94%) Clinical: 27/31 (87%)	Perforation: 1 Bleeding: 1	1/27 (4%)
Barthet et al,[51] 2008	41	Yes	Technical: 40/41 (98%) Clinical: 36/40 (90%)	Bleeding: 3 Infection: 6	—[a]
Lopes et al,[57] 2008	31	Yes	Technical: 31/31 (100%) Clinical: 29/31 (94%)	Pneumoperito- neum: 1 Peritonitis: 1	6/29 (21%)
Penn et al,[59] 2012	20 (used covered SEMS)	Yes	Technical: 20/20 (100%) Clinical: 17/20 (85%)	Infection: 2	3/17 (18%)
Shrode et al,[49] 2012	36	Not mentioned	27 (75%)	—[a]	—[a]

Abbreviation: SEMS, self-expanding metal stents.
[a] Separate figures for transmural drainage alone not provided.

Recently, Shrode and colleagues[49] presented the results of a retrospective analysis of combined drainage in 113 patients with 114 PD disruptions and PFCs (acute pancreatitis in 58 cases and chronic pancreatitis in 56). In patients with partial PD disruptions, combined drainage was associated with increased rate of resolution (80%) compared with complete disruptions treated in a similar manner (57%).

These conflicting results preclude any definite recommendations and consensus statement on the use of combined drainage for pseudocysts. Based on available evidence, it seems clinically reasonable to attempt to bridge the partial PD disruption while treating patients with PFCs by transmural drainage, particularly patients with underlying chronic pancreatitis and known ductal abnormalities.

Transpapillary Drainage

Transpapillary drainage involves insertion of an endoprosthesis through the major or minor papilla into the PD (**Fig. 4**), creating a path of lesser resistance that directs drainage of the pancreatic secretions through the papillary orifice into the duodenum rather than through the PD disruption. The sphincter of Oddi and any ductal strictures/calculi in the downstream duct are the sites of resistance impeding the flow of pancreatic juices into the duodenum. These obstacles can be removed by pancreatic sphincterotomy, stricture dilation, stone removal, and/or stent/NPD insertion. Of note, this route of drainage is effective only if the PFCs are in communication with the PD.

Several observational case studies have demonstrated that transpapillary drainage is safe and effective in patients with communicating pancreatic pseudocysts (**Table 2**).

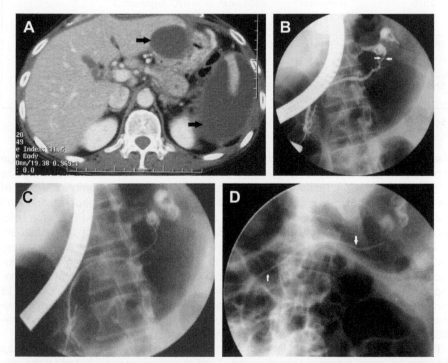

Fig. 4. (*A*) Patient with chronic pancreatitis, and perihepatic and perisplenic pseudocysts (*arrows*). (*B*) ERP: mildly dilated main PD, irregular side branches, and disruption at terminal part of tail end (*arrows*). (*C*) ERP: guide wire negotiated into disruption. (*D*) 5F 15-cm stent placed into disruption (*arrows*).

Table 2
Selected studies on endoscopic transpapillary drainage alone of pancreatic pseudocysts (studies in which results of endoscopic transpapillary drainage alone are given separately)

Authors,[Ref.] Year	No. of Patients	Success	Complication	Recurrence
Kozarek et al,[3] 1991	14	12/14 (86%)	Acute pancreatitis: 1 Stent occlusion: 3 Infection: 2	—[a]
Catalano et al,[62] 1995	21	17/21 (81%)	Acute pancreatitis: 1	—[a]
Binmoeller et al,[52] 1995	33	31/33 (94%)	Acute pancreatitis: 1	5/31 (16%)
Telford et al,[16] 2002	43	25/43 (48%)	Pain abdomen: 1 Acute pancreatitis: 1 Infection: 2	—[a]
Varadarajulu et al,[1] 2005	97	52/97 (55%)	Acute pancreatitis: 1 Stent occlusion: 3 Infection: 1	—[a]
Bhasin et al,[35] 2006	11 (multiple and large pseudocysts)	9/11 (82%)	Infection: 1	None
Barthet et al,[51] 2008	8	8/8 (100%)	None	—[a]
Bhasin et al,[36] 2010	11 (pseudocysts at atypical locations)	11 (100%) additional percutaneous drain 1	NPD block: 1 NPD displaced: 1 Infection: 1	None
Shrode et al,[49] 2012	36	27/31 (75%)	Stent migration: 8 Perforation of side branch by guide wire: 2	—[a]
Bhasin et al,[63] 2012	12 (mediastinal pdeudocysts)	11/11 (100%)	None	None

[a] Separate figures for transpapillary drainage alone not provided.

This route of drainage is physiologic, as it uses the normal anatomic route of drainage of pancreatic juice and does not involve creation of an alternative route of drainage as in transmural drainage. However, the diameter of the PD limits the number and size of the endoprosthesis that can be placed for drainage. Therefore, transpapillary drainage alone is not advisable in patients with large pseudocysts (>6 cm) or PFCs with solid debris, because of the high risk of secondary infection consequent to inadequate drainage.[33,61] However, using NPD, Bhasin and colleagues[35,36] have shown that transpapillary drainage is safe and effective in patients with multiple and large pseudocysts as well as those at distant and atypical locations. The advantage of the transpapillary approach over the transmural drainage is the reduced risk of bleeding or perforation associated with transmural drainage. However, transpapillary drainage raises the risk of infection and stent-induced ductal changes mimicking chronic pancreatitis, especially in patients with acute pancreatitis and normal PD.[33,61,64,65]

There have been attempts to identify the factors that can predict successful outcome following transpapillary drainage. Telford and colleagues[16] studied the efficacy of transpapillary drainage in 43 patients (23 females) with PD disruption of varying etiology. The PD disruption resolved in 25 (58%) patients. The clinical characteristics associated with failure of stent treatment included female gender ($P = .05$), patients with acute pancreatitis ($P = .05$), shorter duration of stenting ($P = .002$) and stent not bridging the disruption ($P = .04$). On logistic regression analysis, only the placement of a bridging stent was associated with a successful outcome. Varadarajulu and colleagues[1] also investigated the role of endoscopic transpapillary drainage with stent placement in 97 patients (63 men) with PD disruption, and reported success in 52 (55%) patients. The factors associated with successful outcome on univariate analysis were partially disrupted PD ($P<.001$), disruption in the body of pancreas ($P = .04$), a bridging stent ($P<.001$), and a longer duration of stent therapy ($P = .03$). However, on multivariate logistic regression analysis, the presence of partial PD disruption and presence of a stent bridging the disruption correlated with successful outcomes. The other case series on patients with multiple pseudocysts as well as pseudocysts at atypical locations have shown that the best results with transpapillary drainage are obtained in the presence of partial PD disruption that can be bridged.[2,35–37]

The current evidence suggests that transpapillary drainage alone is safe and effective for patients with communicating small pseudocysts (<6 cm), and has best results if the PD disruption is partial and is bridged by the endoprosthesis.[42,61] The optimal duration of stent therapy is not clear, as shorter duration is associated with a lack of resolution of PD disruption and, thus, increased risk of recurrences, whereas longer duration of stenting is associated with stent occlusions and stent-induced ductal changes.[1,16,64,65] In the majority of the case series, the stents have been left in place for 4 to 6 weeks and it has been observed that even with this small duration, noticeable ductal changes appear in patients with acute pancreatitis who otherwise have a normal PD in absence of the disruption. Biodegradable stents or recently designed stents that cause less ductal damage may have an increasing role in these clinical situations.[66,67]

PANCREATIC ASCITES AND PLEURAL EFFUSIONS

Pancreatic ascites and pleural effusions occur because of IPFs, which in most patients are secondary to leakage or rupture of a pancreatic pseudocyst that is in turn communicating with a PD disruption. In up to 10% of patients, a fistulous tract may communicate directly with ductal disruption in the absence of a pseudocyst.[69,70] Traditionally these patients have been treated with prolonged conservative medical therapy or surgery.[68–70] The prolonged conservative therapy involving fasting, parenteral nutrition, somatostatin or its analogues, and repeated large-volume paracentesis can lead to resolution of ascites in up to 50% patients.[68,71] Conservative therapy usually fails in patients with severe ductal abnormalities such as strictures or multiple large disruptions, and these patients have been traditionally treated with salvage surgical procedures such as pancreatic resection, cystogastrostomy, or cystojejunostomy that are associated with significant rates of morbidity, mortality, and recurrence.[68,71,72] An alternative and effective treatment plan for pancreatic ascites and pleural effusion is endoscopic transpapillary stent or NPD placement (**Fig. 5**).[68,70–79] As mentioned earlier, by facilitating transpapillary drainage of pancreatic juices, this approach promotes the healing of ductal disruption and its sequelae.

Experience with transpapillary drainage for pancreatic ascites and effusions is limited to case reports and series. Such observational studies have reported the safety and efficacy of transpapillary drainage in patients with PD disruptions manifesting as ascites and effusions (**Table 3**).[68,70–76] Initially, Kozarek and colleagues[73] studied the efficacy of transpapillary stent placement in 4 patients with chronic pancreatitis and pancreatic ascites who had failed prolonged conservative treatment.[73] The ascites resolved in all 4 patients following stent placement. However,

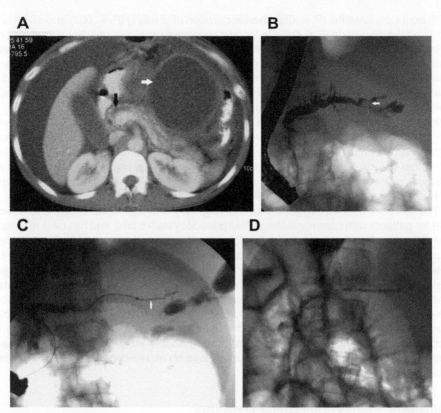

Fig. 5. (*A*) CT: patient with chronic pancreatitis showing dilated main PD (*black arrow*), pseudocyst (*white arrow*), and pancreatic ascites. (*B*) ERP: dilated main PD and side branches. Partial disruption at tail end (*arrow*). (*C*) Guide wire negotiated across disruption (*arrow*). (*D*) 5F 12-cm stent placed across disruption.

ultrasound-guided large-volume paracentesis was done in all patients following stent placement, and 2 of the 4 patients also needed a percutaneous drain. Stent-induced ductal changes were observed in 2 patients. Bracher and colleagues[71] treated 8 patients with pancreatic ascites (6 patients with chronic pancreatitis) with placement of a stent in PD as the initial drainage procedure. There was complete resolution of the ascites within 6 weeks of placement of the stent in 7 of 8 (88%) patients, none of whom needed additional medical, radiologic, or surgical intervention at a mean follow-up period of 14 months. No complications of the procedure were reported. Telford and colleagues[16] also recorded successful resolution of pancreatic ascites in 6 of 7 patients (86%) after endoscopic PD stent placement with a median duration to resolution of 6 weeks.

Bhasin and colleagues[68] described the usefulness of endoscopic transpapillary NPD placement in 10 patients (8 men) with pancreatic ascites and effusion. Of these 10 patients, 4 had only ascites, 4 had pleural effusion alone, and 2 had both ascites and pleural effusion. Following placement of NPD, the ascites and/or pleural effusion resolved in all patients within 4 weeks. All patients had partial PD disruption, and the NPD bridged the disruption in 8 of the 10 (80%) patients. Healing of ductal disruption was demonstrated on nasopancreatogram as early as 2 weeks, and no major complications of the procedure were noted. Pai and colleagues[74] documented the efficacy of

Table 3
Selected studies on endoscopic transpapillary drainage for pancreatic ascites and effusion (studies in which results of endoscopic drainage in patients with pancreatic ascites/effusion are given separately)

Authors,[Ref.] Year	No. of Patients	Success	Complication	Recurrence
Kozarek et al,[73] 1994	4	4/4 (100%) Percutaneous drain in 2	Stent-induced ductal changes: 2	None
Bracher et al,[71] 1999	8	Technical: 8/8 (100%) Clinical: 8/8 (100%) metal stent in 1 patient	None	None
Chebli et al,[72] 2004	11 (4 treated endoscopically)	4/4 (100%)	None	None
Varadarajulu et al,[1] 2005	20	Separate figures for ascites only not given	Separate figures for ascites/ effusion only not given	Separate figures for ascites only not given
Halttunen et al,[80] 2005	25	23/25 (2%)	Separate figures for ascites/effusion only not given	None
Bhasin et al,[68] 2006	10	10/10 (100%)	NPD block: 1 Infection: 1	None
Pai et al,[74] 2009	28	Technical: 27/28 (96%) Clinical: 26/27 (96%)	Severe pain: 2 Fever: 5	None
Kurumboor et al,[75] 2009	11	Technical: 9/11 (82%) Clinical: 5/9 (55%)	Infection: 3	None; recurrent pain in 2
Shrode et al,[49] 2012	3	Separate figures for ascites only not given	Separate figures for ascites/ effusion only not given	Separate figures for ascites only not given

transpapillary stent placement in 28 patients (22 men) with pancreatic ascites and effusion. Of these 28 patients, ascites alone was seen in 15, pleural effusion alone in 6, and both ascites and pleural effusion in 7. Following endoscopic therapy, which consisted of pancreatic sphincterotomy and stent placement, there was complete resolution of ascites and effusion in 26 (92.9%) patients over a period of 3 to 8 (median 5) weeks. Complications included severe abdominal pain caused by worsening pancreatitis (2) and infection (5). Kurumboor and colleagues[75] succeeded in placing transpapillary stent in 9 of 11 cases of pancreatic ascites. Disruption was bridged in 5 cases and ascites healed in all of these. Varadarajulu and colleagues[1] reported endoscopic transpapillary drainage with stent in 20 patients with pancreatic ascites, and reported that the best results with transpapillary drainage are obtained in the presence of partial PD disruption that can be bridged.

EXTERNAL PANCREATIC FISTULAS

As mentioned previously, most cases of EPF occur secondary to iatrogenic (radiologic or surgical) intervention of the PFCs. EPFs have the potential of functioning as high-output fistulas because of the lack of negative feedback control of exocrine pancreatic secretion and, thus, can result in severe electrolyte and nutritional disturbances.[81,82] Established options for management of EPF, as with other consequences of PD disruptions, include conservative medical therapy or surgery.[81,82] The limitations of these therapies have been mentioned previously. Endoscopic transpapillary drainage can also cause closure of EPF by decreasing the intraductal pressure and thus eliminating the transpapillary gradient (**Fig. 6, Table 4**). Before planning endoscopic therapy, complete assessment should be done for the site and type of PD disruption, anatomy of the PD, especially the duct downstream of the disruption, and presence or absence of associated PFCs. An additional investigation that demonstrates the relationship of EPF with PD and is clinically useful, and frequently overlooked, is a fistulogram,[8] which can provide important information and clearly delineate the fistulous tract.

Kozarek and colleagues[83] investigated the role of endoscopic transpapillary PD stent placement in 9 patients with EPF that occurred as a consequence of percutaneous pseudocyst drainage in 4 patients, pancreatic necrosis in 2, complications of pancreatic surgery in 2, and following a perforation of the duct of Santorini at the

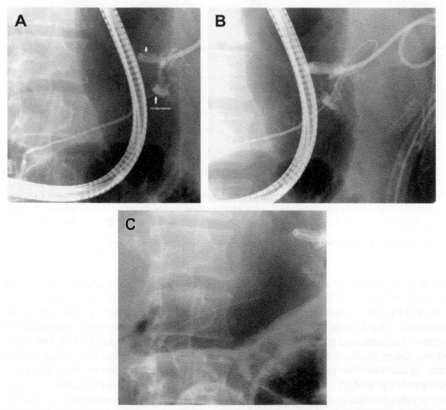

Fig. 6. (*A*) Patient with EPF. Percutaneous catheter noted (*arrow*). PD disruption at tail end with contrast extravasating toward the catheter. (*B*) Guide wire negotiated across disruption. (*C*) 5F stent placed just across PD disruption.

Table 4
Selected studies on endoscopic transpapillary drainage for EPF (studies in which results of endoscopic drainage in patients with EPF are given separately)

Authors,[Ref.] Year	No. of Patients	Success	Complication	Recurrence
Kozarek et al,[83] 1997	9	8/9 (89%)	Stent migration: 1 Infection: 1	None
Boerma et al,[84] 2000	15	Technical: 13/15 (87%) Clinical: 13/13 (100%)	Stent block: 1	None New pseudocyst in 3
Costamagna et al,[85] 2001	16	Technical: 12/16 (75%) Clinical: 11/12 (92%)	None	None
Halttunen et al,[80] 2005	18	13/18 (72%)	Separately for EPF not given	None
Cicek et al,[76] 2006	23	19/23 (83%)	Stent migration: 2	None
Rana et al,[9] 2010	23	Technical: 21/23 (93%) Clinical: 17/21 (81%)	NPD block: 1	None
Goasguen et al,[86] 2009	10	10/10 (100%)	Stent migration: 1 Stent obstruction: 1	One
Bakker et al,[87] 2011	24	Technical: 19/24 (79%) Clinical: 16/19 (84%)	Stent migration: 4 Stent clogging: 2	Residual PFC in 40% of patients at 6 mo

time of minor sphincterotomy in 1. The stents bridged the disruption in 3 patients and fistulas successfully healed in 8 (89%). Boerma and colleagues[84] attempted PD stenting in 15 patients with EPF that developed after operative necrosectomy. A stent was placed in 13 (87%) patients, and in 9 patients it was placed across the disruption. In all 13 patients the drainage from EPF ceased, but 3 patients with nonbridging disruption developed a pseudocyst at the tail end of the pancreas requiring a distal pancreatectomy. The median time of EPF closure was 10 days (range: 2–64 days). Costamagna and colleagues[85] reported the results on 16 patients with postsurgical EPFs using endoscopic transpapillary NPD. Successful outcomes were achieved in 12 (75%) patients, and fistulas healed in 11 of these 12 patients with a mean time to closure of EPF of 8.8 days (range: 2–33 days). Halttunen and colleagues[80] observed a success rate of 72% on 18 patients with EPF and a median time to healing of fistula of 122 days. A stent was placed in 13 of 15 (87%) patients, and in 9 of 13 patients it was placed across the disruption. In all 13 patients the drainage from EPF ceased, but 3 patients with nonbridging disruption developed a pseudocyst at the tail end of the pancreas requiring distal pancreatectomy. The median time of EPF closure was 10 days (range: 2–64 days). Cicek and colleagues[76] performed pancreatic endotherapy in 23 patients with EPF (postsurgical in 22 patients and after percutaneous drainage in 1 patient). Sixteen of these patients had partial PD disruption, and the EPF healed after transpapillary drainage in 15 (94%) of these patients. The EPF healed in all 7 patients with bridged partial disruption, whereas it healed in 8 of 9 patients (89%) with nonbridged partial duct disruption. On the other hand, fistulas closed in only 20% of patients with complete PD disruption. In this study, the investigators used a combination of pancreatic sphincterotomy, pancreatic stent, or NPD as endotherapy.

Rana and colleagues[9] attempted endoscopic transpapillary NPD placement in 23 patients (19 males) with EPF. Sixteen patients had partial PD disruption and 7 had complete PD disruption, and an NPD was placed in 21 (91%) patients. Following the NPD placement, the EPF healed in 17 (73.9%) patients at a mean duration of 5.3 weeks. The EPF closed in all 15 patients with partial duct disruption that was bridged with NPD, whereas it healed in only 2 of 8 (20%) patients with complete PD disruption.

Bakker and colleagues[87] conducted a retrospective analysis of patients with acute pancreatitis with EPF who underwent endoscopic transpapillary stenting (19 patients) or conservative medical therapy (12 patients), and demonstrated that EPF closed in 16 of 19 patients (84%) in the stent group and in 8 of 12 patients (75%) in the conservative management group ($P = .175$). The median time to fistula closure after stenting was 71 days (interquartile range [IQR] 34–142), whereas in the conservative group it was 120 days (IQR 51–175 days; $P = .130$). The same investigators also conducted a literature review for EPF in patients with acute pancreatitis, including 10 studies that reported the results of 281 patients following stent placement. EPF closed in 200 patients (71%) and stent-related complications were reported in only 9% of patients.[87] It was concluded that endoscopic transpapillary treatment in patients with pancreatic fistulas after intervention for infected necrotizing pancreatitis is a feasible and safe alternative to conservative treatment.

The aforementioned studies suggest that EPF can be effectively treated by transpapillary stent placement, with the best results in patients with partial PD disruption that can be bridged. There remain unanswered questions that need to be addressed by future studies:

1. How long should conservative therapy be attempted in patients with EPF before considering endotherapy?
2. What is the role of combined medical (somatostatin or its analogues) and endoscopic therapy?
3. What is role of preoperative stenting in the prevention of postsurgical EPF?

NOVEL ENDOSCOPIC MODALITIES FOR HEALING PANCREATIC DUCTAL DISRUPTION

As discussed earlier, endoscopic transpapillary drainage is currently the treatment of choice for patients with PD disruptions and consequent fistulas. However, some patients may have refractory fistulas that may not heal even after optimal endoscopic management. Many patients with refractory PD disruptions have large disruptions, disruptions located at the tail end of the pancreas, or complete PD disruptions. The endoscopic management of patients with complete PD disruption is discussed in the section on DPDS.

Patients with refractory fistulas may be treated with endoscopic glue or fibrin injection. Fibrin is a physiologic adhesive containing a combination of thrombin, fibrinogen, and calcium, and does not promote foreign-body reaction or inflammation, but the exposure to pancreatic juice leads to its rapid degradation and, therefore, periodic injections are required to keep the fistula closed.[88] In contrast to fibrin, cyanoacrylate glue is a nonbiological compound that is more stable and is not degraded by pancreatic enzymes. Seewald and colleagues[89] assessed the safety and efficacy of endoscopic injection of N-butyl-2-cyanoacrylate into the fistulous tract combined with endoscopic transpapillary drainage in 12 patients with IPF and EPF. The fistulas closed in 8 (67%) patients, with a single injection in 7 of these 8 successfully treated patients. There were no complications, and none of the successfully treated patients had recurrence of the fistula. Another compound that has been used for closure of EPF is Glubran 2. This surgical glue is composed of N-butyl-2-cyanoacrylate and metha-cryloxysulfolane, and has lower toxicity and elicits lesser inflammatory response in comparison with N-butyl-2-cyanoacrylate glue. Mutignani and colleagues[90] used endoscopic injection of Glubran 2 for closure of pancreatic fistula in 4 patients, 3 of whom had failed endoscopic drainage. The PD disruption healed in 3 (75%) patients within 24 hours of the procedure.

Based on the experience of treating 4 patients with pancreatic fistula by endoscopic glue injection, and a literature review of 32 patients in whom pancreatic fistulas were treated with fibrin sealants (n = 11) or cyanoacrylate (n = 21), Labori and colleagues[91] concluded that endoscopic sealing of pancreatic fistulas can be performed safely and effectively. There is also a report of sealing of an EPF by endoscopic deployment of a coil (intravascular use coil made of fibered platinum, 0.035 inches [0.89 mm] in diameter, straight length 50 mm, coiled size 5 × 4 mm; Target Vascular, Boston Scientific, Ireland), but the safety and efficacy of this approach needs further study.[92]

An alternative approach to treating refractory PD disruptions is placement of covered metallic stents. There have been case reports describing successful healing of refractory pancreatic fistulas by endoscopic insertion of self-expanding metallic stents (SEMS).[71,93,94] Although placement of SEMS appears to be an attractive option, stent-induced ductal and parenchymal changes limit its routine use; therefore, it should be used a last resort in difficult cases with no other feasible treatment options.[95]

PANCREATIC DUCT LEAKS WITH DISCONNECTED PANCREATIC DUCT (DISCONNECTED PANCREATIC DUCT SYNDROME)

In severe acute pancreatitis and, rarely, in chronic pancreatitis, trauma, or malignancy, rupture of the main PD can result in a portion of the pancreatic gland becoming isolated from the duct proximal to the obstruction. This process causes leakage of secretions through the injured area to surrounding tissues, resulting in the formation external or internal fistulas and peripancreatic fluid collections.

Disease Characteristics

The most common causes of DPDS are acute pancreatitis (55%), chronic pancreatitis (25%), postsurgical adverse events (15%), and other uncommon causes such as trauma and malignancy.[14,96–98] The median age of patients is 50 years, more than 65% of whom are male. The site of disconnection in more than 80% of cases is the head or neck/body portion of the pancreas.[14,96] While the size of the PFC is not a key factor in determining the likelihood of DPDS, the anatomic location of the fluid collection, particularly into the pancreatic neck, should arouse suspicion of this syndrome. This observation is related to the unique anatomic susceptibility of this region to ischemic necrosis owing to the tenuous vascular supply through the lateral pancreatic arterial branches.

Whereas a disconnected gland can be diagnosed immediately after an inciting event such as trauma, this may not be obvious in patients with pancreatitis. In many patients with severe acute pancreatitis, there is an evolution of inflammation and necrosis over time so that the specific radiologic findings may not be evident early in their hospital course.[99] In 2 series, a DPDS was diagnosed at a median duration of 163 days (range: 3–1095 days) after acute pancreatitis.[14,98] In the authors' experience, by 2 weeks after the initial attack pertinent CT and other radiologic findings of DPDS become evident, therefore the most common reason for delayed diagnosis is a lack of awareness about this disease entity.[100] During this diagnostic delay, patients usually linger with a nonresolving pancreatic pseudocyst or WOPN, a persistent pancreatic fistula, have undergone an ineffective percutaneous drainage procedure, or develop complications such as bleeding or infection caused by fistula management. Unlike other forms of pancreatitis-related complications that can be managed by medical therapies and other minimally invasive procedures for fluid drainage, DPDS will not respond favorably to conventional measures, and unplanned interventions are likely to result in more complications such as an EPF. Therefore, the first and foremost step is to establish a correct diagnosis so that the appropriate treatment can be instituted.

Diagnosis of DPDS

The most important clinical clue is a nonhealing pancreatic fistula or peripancreatic fluid collection that does not resolve with conservative medical management.

CT scan
CT evidence of an intrapancreatic fluid collection or segmental necrosis along the expected course of the main PD with viable upstream pancreatic parenchyma suggests the diagnosis of DPDS (**Fig. 7**). As false positives can occur with CT in the setting of partial duct disruption, a confirmatory diagnosis can be established most reliably only by pancreatography, either an MRCP or ERCP. Another disadvantage of CT is that, unfortunately, many examinations in the setting of severe acute pancreatitis are performed without contrast media because of concerns about exacerbating microvascular necrosis in the pancreas or renal damage. Withholding intravenous contrast significantly limits the ability to differentiate viable from necrotic pancreatic tissue, although the use of contrast is generally safe in most patients.[101]

MRCP
At MRCP, abrupt discontinuity of the main PD at the level of the fluid collection is usually diagnostic of DPDS (**Fig. 8**). However, a focal stenosis or mechanical compression from an acute fluid collection can mimic a disrupted main PD. Administration of intravenous secretin can better delineate the PD's anatomy under such circumstances.

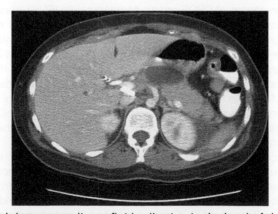

Fig. 7. CT of the abdomen revealing a fluid collection in the head of the pancreas with a viable pancreatic parenchyma in the upstream gland. On pancreatography this patient was found to have a disconnected pancreatic duct syndrome (DPDS).

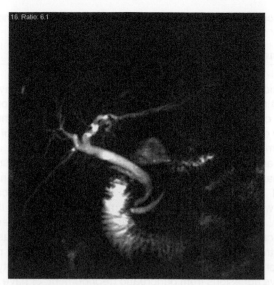

Fig. 8. Secretin-enhanced MRCP revealing a disconnected main PD with enhancement of the upstream gland.

Despite being noninvasive and fairly accurate, it is important to bear in mind that the sensitivity of secretin-enhanced MRCP for showing extravasation at the site of PD disconnection is lower than that of ERCP.[102] It is probable that the ductal pressure with manual injection of contrast material during ERCP cannot be attained with increased exocrine output in response to secretin.

ERCP
At ERCP, an abrupt cutoff of the main PD, with or without contrast extravasation, is diagnostic of DPDS (**Fig. 9**). Inability to traverse this disconnection with a guide wire

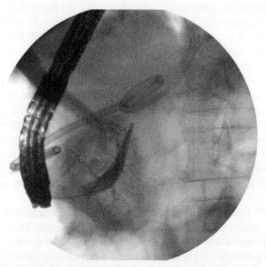

Fig. 9. Endoscopic retrograde cholangiopancreatography revealing a disconnected main PD in a patient with walled-off pancreatic necrosis.

is a priori evidence that the duct is completely "disconnected" and not just focally "disrupted."

Treatment Options

Surgery

Despite its limitations, surgical treatment has remained the mainstay of treatment for DPDS. Treatment may involve removal of the viable upstream disconnected pancreatic segment or creation of a pancreaticojejunostomy to drain this segment. The choice of surgery depends on the age of the patient, the presence of continued retroperitoneal inflammation, the volume of the disconnected segment, and the exocrine and endocrine pancreatic function.[81] In patients in whom the disconnected distal portion of the gland is thought to substantially contribute to pancreatic function, median segment pancreaticojejunostomy is the preferred surgical option. Distal pancreatectomy with or without splenectomy may be performed if the disconnected segment is small. In patients with chronic pancreatitis and persistent pain, in select centers total pancreatectomy with auto–islet cell transplantation has been proposed as an alternative treatment.[103] However, many patients with DPDS, particularly those with underlying chronic pancreatitis, suffer from other comorbidity such as portal hypertension, have adhesions from pancreatic debridement, or have significant endocrine insufficiency that makes surgery a less attractive option.

Endoscopic management

The treatment of DPDS depends on the nature of the clinical presentation, which includes (1) nonresolving peripancreatic fluid collection, (2) percutaneous fistula, and (3) recurrent pancreatitis or persistent abdominal pain. Other rare presentations include GI bleeding secondary to portal hypertension, infection of the fistula, and pancreatic exocrine or endocrine insufficiency.

Nonresolving peripancreatic fluid collection Transmural drainage of the fluid collection by conventional endoscopy or under EUS guidance enables the formation of an enteric fistula that facilitates drainage of the disconnected segment into the enteral lumen. The fistula is kept patent by the placement of transmural stents. Physiologically this approach is logical, as pancreatic secretions should flow into the GI tract whether through the ductal system or via the endoscopic bypass. In patients with infective organized necrosis, the necrotic debris must be removed either by endoscopic necrosectomy, the multiple transluminal gateway technique, or other hybrid approaches.[104] The conventional wisdom has been to remove the transmural stents in 6 to 8 weeks after resolution of the fluid collection is confirmed on a follow-up CT scan. However, this strategy is associated with PFC recurrence in 10% to 30% of patients, usually 1 year after stent removal.[29,47] Recently a new concept was developed by a Belgian group, whereby the transmural stents are left in place indefinitely, even after PFC resolution, so that the stents serve as a conduit between the PFC and, indirectly, the PD and the digestive tract (**Fig. 10**).[46] This approach is particularly beneficial for patients with DPDS, when the main PD segment upstream of the rupture is disconnected and exclusively drains through the fistula that is kept patent by the transmural stent.

In 2 studies,[13,46] none of the patients treated with permanent transmural stents developed a PFC recurrence at a median follow-up of 16 and 28 months, respectively (**Table 5**). Although the rate of spontaneous stent migration is unknown, in one study[13] one-third of these patients had spontaneous stent migration after PFC resolution. It is likely that PFC resolution leads to eventual adherence of the walls of the cavity, which in turn leads to gradual migration of the stent toward the GI lumen. By contrast, stent

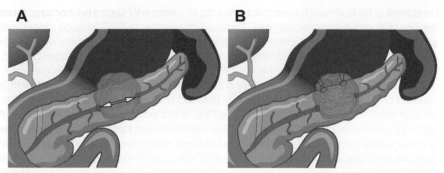

Fig. 10. (A) Illustration of DPDS, with the white arrow revealing the region of ductal rupture. (B) Illustration demonstrating the concept of permanent transmural stent placement by endoscopy for drainage of the upstream gland into the enteral lumen.

retrieval occurring before complete collapse of the cavity might lead to PFC recurrence, particularly if a communication exists between the cavity and the PD. Therefore, the duration of stent placement may be more important than whether the stents are still present or retrieved after an adequate stent-placement period.

The major concern about permanent stents stems from the premise that (1) stent occlusion leads to PFC recurrence and (2) stents may act as a nidus for infectious complications. In one study, although no infectious complications were encountered, at a median follow-up of 28 months stent migration was documented in 13.6% of patients, leading to small-bowel obstruction in 2 and the stent lodging within the PFC in 1.[13] Although the concept of permanent transmural stents seems promising, better endoprostheses with antimigratory properties are needed to keep the transmural tract patent.

Percutaneous fistulas The management of DPDS in the setting of pancreatic fistulas can be challenging. The 2 most important questions to address are (1) is the disconnection "complete" or "partial"? and (2) is there an associated PFC at the site of the disconnected duct?

In patients with a partially disconnected duct, a pancreatic sphincterotomy with placement of a transpapillary PD stent bridging the site of disconnection will resolve the leak in most patients.[1] On the other hand, when the disconnection is complete, the upstream duct cannot be accessed by ERCP and transpapillary interventions are futile. In such cases, EUS-guided and/or percutaneous intervention is needed to treat the fistula.

Table 5
Outcomes of patients treated with permanent indwelling transmural stents for management of pancreatic fluid collections

Authors,[Ref.] Year	No. of Patients	Treatment Success (%)	Median Follow-Up (mo)	Recurrence (%)	Adverse Events (%)
Arvanitakis et al,[46] 2007	15	100	14	0	None
Varadarajulu et al,[104,a] 2011	22	100	28	0	3 cases of stent migration (13.6%)

[a] All patients had a DPDS.

Treatment is fairly straightforward for patients in whom a PFC can be demonstrated at the site of ductal disconnection on CT scan. Endoscopic or EUS-guided placement of permanent indwelling transmural stents will facilitate decompression of the upstream duct in these patients. With diversion of pancreatic flow to a dependent lumen, the fistula eventually heals. A technical challenge in these circumstances is the ability to deploy stents within PFCs that are very small. In the authors' experience, even PFCs measuring only up to 35 mm can be safely drained under EUS guidance with placement of at least 1 7F double-pigtail stent. If a PFC is too small or is not visible, contrast medium or water can be instilled through the percutaneous fistula so as to make the PFC more visible and amenable for transmural stent placement. In patients for whom transmural drainage is not possible because of the lack of visible fluid as a result of prior percutaneous or surgical drainage, and in whom no external drain is in place, a hybrid approach can be undertaken using a combination of techniques to drain the disconnected duct.

In the technique known as outside-in transluminal puncture, the path of the external fistula is first opacified with contrast using a catheter that is inserted via the fistula orifice.[96,97] Under fluoroscopic guidance, a hydrophilic guide wire is then advanced through the catheter to reach the virtual cavity adjacent to the site of disconnection. The catheter is then advanced to the site of disconnection and the hydrophilic wire is exchanged for a stiffer wire, which is manipulated to approximate the stomach or duodenal wall. The gut lumen is then insufflated with air using a duodenoscope. The radiologist then punctures the gastric/duodenal wall under fluoroscopic and endoscopic guidance by using a transjugular intrahepatic portosystemic shunt needle (angled needle/catheter combination; Cook Medical, Winston-Salem, NC). A flexible guide wire is then advanced through the needle, which in turn is captured and retrieved out of the endoscope. If required, a second wire can be advanced by the radiologist by using a 6.5F Lieberman introducer (Cook Medical) over the first working wire, and the second wire can be retrieved with the help of the duodenoscope. With 2 wires secured at both ends, the gut wall can be balloon-dilated to 8 to 10 mm under fluoroscopic guidance. Double-pigtail stents can then be deployed adjacent to the PD disruption with the proximal portions in the gastric or duodenal lumen. Contrast is then injected via the percutaneous drain to ensure adequate diversion into the gastric/duodenal lumen. The drainage catheter is then capped and eventually removed once definitive diversion of pancreatic secretions is confirmed. This approach has an overall treatment success of more than 70% (**Table 6**). The reported procedural adverse events include infection, abdominal pain, fever, and stent migration or fragmentation.[96,97] A second technique is EUS-guided PD drainage. At EUS, the dilated

Table 6
Outcomes of patients treated with the hybrid "outside-in" transluminal puncture technique

Authors,[Ref.] Year	No. of Patients	Treatment Success (%)	Median Follow-Up (mo)	Recurrence (%)	Adverse Events (%)
Arvanitakis et al,[96] 2007	5	4 (80)	18	1 (10)	None
Irani et al,[97] 2012	10	7 (70)	25	3 (30)[a]	3 cases of infection (13.6%)[b]

[a] Three patients had recurrence of pancreatic fluid collections (PFC) at follow-up. Treatment failure in this review was considered to be fistula or PFC recurrence.
[b] Two required percutaneous drains and 1 was managed with antibiotics; 1 patient also had stent fragmentation.

upstream duct is first accessed using a 19-gauge aspiration needle. After injection of contrast to opacify the duct, a 0.035-inch or smaller caliber guide wire (**Fig. 11**) is advanced within the ductal system. The transmural tract is then dilated by using a graded dilation catheter or a cautery-based needle knife system to create a fistula. Once access to the disconnected duct is gained, a double-pigtail stent of suitable

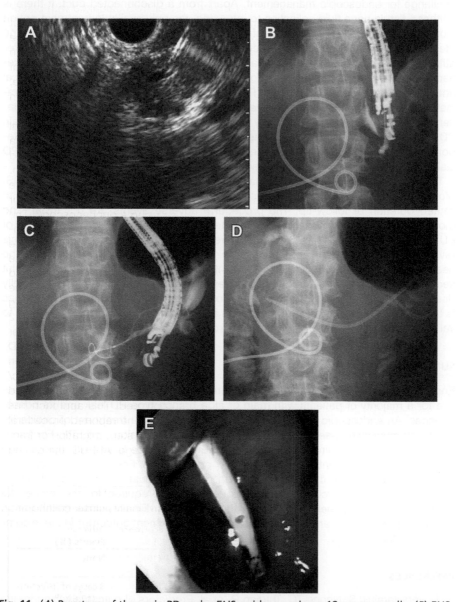

Fig. 11. (*A*) Puncture of the main PD under EUS guidance using a 19-gauge needle. (*B*) EUS-guided pancreatogram revealing DPDS. (*C*) Passage of a guide wire into the main PD following by graded dilation of the transmural tract. (*D*) Fluoroscopic image revealing a plastic stent within the pancreatic ductal system. (*E*) Endoscopic image of the proximal portion of the stent in the stomach. (*Courtesy of* Dr Takao Itoi.)

caliber is deployed to drain the disconnected main PD within the stomach or the duodenal lumen. Experience with this technique for treatment of EPF is limited. Two patients reportedly treated using this approach had successful clinical outcomes following stent placement.[96,105]

Abdominal pain or recurrent pancreatitis This patient cohort presents the greatest challenge for endoscopic management. Apart from a disconnected duct, if there is neither a fistula nor a fluid collection to intervene, the only available treatment option would be internal decompression of the main PD by EUS-guided PD drainage (described above). Data on the efficacy of this technique for treating pain or pancreatitis secondary to DPDS are scant, as most studies are composed of a heterogeneous cohort of patients with chronic pancreatitis–induced strictures, postsurgical anastomotic strictures or fistulas, and PFC.[106,107] In a study of 4 patients with abdominal pain secondary to DPDS, the procedure yielded long-term symptom relief in 3 patients.[108] This procedure is technically not feasible in patients with a nondilated main PD and in those with multiple strictures or stones that preclude stent placement. Reported adverse events with this technique include abdominal pain, perforation, PD leak, pancreatitis, hematoma, and infection.[106]

There is no consensus on the optimal endoscopic approach to treatment of DPDS. Most studies are from expert centers that include a small cohort of patients with limited duration of follow-up. The procedural adverse events are not trivial, and most involve multidisciplinary care. Despite these limitations, with the advent of EUS enormous progress has been made over the past few years. As outlined in this review, several treatment approaches are now possible, thereby precluding the need for a difficult operation in these patients. The main limiting factor at this point seems to be the lack of dedicated accessories to perform these procedures. Specially designed one-step access devices and endoprosthesis with antimigratory properties is the need of the hour. Also, more data with a larger cohort of patients are needed to validate the promising preliminary findings from a few expert centers.

SUMMARY

Endoscopic therapy by placement of a bridging transpapillary endoprosthesis is effective for a majority of patients with main or side-branch type PD leak and its consequences. An endoscopic transpapillary bridging stent is the treatment of choice for small communicating pseudocysts, pancreatic ascites, effusion, and EPF. For pseudocysts, transmural drainage with or without EUS guidance is also efficacious, and is the preferred treatment modality for larger pseudocysts. For DPDS, the treatment must be tailored to the clinical presentation of an individual patient. A combination of endoscopic and percutaneous techniques may be required for the successful nonoperative management of some of these patients. Finally, close collaboration between specialties is paramount to optimizing the treatment outcomes in these complex patients.

REFERENCES

1. Varadarajulu S, Noone TC, Tutuian R, et al. Predictors of outcome in pancreatic duct disruption managed by endoscopic transpapillary stent placement. Gastrointest Endosc 2005;61:568–75.
2. Bhasin DK, Dhavan S, Sriram PV, et al. Endoscopic management of pancreatic diseases. Indian J Gastroenterol 1997;16:151–2.

3. Kozarek RA, Ball TJ, Patterson DJ, et al. Endoscopic transpapillary therapy for disrupted pancreatic duct and peripancreatic fluid collections. Gastroenterology 1991;100:1362–70.
4. Neoptolemos JP, London NJ, Carr-Locke DL. Assessment of the main pancreatic duct integrity by endoscopic retrograde pancreatography in patients with acute pancreatitis. Br J Surg 1993;80:94–9.
5. Kozarek RA. Endoscopic therapy of complete and partial pancreatic duct disruptions. Gastrointest Endosc Clin N Am 1998;8:39–53.
6. Pannegeon V, Pessaux P, Sauvanet A, et al. Pancreatic fistula after distal pancreatectomy: predictive risk factors and value of conservative treatment. Arch Surg 2006;141:1071–6.
7. Fazel A. Postoperative pancreatic leaks and fistulae: the role of the endoscopist. Tech Gastrointest Endosc 2006;8:92–8.
8. Morgan KA, Adams DB. Management of internal and external pancreatic fistulae. Surg Clin North Am 2007;87:1503–13.
9. Rana SS, Bhasin DK, Nanda M, et al. Endoscopic transpapillary drainage for external fistulae developing after surgical or radiological pancreatic interventions. J Gastroenterol Hepatol 2010;25:1087–92.
10. Uomo G, Molino D, Visconti M, et al. The incidence of main pancreatic duct disruption in severe biliary pancreatitis. Am J Surg 1998;176:49–52.
11. Lau ST, Simchuk EJ, Kozarek RA, et al. A pancreatic ductal leak should be sought to direct treatment in patients with acute pancreatitis. Am J Surg 2001; 181:411–5.
12. Banks PA, Bollen TL, Dervenis C, et al, Acute Pancreatitis Classification Working Group. Classification of acute pancreatitis—2012: revision of the Atlanta classification and definitions by international consensus. Gut 2013;62:102–11.
13. Varadarajulu S, Wilcox CM. Endoscopic placement of permanent indwelling transmural stents in disconnected pancreatic duct syndrome: does benefit outweigh the risks? Gastrointest Endosc 2011;74:1408–12.
14. Pelaez-Luna M, Vege SS, Petersen BT, et al. Disconnected pancreatic duct syndrome in severe acute pancreatitis: clinical and imaging characteristics and outcomes in a cohort of 31 cases. Gastrointest Endosc 2008;68:91–7.
15. Rana SS, Bhasin DK, Rao C, et al. Non fluoroscopic endoscopic ultrasound guided transmural drainage of symptomatic non bulging walled of pancreatic necrosis. Dig Endosc 2013;25:47–52. Early online 2012.
16. Telford JJ, Farrell JJ, Saltzman JR, et al. Pancreatic stent placement for duct disruption. Gastrointest Endosc 2002;56:18–24.
17. Kim HS, Lee DK, Kim IW, et al. The role of endoscopic retrograde pancreatography in the treatment of traumatic pancreatic duct injury. Gastrointest Endosc 2001;54:49–55.
18. Barish MA, Yucel EK, Ferrucci JT. Magnetic resonance cholangiopancreatography. N Engl J Med 1999;341:258–64.
19. Freeman ML. Adverse outcomes of ERCP. Gastrointest Endosc 2002;56(Suppl): S273–82.
20. Blero D, Devière J. Endoscopic complications—avoidance and management. Nat Rev Gastroenterol Hepatol 2012;9:162–72.
21. Itoh S, Ikeda M, Ota T, et al. Assessment of the pancreatic and intra pancreatic bile ducts using 0.5-mm collimation and multi planar reformatted images in multi slice CT. Eur Radiol 2003;13:277–85.
22. Anderson SW, Soto JA. Pancreatic duct evaluation: accuracy of portal venous phase 64 MDCT. Abdom Imaging 2009;34:55–63.

23. O'Toole D, Vullierme MP, Ponsot P, et al. Diagnosis and management of pancreatic fistulae resulting in pancreatic ascites or pleural effusions in the era of helical CT and magnetic resonance imaging. Gastroenterol Clin Biol 2007;31: 686–93.

24. Wong YC, Wang LJ, Fang JF, et al. Multidetector-row computed tomography (CT) of blunt pancreatic injuries: can contrast-enhanced multiphasic CT detect pancreatic duct injuries? J Trauma 2008;64:666–72.

25. Drake LM, Anis M, Lawrence C. Accuracy of magnetic resonance cholangiopancreatography in identifying pancreatic duct disruption. J Clin Gastroenterol 2012;46:696–9.

26. Soto JA, Alvarez O, Munera F, et al. Traumatic disruption of the pancreatic duct: diagnosis with MR pancreatography. AJR Am J Roentgenol 2001;176:175–8.

27. Subramanian A, Dente CJ, Feliciano DV. The management of pancreatic trauma in the modern era. Surg Clin North Am 2007;87:1515–32.

28. Gillams AR, Kurzawinski T, Lees WR. Diagnosis of duct disruption and assessment of pancreatic leak with dynamic secretin-stimulated MR cholangiopancreatography. AJR Am J Roentgenol 2006;186:499–506.

29. Alexakis N, Sutton R, Neoptolemos JP. Surgical treatment of pancreatic fistula. Dig Surg 2004;21:262–74.

30. Eckhauser F, Raper SE, Knol JA, et al. Surgical management of pancreatic pseudocysts, pancreatic ascites, and pancreaticopleural fistulae. Pancreas 1991;6(Suppl 1):S66–75.

31. Arvanitakis M, Delhaye M, Chamlou R, et al. Endoscopic therapy for main pancreatic-duct rupture after Silastic-ring vertical gastroplasty. Gastrointest Endosc 2005;62:143–51.

32. Carr-Locke DL, Gregg JA. Endoscopic manometry of pancreatic and biliary sphincter zones in man: basal results in healthy volunteers. Dig Dis Sci 1981; 26:7–15.

33. Baron TH, Harewood GC, Morgan DE, et al. Outcome differences after endoscopic drainage of pancreatic necrosis, acute pancreatic pseudocysts, and chronic pancreatic pseudocysts. Gastrointest Endosc 2002;56:7–17.

34. Hookey LC, Debroux S, Delhaye M, et al. Endoscopic drainage of pancreatic fluid collections in 116 patients: a comparison of etiologies, drainage techniques, and outcomes. Gastrointest Endosc 2006;63:635–43.

35. Bhasin DK, Rana SS, Udawat HP, et al. Management of multiple and large pancreatic pseudocysts by endoscopic transpapillary nasopancreatic drainage alone. Am J Gastroenterol 2006;101:1780–6.

36. Bhasin DK, Rana SS, Nanda M, et al. Endoscopic management of pancreatic pseudocysts at atypical locations. Surg Endosc 2010;24:1085–91.

37. Lakhtakia S, Reddy DN. Pancreatic leaks: endo-therapy first? J Gastroenterol Hepatol 2009;24:1158–60.

38. Beckingham IJ, Krige JE, Bornman PC, et al. Endoscopic management of pancreatic pseudocysts. Br J Surg 1997;84:1638–45.

39. Kahaleh M, Shami VM, Conway MR, et al. Comparison of EUS and conventional endoscopic drainage of pancreatic pseudocyst. Endoscopy 2006;38: 355–9.

40. Varadarajulu S, Wilcox CM, Tamhane A, et al. Role of EUS in drainage of peripancreatic fluid collections not amenable for endoscopic transmural drainage. Gastrointest Endosc 2007;66:1107–19.

41. Nasr JY, Chennat J. Endoscopic ultrasonography-guided transmural drainage of pseudocysts. Tech Gastrointest Endosc 2012;14:195–8.

42. Samuelson AL, Shah RJ. Endoscopic management of pancreatic pseudocysts. Gastroenterol Clin North Am 2012;41:47–62.
43. Giovannini M. Endoscopic ultrasonography-guided pancreatic drainage. Gastrointest Endosc Clin N Am 2012;22:221–30.
44. Varadarajulu S, Lopes TL, Wilcox CM, et al. EUS versus surgical cyst-gastrostomy for management of pancreatic pseudocysts. Gastrointest Endosc 2008;68:649–55.
45. Bhasin DK, Rana SS. Combining transpapillary pancreatic duct stenting with endoscopic transmural drainage for pancreatic fluid collections: two heads are better than one! J Gastroenterol Hepatol 2010;25:433–4.
46. Arvanitakis M, Delhaye M, Bali MA, et al. Pancreatic fluid collections: a randomized controlled trial regarding stent removal after endoscopic transmural drainage. Gastrointest Endosc 2007;65:609–19.
47. Cahen D, Rauws E, Fockens P, et al. Endoscopic drainage of pancreatic pseudocysts: long-term outcome and procedural factors associated with safe and successful treatment. Endoscopy 2005;37:977–83.
48. Trevino JM, Tamhane A, Varadarajulu S. Successful stenting in ductal disruption favorably impacts treatment outcomes in patients undergoing transmural drainage of peripancreatic fluid collections. J Gastroenterol Hepatol 2010;25:526–31.
49. Shrode CW, Macdonough P, Gaidhane M, et al. Multimodality endoscopic treatment of pancreatic duct disruption with stenting and pseudocyst drainage: How efficacious is it? Dig Liver Dis 2013;45:129–33. Early online 2012.
50. Kozarek RA, Brayko CM, Harlan J, et al. Endoscopic drainage of pancreatic pseudocysts. Gastrointest Endosc 1985;31:322–7.
51. Barthet M, Lamblin G, Gasmi M, et al. Clinical usefulness of a treatment algorithm for pancreatic pseudocysts. Gastrointest Endosc 2008;67:245–52.
52. Binmoeller KF, Seifert H, Walter A, et al. Transpapillary and transmural drainage of pancreatic pseudocysts. Gastrointest Endosc 1995;42:219–24.
53. Krüger M, Schneider AS, Manns MP, et al. Endoscopic management of pancreatic pseudocysts or abscesses after an EUS-guided 1-step procedure for initial access. Gastrointest Endosc 2006;63:409–16.
54. Cremer M, Deviere J, Engelholm L. Endoscopic management of cysts and pseudocysts in chronic pancreatitis: long-term follow-up after 7 years of experience. Gastrointest Endosc 1989;35:1–9.
55. Smits ME, Rauws EA, Tytgat GN, et al. The efficacy of endoscopic treatment of pancreatic pseudocysts. Gastrointest Endosc 1995;42:202–7.
56. Sharma SS, Bhargawa N, Govil A. Endoscopic management of pancreatic pseudocyst: a long-term follow-up. Endoscopy 2002;34:203–7.
57. Lopes CV, Pesenti C, Bories E, et al. Endoscopic ultrasound-guided endoscopic transmural drainage of pancreatic pseudocysts. Arq Gastroenterol 2008;45:17–21.
58. Antillon MR, Shah RJ, Stiegmann G, et al. Single-step EUS-guided transmural drainage of simple and complicated pancreatic pseudocysts. Gastrointest Endosc 2006;63:797–803.
59. Penn DE, Draganov PV, Wagh MS, et al. Prospective evaluation of the use of fully covered self-expanding metal stents for EUS-guided transmural drainage of pancreatic pseudocysts. Gastrointest Endosc 2012;76:679–84.
60. Sanchez Cortes E, Maalak A, Le Moine O, et al. Endoscopic cystenterostomy of nonbulging pancreatic fluid collections. Gastrointest Endosc 2002;56:380–6.
61. Baron TH. Endoscopic drainage of pancreatic fluid collections and pancreatic necrosis. Gastrointest Endosc Clin N Am 2003;13:743–64.

62. Catalano MF, Geenen JE, Schmalz MJ, et al. Treatment of pancreatic pseudocysts with ductal communication by transpapillary pancreatic duct endoprosthesis. Gastrointest Endosc 1995;42:214–8.
63. Bhasin DK, Rana SS, Rao C, et al. Clinical presentation, radiological features, and endoscopic management of mediastinal pseudocysts: experience of a decade. Gastrointest Endosc 2012;76:1056–60.
64. Smith MT, Sherman S, Ikenberry SO, et al. Alterations in pancreatic ductal morphology following polyethylene pancreatic stent therapy. Gastrointest Endosc 1996;44:268–75.
65. Sherman S, Hawes RH, Savides TJ, et al. Stent-induced pancreatic ductal and parenchymal changes: correlation of endoscopic ultrasound with ERCP. Gastrointest Endosc 1996;44:276–82.
66. Raju GS, Gomez G, Xiao SY, et al. Effect of a novel pancreatic stent design on short-term pancreatic injury in a canine model. Endoscopy 2006;38:260–5.
67. Bhasin DK, Rana SS. Biodegradable pancreatic stents: are they a disappearing wonder? Gastrointest Endosc 2008;67:1113–6.
68. Bhasin DK, Rana SS, Siyad I, et al. Endoscopic transpapillary nasopancreatic drainage alone to treat pancreatic ascites and pleural effusion. J Gastroenterol Hepatol 2006;21:1059–64.
69. Parekh D, Segal I. Pancreatic ascites and effusion. Risk factors for failure of conservative therapy and the role of octreotide. Arch Surg 1992;127:707–12.
70. Gomez-Cerezo J, Cano AB, Suarez I, et al. Pancreatic ascites: study of therapeutic options by analysis of case reports and case series between the years 1975 and 2000. Am J Gastroenterol 2003;98:568–77.
71. Bracher GA, Manocha AP, DeBanto JR, et al. Endoscopic pancreatic duct stenting to treat pancreatic ascites. Gastrointest Endosc 1999;49:710–5.
72. Chebli JM, Gaburri PD, de Souza AF, et al. Internal pancreatic fistulae: proposal of a management algorithm based on a case series analysis. J Clin Gastroenterol 2004;38:795–800.
73. Kozarek RA, Jiranek GC, Traverso LW. Endoscopic treatment of pancreatic ascites. Am J Surg 1994;168:223–6.
74. Pai CG, Suvarna D, Bhat G. Endoscopic treatment as first-line therapy for pancreatic ascites and pleural effusion. J Gastroenterol Hepatol 2009;24:1198–202.
75. Kurumboor P, Varma D, Rajan M, et al. Outcome of pancreatic ascites in patients with tropical calcific pancreatitis managed using a uniform treatment protocol. Indian J Gastroenterol 2009;28:102–6.
76. Cicek B, Parlak E, Oguz D, et al. Endoscopic treatment of pancreatic fistulae. Surg Endosc 2006;20:1706–12.
77. Miyachi A, Kikuyama M, Kageyama F, et al. Successful treatment of pancreaticopleural fistula by nasopancreatic drainage and endoscopic removal of pancreatic duct calculi: a case report. Gastrointest Endosc 2004;59:454–7.
78. Uchiyama T, Suzuki T, Adachi A, et al. Pancreatic pleural effusion. Case report and review of 113 cases in Japan. Am J Gastroenterol 1992;87:387–91.
79. Neher JR, Brady PG, Pinkas H, et al. Pancreaticopleural fistula in chronic pancreatitis: resolution with endoscopic therapy. Gastrointest Endosc 2000;52:416–8.
80. Halttunen J, Weckman L, Kemppainen E, et al. The endoscopic management of pancreatic fistulae. Surg Endosc 2005;19:559–62.
81. Howard TJ, Stonerock CE, Sarkar J, et al. Contemporary treatment strategies for external pancreatic fistulae. Surgery 1998;124:627–33.
82. Lansden FT, Adams DB, Anderson MC. Treatment of external pancreatic fistulae with somatostatin. Am Surg 1989;55:695–8.

83. Kozarek RA, Ball TJ, Patterson DJ, et al. Transpapillary stenting for pancreatico-cutaneous fistulae. J Gastrointest Surg 1997;1:357–61.
84. Boerma D, Rauws AJ, van Gulik TM, et al. Endoscopic stent placement for pan-creaticocutaneous fistula after surgical drainage of the pancreas. Br J Surg 2000;87:1506–9.
85. Costamagna G, Mutignani M, Ingrosso M, et al. Endoscopic treatment of post-surgical external pancreatic fistulae. Endoscopy 2001;33:317–22.
86. Goasguen N, Bourrier A, Ponsot P, et al. Endoscopic management of pancreatic fistula after distal pancreatectomy and enucleation. Am J Surg 2009;197:715–20.
87. Bakker OJ, van Baal MC, van Santvoort HC, et al, Dutch Pancreatitis Study Group. Endoscopic transpapillary stenting or conservative treatment for pancre-atic fistulae in necrotizing pancreatitis: multicenter series and literature review. Ann Surg 2011;253:961–7.
88. Engler S, Dorlars D, Riemann JF. Endoscopic fibrin gluing of pancreatic duct fis-tula following acute pancreatitis. Dtsch Med Wochenschr 1996;121:1396–400.
89. Seewald S, Brand B, Groth S, et al. Endoscopic sealing of pancreatic fistula by using N-butyl-2-cyanoacrylate. Gastrointest Endosc 2004;59:463–70.
90. Mutignani M, Tringali A, Khodadadian E, et al. External pancreatic fistulae resis-tant to conventional endoscopic therapy: endoscopic closure with N-butyl-2-cyanoacrylate (Glubran 2). Endoscopy 2004;36:738–42.
91. Labori KJ, Trondsen E, Buanes T, et al. Endoscopic sealing of pancreatic fistulae: four case reports and review of the literature. Scand J Gastroenterol 2009;44:1491–6.
92. Lüthen R, Jaklin P, Cohnen M. Permanent closure of a pancreatic duct leak by endoscopic coiling. Endoscopy 2007;39(Suppl 1):E21–2.
93. Gane E, Fata'ar S, Hamilton I. Management of a persistent pancreatic fistula secondary to a ruptured pseudocyst with endoscopic insertion of an expand-able metal stent. Endoscopy 1994;26:254–6.
94. Baron TH, Ferreira LE. Covered expandable metal stent placement for treatment of a refractory pancreatic duct leak. Gastrointest Endosc 2007;66:1239–41.
95. Yamakado K, Nakatsuka A, Kihira N, et al. Metallic stent placement in the pancreatic duct: an experimental study in the normal dog pancreas. J Vasc In-terv Radiol 2003;14:357–62.
96. Arvanitakis M, Delhaye M, Bali MA, et al. Endoscopic treatment of external pancreatic fistulas: when draining the main pancreatic duct is not enough. Am J Gastroenterol 2007;102:516–24.
97. Irani S, Gluck M, Ross A, et al. Resolving external pancreatic fistulas in patients with disconnected pancreatic duct syndrome: using rendezvous techniques to avoid surgery (video). Gastrointest Endosc 2012;76:586–93.
98. Tann M, Maglinte D, Howard TJ, et al. Disconnected pancreatic duct syndrome: imaging findings and therapeutic implications in 26 surgically corrected patients. J Comput Assist Tomogr 2003;27:577–82.
99. Beger HG, Rau B, Mayer J, et al. Natural course of acute pancreatitis. World J Surg 1997;21:130–5.
100. Sandrasegaran K, Tann M, Jennings SG, et al. Disconnection of the pancreatic duct: an important but over-looked complication of severe acute pancreatitis. Radiographics 2007;27:1389–400.
101. Uhl W, Roggo A, Kirscchstein T, et al. Influence of contrast enhanced computed tomography on course and outcomes in patients with acute pancreatitis. Pancreas 2002;24:191–7.

102. Aksik MF, Sandrasegaran K, Aisen AA, et al. Dynamic secretin-enhanced MR cholangiopancreatography. Radiographics 2006;26:665–77.
103. Sutherland DE, Radosevich DM, Bellin MD, et al. Total pancreatectomy and islet autotransplantation for chronic pancreatitis. J Am Coll Surg 2012;214:409–24.
104. Varadarajulu S, Bang JY, Phadnis MA, et al. Endoscopic transmural drainage of peripancreatic fluid collections: outcomes and predictors of treatment success in 211 consecutive patients. J Gastrointest Surg 2011;15:2080–8.
105. Will U, Fueldner F, Goldmann B, et al. Successful transgastric pancreaticography and endoscopic ultrasound-guided drainage of a disconnected pancreatic tail syndrome. Therap Adv Gastroenterol 2011;4:213–8.
106. Tessier G, Bories E, Arvanitakis M, et al. EUS-guided pancreaticogastrostomy and pancreaticobulbostomy for the treatment of pain with pancreatic ductal dilation inaccessible to transpapillary endoscopic therapy. Gastrointest Endosc 2007;65:233–41.
107. Varadarajulu S, Trevino JM. Review of EUS-guided pancreatic duct drainage (with video). Gastrointest Endosc 2009;69(Suppl 2):S200–2.
108. Francois E, Kahaleh M, Giovannini M, et al. EUS-guided pancreaticogastrostomy. Gastrointest Endosc 2002;56:128–33.

Autoimmune Pancreatitis
Role of Endoscopy in Diagnosis and Treatment

Sung-Hoon Moon, MD[a], Myung-Hwan Kim, MD, PhD[b],*

KEYWORDS

- Autoimmune pancreatitis • IgG4-related disease • Pancreatic cancer
- Endoscopic ultrasonography • Endoscopic retrograde cholangiopancreatography
- Endoscopy

KEY POINTS

- Autoimmune pancreatitis (AIP) is a rarer disease than are pancreatobiliary malignancies.
- Patients with indeterminate computed tomography findings for AIP (pancreatic mass, focal/segmental pancreatic enlargement, and cutoff/dilatation of the main pancreatic duct) require exclusion of malignancy as a prerequisite for further workup to diagnose AIP. The recommended first-line procedure to exclude malignancy is endoscopic ultrasonography-guided fine-needle aspiration in cases in which sampling of a suspected pancreatic cancer is indicated, whereas endoscopic retrograde cholangiopancreatography (ERCP)-guided sampling is recommended in cases in which sampling of a suspected bile duct cancer is indicated, especially when ERCP is needed to relieve biliary obstruction.
- ERCP is not mandatory for all cases with suspected AIP. Diagnostic endoscopic retrograde pancreatography is useful in the setting of indeterminate CT imaging for AIP or seronegative AIP without other organ involvement.

INTRODUCTION

Autoimmune pancreatitis (AIP) is a peculiar type of chronic pancreatitis in which pathogenesis involves an autoimmune mechanism.[1,2] AIP responds dramatically to corticosteroid therapy, but it otherwise mimics pancreatobiliary malignancies.[1,3,4] The diagnosis of AIP may be challenging and requires a full workup in some cases. Major pancreatic resections including pancreaticoduodenectomy continue to be performed for this benign disease, although surgeries for AIP have been dwindling as clinical experience increases.[5–8] A higher awareness of AIP would mean that fewer

[a] Department of Internal Medicine, Hallym University Sacred Heart Hospital, Hallym University College of Medicine, 896 Pyeongchon-dong, Dongan-gu, Anyang 431-070, South Korea; [b] Department of Internal Medicine, Asan Medical Center, University of Ulsan College of Medicine, Asanbyeongwon-Gil 86, Songpa-Gu, Seoul 138-736, South Korea
* Corresponding author.
E-mail address: mhkim@amc.seoul.kr

Gastrointest Endoscopy Clin N Am 23 (2013) 893–915
http://dx.doi.org/10.1016/j.giec.2013.06.005
1052-5157/13/$ – see front matter © 2013 Elsevier Inc. All rights reserved.

patients with AIP would undergo operations.[9] However, clinicians must also remain aware that AIP is a rarer disease than are pancreatobiliary malignancies.[3,10,11] Overenthusiasm to diagnose AIP should be avoided, because giving corticosteroids to patients with resectable pancreatic adenocarcinoma creates a more fearful scenario than does performing a surgical pancreatic resection in patients with AIP.[9,12–14]

A set of international consensus diagnostic criteria and algorithms (ICDC) for AIP has been recently proposed, based on a consensus of expert opinion, for the nonsurgical diagnosis of AIP and to avoid misdiagnosis of pancreatobiliary malignancies as AIP.[1] According to the ICDC, endoscopic evaluations including endoscopic ultrasonography (EUS) and endoscopic retrograde cholangiopancreatography (ERCP), are important for the diagnosis of AIP and for the differentiation of AIP from pancreatic cancer.[13,15] Endoscopy also has a role in the treatment of AIP by relieving cholestasis in the acute phase of disease, and also in the assessment of steroid responsiveness.

This review addresses the role of endoscopy in the diagnosis and treatment of AIP and provides a diagnostic process for patients with suspected AIP. We answer the following questions: When should AIP be suspected? When can AIP be diagnosed without endoscopic examination? Which endoscopic approaches are appropriate in suspected AIP, and when? Is there a role for diagnostic endoscopic retrograde pancreatography (ERP) for AIP? What are the roles of endoscopic biopsies and IgG4 immunostaining in the diagnosis of AIP? What is the proper use of the steroid trial in the diagnosis of AIP in patients with indeterminate computed tomography (CT) imaging? Should biliary stenting be performed in patients with AIP with obstructive jaundice?

WHEN SHOULD AIP BE SUSPECTED?

The frequent acute presentations of AIP are obstructive jaundice, no or mild abdominal pain, anorexia, and new-onset diabetes mellitus.[2,16–18] Serum biochemical tests usually show abnormal levels of pancreatic or biliary enzymes, and even increased levels of cancer antigen 19-9.[16,19,20] Most patients with AIP are older than 50 years, and male predominance is usually noted.[3,5,18,21,22] These are all also the features of patients with pancreatic cancer, which complicates the differentiation of AIP from pancreatic cancer solely based on clinical manifestation and blood biochemistry.

In clinical practice, these clinical manifestations routinely lead to performance of imaging studies, especially abdominal CT scans. The typical image of AIP on CT scan is diffuse enlargement of the pancreas with a capsulelike rim and delayed homogeneous enhancement, lacking upstream duct dilatation (**Fig. 1**).[23,24] However, only 20% to 40% of patients with AIP show this typical imaging,[17,18,22,25] whereas the remainder show the indeterminate (atypical) imaging features of AIP such as a low-density pancreatic mass, focal/segmental pancreatic enlargement, and dilatation/cutoff of the main pancreatic duct (see **Fig. 1**). The diagnosis of AIP therefore requires a high index of suspicion based on imaging findings. Clinicians as well as radiologists must be aware of the imaging features for suspicion of AIP rather than pancreatic cancer (**Table 1**).[3,4,26]

TWO SUBTYPES OF AIP

The increasing number of reported AIP cases had resulted in identification of several clinical, serologic, and histopathologic features that distinguish the 2 subtypes of the disease. Type 1 and type 2 AIP correspond roughly to lymphoplasmacytic sclerosing pancreatitis and idiopathic duct-centric chronic pancreatitis, respectively.[13,27] There is a difference in the prevalence of 2 subtypes. Type 2 AIP seems to be common in the United States and Europe but rare in East Asia.[22] Type 1 AIP is regarded as the

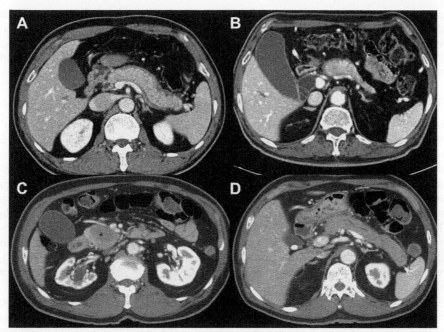

Fig. 1. Typical (*A*) and indeterminate CT findings (*B–D*) for AIP. (*A*) Diffuse enlargement of the pancreas with a low-density capsulelike rim. (*B*) Segmental enlargement of the pancreas. (*C, D*) A discrete pancreatic mass (*asterisk*) on pancreatic head with enlargement of pancreatic body/tail and minimal upstream dilatation.

pancreatic manifestation of systemic IgG4-related disease, whereas type 2 AIP is not.[27–29] Compared with patients with type 2 AIP, patients with type 1 AIP are older, have increased serum IgG4 levels, and show a strong association with sclerosing cholangitis, sialadenitis, and retroperitoneal fibrosis.[8,30–32] In contrast, patients with

Table 1	
Imaging findings suggestive of AIP versus pancreatic cancer	
Findings Suggestive of AIP	**Findings Suggestive of Pancreatic Cancer**
Diffuse pancreatic enlargement with a capsulelike low-density rim	Parenchymal atrophy above the stricture
Delayed homogeneous enhancement	Heterogeneous/poor enhancement
Absent or minimal upstream duct dilatation despite a discrete pancreatic mass	Marked upstream duct dilatation
Double duct sign without a discrete pancreatic mass on CT in a patient with obstructive jaundice	A visible mass
Multifocal strictures of main pancreatic duct with normal-looking intervening duct	A single localized stricture
Other organ involvement such as proximal bile duct stricture, salivary glands enlargement, renal involvement, or retroperitoneal fibrosis	Multiple hepatic nodules suggestive of liver metastasis
Absence of exophytic mass and smooth pancreatic contour	Exophytic mass and irregular pancreatic contour

type 2 AIP are younger, have normal serum IgG4 levels, and show an association with inflammatory bowel disease.[8,22,29,31] In seronegative AIP cases without other organ involvement, determination of the AIP subtype may not be possible without the aid of histopathology because a proportion of histologically confirmed type 1 AIP can also show seronegativity and no other organ involvement.[1,33]

WHEN CAN AIP BE DIAGNOSED WITHOUT ENDOSCOPIC EXAMINATION?

Diagnosis of AIP can be made when resected pancreata reveals the typical histopathologic features of AIP; however, AIP is usually diagnosed by a combination of the 5 cardinal features of AIP: imaging, serology, other organ involvement, histology, and response to steroids. In patients with typical imaging findings of AIP (diffuse pancreatic enlargement with or without a rim, delayed homogeneous enhancement, and no main pancreatic duct dilatation), AIP can be diagnosed by the presence of positive serology or other organ involvement, without the aid of endoscopic examination (**Fig. 2**). As a serologic marker, increased serum IgG4 level is suggestive of AIP.[34] According to the ICDC, other organ involvement in AIP is defined by radiologic evidence (hilar/intrahepatic biliary stricture, retroperitoneal fibrosis, and renal involvement), physical evidence (bilaterally enlarged salivary glands), and compatible histology of extrapancreatic organs.[1]

Contrary to typical imaging, in patients with indeterminate findings of AIP (pancreatic mass, focal/segmental pancreatic enlargement, and cutoff/dilatation of the main pancreatic duct), exclusion of pancreatic cancer is the prerequisite for the diagnosis of AIP and more collateral evidence of AIP is needed to proceed to further evaluation for AIP (see **Fig. 2**). As many as 10% of patients with pancreatic cancer have increased serum IgG4 levels; consequently, increase of serum IgG4 levels alone should not be accepted as diagnostic of AIP in patients with indeterminate imaging.[3,34,35] These levels instead serve as a useful first screen to determine those patients who need further evaluation for possibility of AIP.[34] Investigation of patients with indeterminate imaging findings might be difficult and requires a substantial amount of experience. These patients should be referred to a tertiary center that has clinicians and radiologists who are familiar with both AIP and pancreatic cancer.[12]

APPROPRIATE ENDOSCOPIC APPROACHES IN SUSPECTED AIP: WHEN AND WHICH?

Various endoscopic tools are now used for diagnostic purposes in patients with AIP and for the differentiation of AIP from pancreatic cancer (**Table 2**). The diversity of diagnostic algorithms for AIP in individual countries may reflect differences in practice patterns in the usage of various tests and differences in local expertise. Endoscopists need to be fully aware of the strengths (and weaknesses) of the various endoscopic examinations and to use these tools properly for individual clinical situations.[13] We submit the following recommendations, but the type and sequence of endoscopic workup may vary from center to center depending on local facilities, expertise, and subspecialty background of a treating physician.

Cases with Typical CT Imaging for AIP

Patients with typical CT imaging require endoscopic examination when no collateral evidence of AIP is present, based on serology or other organ involvement. According to the ICDC, pancreatic core biopsy (preferably EUS-guided) is recommended for these patients to obtain pancreatic tissue for the diagnosis of AIP.[1] In centers that routinely perform ERP to diagnose AIP, ERCP may be an alternative choice for obtaining pancreatograms and biopsy specimens from the major duodenal papilla or bile

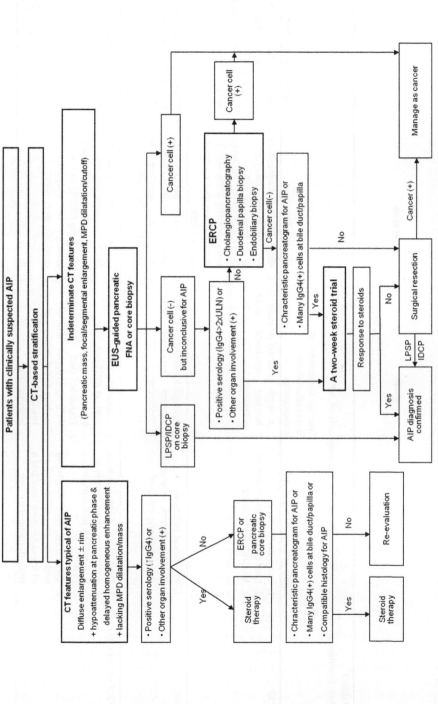

Fig. 2. A practical approach to the diagnosis of AIP. IDCP, idiopathic chronic duct-centric pancreatitis; LPSP, lymphoplasmacytic sclerosing pancreatitis; MPD, main pancreatic duct.

Table 2
Armamentarium of endoscopic examination for the diagnosis of AIP

	Findings Suggestive of AIP	Findings Suggestive of Pancreaticobiliary Malignancies	Strengths of the Test	Limitations of the Test
ERP	1. Long stricture 2. Lack of upstream dilatation 3. Multifocal strictures	1. A single localized stricture 2. Marked upstream duct dilatation	1. Helpful in the diagnosis of AIP with atypical imaging or seronegative AIP 2. High sensitivity (70%–90%) and specificity (80%–90%) in the centers that routinely perform ERP	1. Low sensitivity in the centers that do not routinely perform ERP 2. Concern of post-ERCP pancreatitis
ERC	1. Multifocal strictures 2. Mild proximal dilatation despite a long stricture	1. A single localized stricture 2. Marked proximal duct dilatation	1. ERCP is usually performed to relieve biliary obstruction 2. Allows tissue sampling from ampulla or bile duct	1. In cases with isolated stricture of intrapancreatic CBD, ERC finding of AIP is similar to that of pancreatic or CBD cancer
IDUS of the bile duct	1. Thickening of the bile duct wall (>1 mm) on IDUS in a nonstenotic bile duct on ERC 2. Concentric wall thickening with smooth configuration of the outermost layer and a smooth luminal surface	1. Thickening of the bile duct wall on IDUS only in a stenotic bile duct on ERC 2. Eccentric wall thickening with an irregular luminal surface and disruption of the layer structure of the bile duct wall	1. Can be performed during ERCP in a single session 2. High sensitivity (85%) and specificity (100%) in the setting of AIP with thickened bile duct wall	1. Expertise in ERCP and EUS is required

EUS	1. Diffuse hypoechoic pancreatic enlargement 2. Concentric bile duct wall thickening (homogeneous regular thickening with a hypoechoic intermediate layer and hyperechoic outer and inner layer)	1. Hypoechoic pancreatic mass	1. Can examine the pancreas in real time 2. Allows EUS-FNA or core biopsy	1. Diverse spectrum of EUS morphologic findings in AIP
EUS elastography	1. Hard (blue) area including mass and surrounding pancreatic parenchyma	1. Hard area confined to the site of the low-echoic tumor	1. Noninvasive measurement of tissue stiffness 2. Might increase the yield of EUS-FNA for diagnosing malignancy	1. Subjective color interpretation 2. Needs special equipment and expertise
Contrast-enhanced (harmonic) EUS	1. Hypervascularization of pseudotumor	1. Hypovascular mass	1. Real-time perfusion imaging 2. Might increase the yield of EUS-FNA for diagnosing malignancy	1. Needs special equipment and expertise

Abbreviations: CBD, common bile duct; ERC, endoscopic retrograde cholangiography; FNA, fine-needle aspiration; IDUS, intraductal ultrasonography.

ducts for the purpose of IgG4 immunostaining. In cases with typical CT imaging but no collateral evidence, the diagnosis of AIP can be made when pancreatic biopsy specimens show compatible histology for AIP, or when biopsy specimens from the major duodenal papilla or bile ducts show positive IgG4 immunostaining.

Cases with Indeterminate CT Imaging for AIP

Patients with indeterminate CT findings for AIP require exclusion of malignancy as a prerequisite of further workup to diagnose AIP; EUS should be considered as a first step. EUS is superior to other radiologic modalities, including CT scans, for the detection of a pancreatic mass, because it has the negative predictive value for pancreatic tumor detection of nearly 100%.[36-38] When a pancreatic mass is detected, real-time EUS can guide cytology/biopsy, allowing distinction of benign from malignant masses.[13]

ERCP
ERP

Characteristic ERP features of AIP that are useful in the differential diagnosis of AIP and pancreatic cancer are: (1) a long (>one-third the length of the pancreatic duct) stricture; (2) lack of upstream dilatation from the stricture (<5 mm); and (3) multifocal strictures with intervening normal-looking duct (**Fig. 3**).[39] In contrast, the typical ERP appearance of pancreatic cancer is a single focal stricture associated with marked upstream duct dilatation.[40] The sensitivity and specificity of ERP for differentiating AIP from pancreatic cancer are 33% to 91% and 80% to 90%, respectively.[26,39,41,42] The use of ERP shows poor sensitivity in centers that do not routinely perform ERP to diagnose AIP.[39]

The fear of post-ERCP pancreatitis causes Western endoscopists, in general, to avoid injecting the pancreatic duct in patients with obstructive jaundice.[1,13] However, AIP is a form of chronic pancreatitis that has the characteristic of protecting against ERCP-induced pancreatitis, perhaps because of fibrosis and decreases in enzymatic activity.[41,43] No complication of ERCP-induced pancreatitis has been reported in AIP studies.[41,44,45]

Magnetic resonance cholangiopancreatography (MRCP) is not equivalent for showing pancreatic ductal narrowing in patients with AIP because MRCP may not accurately depict diffusely narrowed main pancreatic duct that is thinner than normal

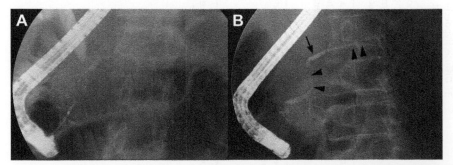

Fig. 3. (A) Typical finding of diffuse irregular narrowing (thinner than normal diameter) of the main pancreatic duct on ERP in a patient with AIP. Narrowing of distal CBD is also seen. (B) Typical finding of multifocal strictures (*arrowheads*) with intervening normal-looking duct (*arrow*) on ERP in a patient with AIP.

diameter, in patients with AIP.[46,47] Secretin-stimulated MRCP may improve the visualization of the narrow pancreatic duct and may be useful in examining patients with suspected AIP.[13,48]

Endoscopic Retrograde Cholangiography

Patients with AIP commonly show the co-occurrence of bile duct abnormalities with strictures of the common bile duct (CBD) and occasionally the proximal bile duct. However, cholangiographic findings of isolated strictures of intrapancreatic CBD in patients with AIP are similar to those of patients with biliary stricture associated with pancreatic cancer or distal CBD cancer. Unlike intrapancreatic CBD strictures, intrahepatic or hilar bile duct strictures associated with pancreatic lesions give important clues to the diagnosis of AIP, because proximal bile duct strictures are rarely detected in pancreatic cancer. For these strictures, multifocal strictures and mild proximal duct dilatation despite a long stricture are characteristic findings of AIP, whereas a single localized stricture with marked proximal duct dilatation, is a characteristic of cholangiocarcinoma.[13,49]

MRCP permits the noninvasive acquisition of cross-sectional magnetic resonance images of the pancreas as well as of the pancreatic and biliary ducts. Moreover, MRCP has been shown to be comparable with endoscopic retrograde cholangiography (ERC) for the evaluation of bile ductal abnormalities, including sclerosing cholangitis.[50] MRCP may therefore be recommended as a first step for the evaluation of suspected AIP associated with IgG4-related sclerosing cholangitis.

IS THERE A ROLE FOR DIAGNOSTIC ERP FOR AIP?

Substantial differences have been noted between American and Asian diagnostic strategies.[14] Asian pancreatologists usually perform diagnostic ERP in most patients with suspected AIP, whereas American pancreatologists rarely use this procedure.[1,14] However, the American strategy for distinguishing AIP from pancreatic cancer dictates that approximately 30% of cases of AIP needed pancreatic core biopsy, resection, or steroid trial for the diagnosis of AIP, because of seronegativity and lack of other organ involvement.[3,14]

A tailored approach for the use of ERP was reported in a recent study comparing CT alone and CT with additional ERP for the diagnosis of AIP.[41] When patients with AIP were divided into 2 subgroups according to CT features (typical vs indeterminate), an additional ERP increased the sensitivity and specificity for distinguishing AIP from pancreatic cancer if the CT features were indeterminate. On the other hand, when the findings on CT were typical for AIP, little incremental benefit was gained from an additional ERP.[41] That study also revealed that the use of ERP could obviate pancreatic core biopsy to diagnose AIP in 17 (63%) of 27 patients with AIP, who would otherwise have undergone pancreatic core biopsy based on negative serology and lack of other organ involvement.[41] In addition, there were no cases of ERP-induced pancreatitis in 84 patients with AIP.[41] Diagnostic ERP may therefore be useful in the setting of indeterminate CT imaging for AIP or seronegative AIP without other organ involvement.

A recent study reported that the typical pancreatographic abnormalities seen in type 1 AIP were also seen in type 2 AIP with similar frequencies.[51] Type 2 AIP potentially benefits the most from diagnostic ERP because patients with type 2 AIP typically have normal levels of serum IgG4 and negative tissue IgG4.[52] However, 1 role of ERCP (namely, obtaining biopsy specimens from the bile duct/ampulla for IgG4 immunostaining) may be limited in the diagnosis of type 2 AIP because type 2 AIP is distinct from IgG4-related disease.

EUS

EUS imaging includes conventional EUS imaging, EUS elastography, contrast-enhanced EUS, and intraductal ultrasonography (IDUS). Although this type of imaging cannot be used as the sole basis to make a diagnosis of AIP, it can aid in gathering extra arguments for differentiating AIP from pancreatic cancer and can guide aspiration/biopsy.

Conventional EUS Imaging

EUS can reveal pancreatic parenchymal and ductal features in substantial detail.[53] Diffuse hypoechoic pancreatic enlargement, sometimes with hyperechoic inclusions, is the characteristic morphologic finding for AIP.[53–55] According to Hoki and colleagues,[53] diffuse hypoechoic area, diffuse enlargement, peripancreatic hypoechoic margin, and bile duct wall thickening are more frequently found in AIP than in pancreatic cancer. A finding of a peripancreatic hypoechoic margin corresponds to a capsulelike low-density rim on CT.[53] Concentric bile duct wall thickening is another characteristic finding for AIP, sometimes depicted as a homogeneous, regular thickening with a hypoechoic intermediate layer and hyperechoic outer and inner layers (3-layer type).[53,55,56] However, in AIP, the EUS morphologic spectrum is diverse and may show a mass lesion mimicking pancreatic cancer.[54,57]

EUS Elastography/Contrast-Enhanced (Harmonic) EUS

Elastography is a technology that shows the relative stiffness of the examined lesion compared with the surrounding tissue.[58] The stiffness is estimated by analyzing back-scattered ultrasound (US) signals while the probe is compressing the tissue.[58,59] Soft tissue is displayed as red, intermediate areas as green, and hard areas as blue.[59] Malignant tumors are basically harder than benign tumors or normal tissue.[58] According to a recent meta-analysis, which analyzed 13 studies involving a total of 1042 patients,[60] the pooled sensitivity and specificity of EUS elastography for differentiating benign from malignant pancreatic masses were 95% and 69%, respectively. Differentiation of mass-forming AIP from pancreatic cancer by EUS elastography relies more on the stiffness of the surrounding pancreas, rather than that of the mass lesion itself. A study by Dietrich and colleagues[61] revealed that elastographic imaging of patients with pancreatic cancer showed a markedly hard (blue) area confined to the site of the low-echoic tumor area, whereas in patients with AIP, the hard area was not restricted to the mass lesion but also included the surrounding pancreatic parenchyma.

Contrast-enhanced (harmonic) EUS may provide images of microcirculation and parenchymal perfusion through the use of a contrast agent and Doppler mode/harmonic detection mode.[58] The contrast agent creates encapsulated gas microbubbles, which produce a strong back-scattered acoustic signal when hit by a US wave. Contrast-enhanced EUS may be performed by using color or power Doppler or, more appropriately, by using a dedicated contrast harmonic imaging mode.[58,62] Mass-forming AIP can be differentiated from pancreatic cancer by contrast-enhanced (harmonic) EUS, because a pseudotumor caused by AIP typically appears as hypervascularization, whereas a hypoechoic tumor caused by pancreatic cancer appears as a hypovascular mass (**Figs. 4** and **5**).[63–65] A recent meta-analysis analyzing 12 studies involving 1139 patients showed that the pooled sensitivity of contrast-enhanced EUS for the differential diagnosis of pancreatic adenocarcinoma was 94%, and the specificity was 89%.[62]

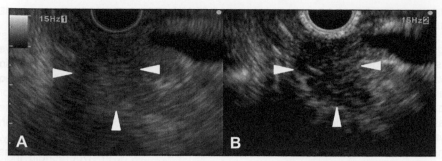

Fig. 4. (*A*) Conventional EUS imaging of a 73-year-old patient with pancreatic cancer shows low-echoic mass in pancreas (*arrowheads*). (*B*) Contrast-enhanced harmonic EUS shows hypoenhancement in the mass (*arrowheads*).

Diagnosis of malignancy with these new EUS techniques may also have the potential of selecting the most suspicious area of a lymph node/tumor, thereby guiding the fine-needle aspiration (FNA)/biopsy more specifically and increasing the diagnostic yield of EUS-guided tissue sampling.[66–68]

IDUS of the Bile Duct Wall

Biliary involvement of AIP presents radiographically as bile duct strictures with ductal wall thickening.[13,49,69] Evaluation of the thickening of the bile duct wall may provide supplemental information for differentiating AIP from pancreatobiliary malignancies. Transpapillary IDUS can be performed during ERCP in a single session. Once the IDUS probe (scanning frequency of 20 MHz) is inserted into the bile duct along the guidewire, IDUS provides high-resolution images of the layer structure of the bile duct wall, which normally has an inner hypoechoic and outer hyperechoic layer.[13] The IDUS findings for AIP are concentric bile duct wall thickening with smooth configuration of the outermost layer and a smooth luminal surface.[55,70–72] In contrast, those for cholangiocarcinoma include eccentric wall thickening with an irregular luminal surface, disruption of the layer structure of the bile duct wall, and a hypoechoic mass with irregular margins. Naitoh and colleagues[71] reported that the most specific IDUS finding for differentiating AIP from cholangiocarcinoma was thickening of the bile duct wall (exceeding 1 mm) in a bile duct that is nonstenotic on ERC (specificity 100%, sensitivity 85%).

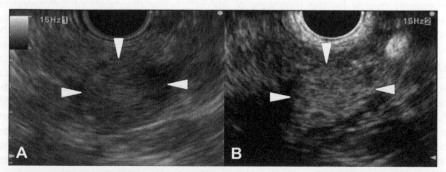

Fig. 5. (*A*) Conventional EUS imaging of a 78-year-old patient with AIP shows low-echoic mass in pancreas (*arrowheads*). (*B*) Contrast-enhanced harmonic EUS shows a homogeneous isoenhancement in the mass (*arrowheads*).

WHAT ARE THE ROLES OF ENDOSCOPIC BIOPSIES AND IGG4 IMMUNOSTAINING IN THE DIAGNOSIS OF AIP?

Addition of diagnostic sample acquisition at EUS/ERCP might obviate further invasive testing, thereby making EUS/ERCP the cornerstone procedures for endoscopic evaluation that differentiates AIP from pancreatobiliary malignancies. EUS-guided sampling techniques for differentiation include (1) EUS-guided FNA (EUS-FNA) for pancreatic mass and for biliary stricture and (2) EUS-guided core biopsy for the pancreas. ERCP-guided sampling techniques include (1) bile duct biopsy and brush cytology, (2) pancreatic duct biopsy and brush cytology, and (3) ampullary biopsy. The role of pathologic examination is 2-fold in the diagnosis of AIP, especially in cases with indeterminate imaging. The first is the exclusion of malignancy and the second is the acquisition of pathologic evidence for AIP (**Table 3**).[73] The recommended first-line procedure to exclude malignancy is EUS-FNA in cases in which sampling of a suspected pancreatic cancer is indicated, whereas ERCP-guided sampling is recommended in cases in which sampling of a suspected bile duct cancer is indicated, particularly when ERCP is needed to relieve obstructive jaundice.[74–77]

Histopathologic confirmative diagnosis of AIP is often difficult because of the small endoscopic biopsy specimen. Given the nature of AIP (specifically, type 1 AIP) as part of a systemic IgG4-related fibroinflammatory disease, IgG4 immunostaining of the pancreatic/extrapancreatic tissue is often used to support the diagnosis of AIP.[3,78] Positive IgG4 immunostaining of the pancreatic/extrapancreatic tissue is found independently of the presence of increased serum IgG4 levels.[78] The cutoff for the number of IgG4-positive plasma cells in a biopsy/surgical specimen has recently been proposed by international consensus.[79] The consensus statement asserts that the appropriate cutoff point may vary from organ to organ: (1) more than 10 IgG4-positive plasma cells per high-power field (HPF) for pancreatic biopsy, bile duct biopsy, and liver biopsy specimens; (2) more than 50 IgG4-positive plasma cells/HPF for surgical specimens of the pancreas, bile duct, and liver; and (3) more than 100 IgG4-positive plasma cells/HPF for a lymph node, salivary gland, and lacrimal gland.[79] The sensitivities of positive IgG4 immunostaining (>10 IgG4-positive plasma cells/HPF) reported in the literature vary widely in pancreatic tissue (41%–88%) as well as in extrapancreatic tissue (18%–88%, see **Table 3**).[45,51,71,80–88] The sensitivity of positive IgG4 immunostaining may depend on: (1) the disease activity and stage; (2) the size of the acquired tissue; and (3) the proportion of type 2 AIP. The occasional presence of positive tissue IgG4 has been reported to be as much as 12% in pancreatobiliary malignancies.[71,78,88,89] The result of positive IgG4 immunostaining in isolation does not necessarily qualify for the diagnosis of AIP.[3,78,79] The diagnosis of AIP requires cautious correlation with the histopathologic features in the sample, as well as with the other cardinal features of AIP.[3,79]

EUS-FNA and Core Biopsy for Pancreatic Lesions

When a pancreatic mass is detected during a diagnostic workup, EUS-FNA is the first-line procedure for exclusion of malignancy.[75] A recent review article that analyzed 28 studies involving 4225 patients[90] documented that EUS-FNA provides a median sensitivity of 83%, specificity of 100%, negative predictive value of 72%, and diagnostic accuracy of 88% in distinguishing benign pancreatic disease from pancreatic cancer. These diagnostic sensitivities of EUS-FNA are higher than the sensitivity (47%–67%, mean 52%, 3 studies involving 124 patients) of ERCP-guided transpapillary pancreatic duct biopsy/cytology.[91–93] Even compared with transabdominal US/CT-guided pancreatic FNA (sensitivity, 60%–80%), EUS-FNA has a higher diagnostic

Table 3
Armamentarium of endoscopic sampling techniques for differentiation of AIP from pancreatobiliary malignancies

	Primary Role for Differentiation	Sensitivity for Diagnosing Pancreatobiliary Malignancy	Sensitivity for Diagnosing AIP	Positive IgG4 Immunostaining in Patients with AIP	Positive IgG4 Immunostaining in Patients with Pancreatobiliary Malignancy
EUS-FNA for the pancreatic lesion[90,97,104–107]	Exclusion of malignancy	83% (in 4225 patients)	Variable	N-A	N-A
EUS-FNA for biliary stricture[113]	Exclusion of malignancy	84% (in 284 patients)	N-A	N-A	N-A
EUS-guided core biopsy of the pancreatic lesion[51,57,78,80,82,85,88,89]	Tissue diagnosis of AIP	Similar to that of EUS-FNA (for nontransduodenal routes)	68% (in 117 patients)[a]	51% (in 135 patients)[a]	9% (in 55 patients with pancreatic cancer)[a]
ERCP-guided endobiliary biopsy/brush cytology for the bile duct[45,71,81,82,87,109,111]	Exclusion of malignancy Tissue acquisition for IgG4 immunostaining	Biopsy: 63% (in 127 patients) Brush cytology: 59% (in 306 patients)	0% (in 85 patients)	48% (in 85 patients)	2% (in 51 patients with cholangiocarcinoma)
ERCP-guided intraductal biopsy/brush cytology for the pancreatic duct[91–93]	Exclusion of malignancy	52% (in 124 patients)	N-A	N-A	N-A
Ampullary biopsy[45,83,84,86]	Tissue acquisition for IgG4 immunostaining	N-A	N-A	60% (in 85 patients)	3% (in 92 patients with pancreatobiliary malignancies)

Abbreviations: FNA, fine-needle aspiration; N-A, not available.
[a] The number included some percutaneous or surgical approaches.

sensitivity, particularly for small lesions, and it also has an advantage of a lower risk of peritoneal seeding.[75,94–96] Although cytopathologic examination of EUS-FNA specimens allows detection of malignancy, a pancreatic tissue specimen is still required for the histopathologic diagnosis of AIP.[3,57,75,85,97]

Potential advantages of pancreatic tissue sampling include preservation of tissue architecture and reliable immunostaining.[75] Pancreatic biopsies with IgG4 immunostaining showed moderate sensitivities (47%–81%, mean 68%, 5 studies involving 117 patients) for the histologic diagnosis of AIP.[51,57,80,82,85] EUS-guided core biopsy of the pancreas is usually performed to obtain tissue for unique histopathologic and immunochemical characteristics of AIP.[57,85] Transabdominal US/CT-guided pancreatic biopsy can be considered as an alternative to EUS-guided core biopsy, especially in centers with limited EUS expertise.[13,80,82] Until now, EUS-guided core biopsy has been available in only a few specialized centers, and it has shown a high failure rate when the lesions are located on the pancreatic head.[68] EUS-guided core biopsy is expected to become more widespread and more successful even for the pancreatic head, with the availability of a newly developed fine-needle biopsy needle (ProCore reverse bevel technology; Cook Endoscopy, Winston-Salem, NC).[13,98,99]

Some groups suggested that tissue samples adequate for histopathologic assessment can be obtained with standard EUS-FNA needle.[68,100–103] Several recent studies using conventional 19-gauge or 22-gauge FNA needles showed that EUS-guided FNA biopsy can provide tissue samples adequate for the histopathologic diagnosis of AIP, with a surprisingly low rate (7%–9%) of impossible histopathologic analysis.[104–106] On the contrary, another recent study reported that EUS-FNA biopsy using a 22-gauge FNA needle provided tissue samples that were adequate for the histopathologic diagnosis of pancreatic cancer, but were inadequate for the histopathologic diagnosis of AIP (0% in 21 patients).[107] Further studies may be needed to confirm the ability for reliable tissue acquisition by conventional EUS-FNA needle and its diagnostic efficacy for AIP.

ERCP-guided Bile Duct Biopsy and Brush Cytology

When a pathologic diagnosis is required in the setting of suspected biliary malignancy, ERCP-guided sampling for bile duct stricture is recommended as the first-line procedure, particularly for patients with obstructive jaundice.[76,108] Recent studies indicated that the sensitivities of endobiliary biopsy and brush cytology for distinguishing benign biliary disease from cholangiocarcinoma were 63% (6 studies involving 127 patients) and 59% (18 studies involving 306 patients), respectively.[74,109] This sensitivity may be increased with the combination of the 2 techniques.[74,110] Even in the biliary stricture associated with pancreatic cancer, endobiliary biopsy and brush cytology showed a fair sensitivity of 46% (6 studies involving 104 patients) and 41% (18 studies involving 508 patients), respectively, for diagnosing malignancy.[74,109]

Contrary to the pancreas biopsy specimen obtained by EUS guidance, the small endobiliary biopsy specimen via ERCP does not show the full spectrum of AIP histology (0% in 85 patients with AIP).[45,71,81,82,87,111] However, IgG4 immunostaining of an endobiliary biopsy specimen may provide further histologic support for the diagnosis of AIP. The mean sensitivity and specificity for IgG4 immunostaining of endobiliary biopsies to differentiate AIP from malignancy were 48% and 98% (6 studies involving 85 patients with AIP and 51 patients with pancreatobiliary malignancies), respectively.[45,71,81,82,87,111]

EUS-FNA for the Bile Duct Lesions

Although ERCP-guided approaches for biliary stricture are well established, alternative sampling techniques may be required when ERCP-guided sampling does not provide a definitive diagnosis because of its moderate sensitivity.[108,112] EUS-FNA shows high sensitivity for diagnosis of cholangiocarcinoma in patients with previous negative imaging and nondiagnostic ERCP-guided sampling.[77] EUS-FNA also has an advantage of identifying and sampling regional and distant lymph nodes. A recent meta-analysis (9 studies involving 284 patients) showed that EUS-FNA had a pooled sensitivity of 84% and specificity of 100% for differentiating between benign and malignant biliary strictures.[113] However, EUS-FNA for indeterminate biliary stricture may show a lower yield when bile duct wall thickening rather than a mass is visualized by EUS.[77] Because IgG4-related sclerosing cholangitis usually presents as bile ductal wall thickening, high sensitivity of EUS-FNA for diagnosis of cholangiocarcinoma may be limited in the setting of suspected AIP with sclerosing cholangitis. In the evaluation of biliary strictures, EUS-FNA may be recommended in the absence of obstructive jaundice or when ERCP-guided sampling is nondiagnostic.[108]

Ampullary Biopsy

The ampulla (major duodenal papilla) is often involved in AIP because its structure corresponds anatomically to the junction of the CBD and the main pancreatic duct.[114] Duodenoscopic biopsy of the ampulla may be an easy and safe method for obtaining tissue for IgG4 immunostaining, particularly when pancreatic tissue is not available because IgG4 immunostaining positivity of the ampulla may be well correlated with that of the pancreas.[86] The mean sensitivity and specificity for IgG4 immunostaining of ampullary biopsies to differentiate AIP from malignancy were 60% and 97% (4 studies involving 85 patients with AIP and 92 patients with pancreatobiliary malignancy), respectively.[45,83,84,86]

WHAT IS THE PROPER USE OF THE STEROID TRIAL IN THE DIAGNOSIS OF AIP IN PATIENTS WITH INDETERMINATE CT IMAGING?
Careful Patient Selection by Specialists in Pancreatology

Patients with suspected AIP and a continued need for differentiation from pancreatic cancer because of indeterminate CT imaging occasionally cannot be diagnosed even after a thorough investigation, including imaging, serology, endoscopic examinations, and biopsies. In these select cases with diagnostic uncertainty, steroid responsiveness is a reliable test to confirm the diagnosis of AIP and differentiate it from pancreatic cancer.[4,115] A steroid trial (steroid use as a diagnostic trial) should be differentiated from steroid therapy, in which corticosteroids are given to the patients already diagnosed with AIP. A steroid trial should not be used as a substitute for a thorough search for cause, and its use should be restricted to patients with considerable collateral evidence for AIP and only after negative investigations for pancreatobiliary malignancies.[1,4] The investigations for exclusion of pancreatobiliary malignancies should include EUS (with FNA in cases of depicted pancreatobiliary mass/lymph node) and ERCP-guided endobiliary biopsy in cases of biliary stricture. Repeat sampling (mostly EUS-FNA) may be warranted in patients with continued suspicion of pancreatobiliary malignancies, despite indeterminate or negative findings at initial EUS-FNA or ERCP-guided biopsy.[116,117]

Objective Indices for Steroid Responsiveness

Indices for steroid responsiveness must be objectively monitored and interpreted with caution. The ICDC stipulate that response to steroids be evaluated by radiologically demonstrable resolution or marked improvement in pancreatic/extrapancreatic manifestations.[1] Serum IgG4 levels cannot be used as a marker for steroid responsiveness, because increased serum IgG4 levels, even in patients with pancreatic cancer, can decrease with the administration of corticosteroids.[1,10] Improvement of pancreatic swelling should also be interpreted with caution, because pancreatic swelling that developed from obstructive pancreatitis associated with pancreatic cancer may also be relieved by the administration of corticosteroids because of anti-inflammatory effect of corticosteroids.[1,4] We use the stringent definition of positive steroid responsiveness as relief of the main pancreatic ductal narrowing and, if present, resolution or measurable reduction of the pancreatic mass as well.[4]

Assessment of Steroid Responsiveness After a 2-Week Steroid Trial

Steroid responsiveness should be assessed 2 weeks after the initiation of steroids.[1,3,4] If the response to steroids is negative or equivocal, surgical exploration should be conducted.[4] The reasons for assessing steroid responsiveness after a 2-week steroid trial are as follows: (1) radiologic improvement of AIP can occur as early as 1 to 2 weeks after steroid therapy; (2) given the error inherent in EUS-FNA or ERCP-guided intraductal biopsy/cytology, possible cancer progression in resectable patients during a steroid trial is a concern; and (3) glucocorticoid courses of less than 3 weeks' duration may be discontinued without tapering because they have an insignificant effect on the hypothalamic-pituitary-adrenal axis.[4,44,118,119] Our group suggested that a 2-week delay in operation may not adversely affect the surgical outcome of potentially resectable pancreatic cancer.[4] If the tumor becomes unresectable during this delay, then earlier surgery probably would not have dramatically changed the prognosis of such an aggressive tumor.[12]

SHOULD BILIARY STENTING BE PERFORMED IN PATIENTS WITH AIP WITH OBSTRUCTIVE JAUNDICE?

Obstructive jaundice is the most common initial presentation (50%–75%) of AIP.[18,22] Although some cases show relief of jaundice by steroid therapy alone without stent placement, a plastic biliary stent is mostly placed for jaundiced patients with AIP (usually total bilirubin >3 mg/dL) during the workup of jaundice before the initiation of steroid therapy.[5,15,21,81,120–124] The reasons for this practice are as follows: (1) steroid treatment may trigger or worsen cholangitis in patients with unresolved biliary obstruction[122]; (2) biliary strictures in AIP may require a longer duration of steroid therapy to respond[49,81,125]; and (3) there may be diagnostic uncertainty in case of indeterminate pancreatic imaging. Most biliary stents can be removed after 1 to 2 months, depending on the improvement of biliary stricture or liver biochemistry.[2,21,81,121,124,126] In rare cases, placement of multiple biliary stents is required for adequate remodeling of bile duct strictures.[125,126]

ACKNOWLEDGMENTS

The authors thank Dr Masayuki Kitano (Kinki University School of Medicine, Japan) for providing figures of contrast-enhanced EUS.

REFERENCES

1. Shimosegawa T, Chari ST, Frulloni L, et al. International consensus diagnostic criteria for autoimmune pancreatitis: guidelines of the International Association of Pancreatology. Pancreas 2011;40:352–8.
2. Kim KP, Kim MH, Song MH, et al. Autoimmune chronic pancreatitis. Am J Gastroenterol 2004;99:1605–16.

3. Chari ST, Takahashi N, Levy MJ, et al. A diagnostic strategy to distinguish auto-immune pancreatitis from pancreatic cancer. Clin Gastroenterol Hepatol 2009;7: 1097–103.
4. Moon SH, Kim MH, Park DH, et al. Is a 2-week steroid trial after initial negative investigation for malignancy useful in differentiating autoimmune pancreatitis from pancreatic cancer? A prospective outcome study. Gut 2008;57:1704–12.
5. Detlefsen S, Zamboni G, Frulloni L, et al. Clinical features and relapse rates after surgery in type 1 autoimmune pancreatitis differ from type 2: a study of 114 surgically treated European patients. Pancreatology 2012;12:276–83.
6. van Heerde MJ, Biermann K, Zondervan PE, et al. Prevalence of autoimmune pancreatitis and other benign disorders in pancreatoduodenectomy for pre-sumed malignancy of the pancreatic head. Dig Dis Sci 2012;57:2458–65.
7. Zyromski NJ. Autoimmune pancreatitis (AIP) masquerading as pancreatic cancer: cutting is not a crime... for now. Dig Dis Sci 2012;57:2246–7.
8. Sah RP, Chari ST, Pannala R, et al. Differences in clinical profile and relapse rate of type 1 versus type 2 autoimmune pancreatitis. Gastroenterology 2010;139: 140–8.
9. Learn PA, Grossman EB, Do RK, et al. Pitfalls in avoiding operation for autoim-mune pancreatitis. Surgery 2011;150:968–74.
10. Gardner TB, Levy MJ, Takahashi N, et al. Misdiagnosis of autoimmune pancre-atitis: a caution to clinicians. Am J Gastroenterol 2009;104:1620–3.
11. Nishimori I, Tamakoshi A, Otsuki M. Prevalence of autoimmune pancreatitis in Japan from a nationwide survey in 2002. J Gastroenterol 2007;42(Suppl 18):6–8.
12. Levy P, Hammel P, Ruszniewski P. Diagnostic challenge in autoimmune pancre-atitis: beware of shipwreck! Gut 2008;57:1646–7.
13. Moon SH, Kim MH. The role of endoscopy in the diagnosis of autoimmune pancreatitis. Gastrointest Endosc 2012;76:645–56.
14. Sugumar A, Chari ST. Distinguishing pancreatic cancer from autoimmune pancreatitis: a comparison of two strategies. Clin Gastroenterol Hepatol 2009; 7:S59–62.
15. Maillette de Buy Wenniger L, Rauws EA, Beuers U. What an endoscopist should know about immunoglobulin-G4-associated disease of the pancreas and biliary tree. Endoscopy 2012;44:66–73.
16. Okazaki K, Kawa S, Kamisawa T, et al. Japanese consensus guidelines for man-agement of autoimmune pancreatitis: I. Concept and diagnosis of autoimmune pancreatitis. J Gastroenterol 2010;45:249–65.
17. Chari ST, Smyrk TC, Levy MJ, et al. Diagnosis of autoimmune pancreatitis: the Mayo Clinic experience. Clin Gastroenterol Hepatol 2006;4:1010–6.
18. Kamisawa T, Kim MH, Liao WC, et al. Clinical characteristics of 327 Asian patients with autoimmune pancreatitis based on Asian diagnostic criteria. Pancreas 2011;40:200–5.
19. Kamisawa T, Egawa N, Nakajima H, et al. Clinical difficulties in the differentiation of autoimmune pancreatitis and pancreatic carcinoma. Am J Gastroenterol 2003;98:2694–9.
20. Wakabayashi T, Kawaura Y, Satomura Y, et al. Clinical and imaging features of autoimmune pancreatitis with focal pancreatic swelling or mass formation: com-parison with so-called tumor-forming pancreatitis and pancreatic carcinoma. Am J Gastroenterol 2003;98:2679–87.
21. Church NI, Pereira SP, Deheragoda MG, et al. Autoimmune pancreatitis: clinical and radiological features and objective response to steroid therapy in a UK series. Am J Gastroenterol 2007;102:2417–25.

22. Kamisawa T, Chari ST, Giday SA, et al. Clinical profile of autoimmune pancreatitis and its histological subtypes: an international multicenter survey. Pancreas 2011;40:809–14.
23. Sahani DV, Kalva SP, Farrell J, et al. Autoimmune pancreatitis: imaging features. Radiology 2004;233:345–52.
24. Sugumar A. Diagnosis and management of autoimmune pancreatitis. Gastroenterol Clin North Am 2012;41:9–22.
25. Nakazawa T, Ohara H, Sano H, et al. Difficulty in diagnosing autoimmune pancreatitis by imaging findings. Gastrointest Endosc 2007;65:99–108.
26. Kamisawa T, Imai M, Yui Chen P, et al. Strategy for differentiating autoimmune pancreatitis from pancreatic cancer. Pancreas 2008;37:e62–7.
27. Deshpande V, Gupta R, Sainani N, et al. Subclassification of autoimmune pancreatitis: a histologic classification with clinical significance. Am J Surg Pathol 2011;35:26–35.
28. Kamisawa T, Okamoto A. Autoimmune pancreatitis: proposal of IgG4-related sclerosing disease. J Gastroenterol 2006;41:613–25.
29. Park DH, Kim MH, Chari ST. Recent advances in autoimmune pancreatitis. Gut 2009;58:1680–9.
30. Kim MH, Moon SH, Park DH. Are all pancreatic lesions responsive to steroid therapy autoimmune pancreatitis? Gut 2009;58:1031–2 [author reply].
31. Notohara K, Burgart LJ, Yadav D, et al. Idiopathic chronic pancreatitis with periductal lymphoplasmacytic infiltration: clinicopathologic features of 35 cases. Am J Surg Pathol 2003;27:1119–27.
32. Sugumar A, Kloppel G, Chari ST. Autoimmune pancreatitis: pathologic subtypes and their implications for its diagnosis. Am J Gastroenterol 2009;104:2308–10 [quiz: 11].
33. Balasubramanian G, Sugumar A, Smyrk TC, et al. Demystifying seronegative autoimmune pancreatitis. Pancreatology 2012;12:289–94.
34. Ghazale A, Chari ST, Smyrk TC, et al. Value of serum IgG4 in the diagnosis of autoimmune pancreatitis and in distinguishing it from pancreatic cancer. Am J Gastroenterol 2007;102:1646–53.
35. Raina A, Krasinskas AM, Greer JB, et al. Serum immunoglobulin G fraction 4 levels in pancreatic cancer: elevations not associated with autoimmune pancreatitis. Arch Pathol Lab Med 2008;132:48–53.
36. Catanzaro A, Richardson S, Veloso H, et al. Long-term follow-up of patients with clinically indeterminate suspicion of pancreatic cancer and normal EUS. Gastrointest Endosc 2003;58:836–40.
37. DeWitt J, Kahaleh M. The role of endoscopy in the evaluation of suspected pancreatic malignancy. Clinical Update, ASGE 2008;16:1–4.
38. Klapman JB, Chang KJ, Lee JG, et al. Negative predictive value of endoscopic ultrasound in a large series of patients with a clinical suspicion of pancreatic cancer. Am J Gastroenterol 2005;100:2658–61.
39. Sugumar A, Levy MJ, Kamisawa T, et al. Endoscopic retrograde pancreatography criteria to diagnose autoimmune pancreatitis: an international multicentre study. Gut 2011;60:666–70.
40. Inoue K, Ohuchida J, Ohtsuka T, et al. Severe localized stenosis and marked dilatation of the main pancreatic duct are indicators of pancreatic cancer instead of chronic pancreatitis on endoscopic retrograde balloon pancreatography. Gastrointest Endosc 2003;58:510–5.
41. Kim JH, Kim MH, Byun JH, et al. Diagnostic strategy for differentiating autoimmune pancreatitis from pancreatic cancer: is an endoscopic retrograde pancreatography essential? Pancreas 2012;41:639–47.

42. Nishino T, Oyama H, Toki F, et al. Differentiation between autoimmune pancreatitis and pancreatic carcinoma based on endoscopic retrograde cholangiopancreatography findings. J Gastroenterol 2010;45:988–96.
43. Freeman ML, DiSario JA, Nelson DB, et al. Risk factors for post-ERCP pancreatitis: a prospective, multicenter study. Gastrointest Endosc 2001;54: 425–34.
44. Horiuchi A, Kawa S, Hamano H, et al. ERCP features in 27 patients with autoimmune pancreatitis. Gastrointest Endosc 2002;55:494–9.
45. Kawakami H, Zen Y, Kuwatani M, et al. IgG4-related sclerosing cholangitis and autoimmune pancreatitis: histological assessment of biopsies from Vater's ampulla and the bile duct. J Gastroenterol Hepatol 2010;25:1648–55.
46. Kamisawa T, Tu Y, Egawa N, et al. Can MRCP replace ERCP for the diagnosis of autoimmune pancreatitis? Abdom Imaging 2009;34:381–4.
47. Park SH, Kim MH, Kim SY, et al. Magnetic resonance cholangiopancreatography for the diagnostic evaluation of autoimmune pancreatitis. Pancreas 2010; 39:1191–8.
48. Carbognin G, Girardi V, Biasiutti C, et al. Autoimmune pancreatitis: imaging findings on contrast-enhanced MR, MRCP and dynamic secretin-enhanced MRCP. Radiol Med 2009;114:1214–31.
49. Nishino T, Toki F, Oyama H, et al. Biliary tract involvement in autoimmune pancreatitis. Pancreas 2005;30:76–82.
50. Vitellas KM, Enns RA, Keogan MT, et al. Comparison of MR cholangiopancreatographic techniques with contrast-enhanced cholangiography in the evaluation of sclerosing cholangitis. AJR Am J Roentgenol 2002;178: 327–34.
51. Song TJ, Kim JH, Kim MH, et al. Comparison of clinical findings between histologically confirmed type 1 and type 2 autoimmune pancreatitis. J Gastroenterol Hepatol 2012;27:700–8.
52. Lerch MM, Mayerle J. The benefits of diagnostic ERCP in autoimmune pancreatitis. Gut 2011;60:565–6.
53. Hoki N, Mizuno N, Sawaki A, et al. Diagnosis of autoimmune pancreatitis using endoscopic ultrasonography. J Gastroenterol 2009;44:154–9.
54. Farrell JJ, Garber J, Sahani D, et al. EUS findings in patients with autoimmune pancreatitis. Gastrointest Endosc 2004;60:927–36.
55. Hyodo N, Hyodo T. Ultrasonographic evaluation in patients with autoimmune-related pancreatitis. J Gastroenterol 2003;38:1155–61.
56. De Lisi S, Buscarini E, Arcidiacono PG, et al. Endoscopic ultrasonography findings in autoimmune pancreatitis: be aware of the ambiguous features and look for the pivotal ones. JOP 2010;11:78–84.
57. Levy MJ, Wiersema MJ, Chari ST. Chronic pancreatitis: focal pancreatitis or cancer? Is there a role for FNA/biopsy? Autoimmune pancreatitis. Endoscopy 2006;38(Suppl 1):S30–5.
58. Fusaroli P, Saftoiu A, Mancino MG, et al. Techniques of image enhancement in EUS (with videos). Gastrointest Endosc 2011;74:645–55.
59. Pedrosa MC, Barth BA, Desilets DJ, et al. Enhanced ultrasound imaging. Gastrointest Endosc 2011;73:857–60.
60. Pei Q, Zou X, Zhang X, et al. Diagnostic value of EUS elastography in differentiation of benign and malignant solid pancreatic masses: a meta-analysis. Pancreatology 2012;12:402–8.
61. Dietrich CF, Hirche TO, Ott M, et al. Real-time tissue elastography in the diagnosis of autoimmune pancreatitis. Endoscopy 2009;41:718–20.

62. Gong TT, Hu DM, Zhu Q. Contrast-enhanced EUS for differential diagnosis of pancreatic mass lesions: a meta-analysis. Gastrointest Endosc 2012;76:301–9.
63. Hocke M, Ignee A, Dietrich CF. Contrast-enhanced endoscopic ultrasound in the diagnosis of autoimmune pancreatitis. Endoscopy 2011;43:163–5.
64. Kitano M, Kudo M, Yamao K, et al. Characterization of small solid tumors in the pancreas: the value of contrast-enhanced harmonic endoscopic ultrasonography. Am J Gastroenterol 2012;107:303–10.
65. Kitano M, Sakamoto H, Komaki T, et al. New techniques and future perspective of EUS for the differential diagnosis of pancreatic malignancies: contrast harmonic imaging. Dig Endosc 2011;23(Suppl 1):46–50.
66. Giovannini M, Thomas B, Erwan B, et al. Endoscopic ultrasound elastography for evaluation of lymph nodes and pancreatic masses: a multicenter study. World J Gastroenterol 2009;15:1587–93.
67. Napoleon B, Alvarez-Sanchez MV, Gincoul R, et al. Contrast-enhanced harmonic endoscopic ultrasound in solid lesions of the pancreas: results of a pilot study. Endoscopy 2010;42:564–70.
68. Polkowski M, Larghi A, Weynand B, et al. Learning, techniques, and complications of endoscopic ultrasound (EUS)-guided sampling in gastroenterology: European Society of Gastrointestinal Endoscopy (ESGE) Technical Guideline. Endoscopy 2012;44:190–206.
69. Nakazawa T, Naitoh I, Hayashi K, et al. Diagnostic criteria for IgG4-related sclerosing cholangitis based on cholangiographic classification. J Gastroenterol 2012;47:79–87.
70. Kawa S, Okazaki K, Kamisawa T, et al. Japanese consensus guidelines for management of autoimmune pancreatitis: II. Extrapancreatic lesions, differential diagnosis. J Gastroenterol 2010;45:355–69.
71. Naitoh I, Nakazawa T, Ohara H, et al. Endoscopic transpapillary intraductal ultrasonography and biopsy in the diagnosis of IgG4-related sclerosing cholangitis. J Gastroenterol 2009;44:1147–55.
72. Hirano K, Tada M, Isayama H, et al. Endoscopic evaluation of factors contributing to intrapancreatic biliary stricture in autoimmune pancreatitis. Gastrointest Endosc 2010;71:85–90.
73. Finkelberg DL, Sahani D, Deshpande V, et al. Autoimmune pancreatitis. N Engl J Med 2006;355:2670–6.
74. Dumonceau JM. Sampling at ERCP for cyto- and histopathological examination. Gastrointest Endosc Clin N Am 2012;22:461–77.
75. Dumonceau JM, Polkowski M, Larghi A, et al. Indications, results, and clinical impact of endoscopic ultrasound (EUS)-guided sampling in gastroenterology: European Society of Gastrointestinal Endoscopy (ESGE) Clinical Guideline. Endoscopy 2011;43:897–912.
76. Rosch T, Hofrichter K, Frimberger E, et al. ERCP or EUS for tissue diagnosis of biliary strictures? A prospective comparative study. Gastrointest Endosc 2004;60:390–6.
77. Khashab MA, Fockens P, Al-Haddad MA. Utility of EUS in patients with indeterminate biliary strictures and suspected extrahepatic cholangiocarcinoma (with videos). Gastrointest Endosc 2012;76:1024–33.
78. Deheragoda MG, Church NI, Rodriguez-Justo M, et al. The use of immunoglobulin g4 immunostaining in diagnosing pancreatic and extrapancreatic involvement in autoimmune pancreatitis. Clin Gastroenterol Hepatol 2007;5:1229–34.
79. Deshpande V, Zen Y, Chan JK, et al. Consensus statement on the pathology of IgG4-related disease. Mod Pathol 2012;25:1181–92.

80. Detlefsen S, Mohr Drewes A, Vyberg M, et al. Diagnosis of autoimmune pancre-atitis by core needle biopsy: application of six microscopic criteria. Virchows Arch 2009;454:531–9.

81. Ghazale A, Chari ST, Zhang L, et al. Immunoglobulin G4-associated cholan-gitis: clinical profile and response to therapy. Gastroenterology 2008;134: 706–15.

82. Hirano K, Fukushima N, Tada M, et al. Diagnostic utility of biopsy specimens for autoimmune pancreatitis. J Gastroenterol 2009;44:765–73.

83. Kamisawa T, Tu Y, Egawa N, et al. A new diagnostic endoscopic tool for autoim-mune pancreatitis. Gastrointest Endosc 2008;68:358–61.

84. Kubota K, Kato S, Akiyama T, et al. Differentiating sclerosing cholangitis caused by autoimmune pancreatitis and primary sclerosing cholangitis according to endoscopic duodenal papillary features. Gastrointest Endosc 2008;68: 1204–8.

85. Mizuno N, Bhatia V, Hosoda W, et al. Histological diagnosis of autoimmune pancreatitis using EUS-guided trucut biopsy: a comparison study with EUS-FNA. J Gastroenterol 2009;44:742–50.

86. Moon SH, Kim MH, Park do H, et al. IgG4 immunostaining of duodenal papillary biopsy specimens may be useful for supporting a diagnosis of autoimmune pancreatitis. Gastrointest Endosc 2010;71:960–6.

87. Oh HC, Kim MH, Lee KT, et al. Clinical clues to suspicion of IgG4-associated sclerosing cholangitis disguised as primary sclerosing cholangitis or hilar chol-angiocarcinoma. J Gastroenterol Hepatol 2010;25:1831–7.

88. Zhang L, Notohara K, Levy MJ, et al. IgG4-positive plasma cell infiltration in the diagnosis of autoimmune pancreatitis. Mod Pathol 2007;20:23–8.

89. Bang SJ, Kim MH, Kim do H, et al. Is pancreatic core biopsy sufficient to diag-nose autoimmune chronic pancreatitis? Pancreas 2008;36:84–9.

90. Hartwig W, Schneider L, Diener MK, et al. Preoperative tissue diagnosis for tumours of the pancreas. Br J Surg 2009;96:5–20.

91. Uchida N, Kamada H, Tsutsui K, et al. Utility of pancreatic duct brushing for diagnosis of pancreatic carcinoma. J Gastroenterol 2007;42:657–62.

92. Vandervoort J, Soetikno RM, Montes H, et al. Accuracy and complication rate of brush cytology from bile duct versus pancreatic duct. Gastrointest Endosc 1999;49:322–7.

93. Volmar KE, Vollmer RT, Routbort MJ, et al. Pancreatic and bile duct brushing cytology in 1000 cases: review of findings and comparison of preparation methods. Cancer 2006;108:231–8.

94. Horwhat JD, Paulson EK, McGrath K, et al. A randomized comparison of EUS-guided FNA versus CT or US-guided FNA for the evaluation of pancreatic mass lesions. Gastrointest Endosc 2006;63:966–75.

95. Volmar KE, Vollmer RT, Jowell PS, et al. Pancreatic FNA in 1000 cases: a com-parison of imaging modalities. Gastrointest Endosc 2005;61:854–61.

96. Micames C, Jowell PS, White R, et al. Lower frequency of peritoneal carcinoma-tosis in patients with pancreatic cancer diagnosed by EUS-guided FNA vs. percutaneous FNA. Gastrointest Endosc 2003;58:690–5.

97. Deshpande V, Mino-Kenudson M, Brugge WR, et al. Endoscopic ultrasound guided fine needle aspiration biopsy of autoimmune pancreatitis: diagnostic criteria and pitfalls. Am J Surg Pathol 2005;29:1464–71.

98. Iglesias-Garcia J, Poley JW, Larghi A, et al. Feasibility and yield of a new EUS histology needle: results from a multicenter, pooled, cohort study. Gastrointest Endosc 2011;73:1189–96.

99. Salah W, Naem M, Faulx A, et al. Abdominal pain and a pancreatic head mass: a diagnostic dilemma and the role of EUS in tissue sampling. Am J Gastroenterol 2012;107:S329.

100. Moller K, Papanikolaou IS, Toermer T, et al. EUS-guided FNA of solid pancreatic masses: high yield of 2 passes with combined histologic-cytologic analysis. Gastrointest Endosc 2009;70:60–9.

101. Iglesias-Garcia J, Dominguez-Munoz E, Lozano-Leon A, et al. Impact of endoscopic ultrasound-guided fine needle biopsy for diagnosis of pancreatic masses. World J Gastroenterol 2007;13:289–93.

102. Voss M, Hammel P, Molas G, et al. Value of endoscopic ultrasound guided fine needle aspiration biopsy in the diagnosis of solid pancreatic masses. Gut 2000; 46:244–9.

103. Larghi A, Verna EC, Ricci R, et al. EUS-guided fine-needle tissue acquisition by using a 19-gauge needle in a selected patient population: a prospective study. Gastrointest Endosc 2011;74:504–10.

104. Ishikawa T, Itoh A, Kawashima H, et al. Endoscopic ultrasound-guided fine needle aspiration in the differentiation of type 1 and type 2 autoimmune pancreatitis. World J Gastroenterol 2012;18:3883–8.

105. Iwashita T, Yasuda I, Doi S, et al. Use of samples from endoscopic ultrasound-guided 19-gauge fine-needle aspiration in diagnosis of autoimmune pancreatitis. Clin Gastroenterol Hepatol 2012;10:316–22.

106. Kanno A, Ishida K, Hamada S, et al. Diagnosis of autoimmune pancreatitis by EUS-FNA by using a 22-gauge needle based on the International Consensus Diagnostic Criteria. Gastrointest Endosc 2012;76:594–602.

107. Imai K, Matsubayashi H, Fukutomi A, et al. Endoscopic ultrasonography-guided fine needle aspiration biopsy using 22-gauge needle in diagnosis of autoimmune pancreatitis. Dig Liver Dis 2011;43:869–74.

108. Pavey DA, Gress FG. The role of EUS-guided FNA for the evaluation of biliary strictures. Gastrointest Endosc 2006;64:334–7.

109. Tamada K, Ushio J, Sugano K. Endoscopic diagnosis of extrahepatic bile duct carcinoma: advances and current limitations. World J Clin Oncol 2011;2: 203–16.

110. de Bellis M, Sherman S, Fogel EL, et al. Tissue sampling at ERCP in suspected malignant biliary strictures (Part 2). Gastrointest Endosc 2002;56:720–30.

111. Raina A, Yadav D, Krasinskas AM, et al. Evaluation and management of autoimmune pancreatitis: experience at a large US center. Am J Gastroenterol 2009; 104:2295–306.

112. Anderson MA, Appalaneni V, Ben-Menachem T, et al. The role of endoscopy in the evaluation and treatment of patients with biliary neoplasia. Gastrointest Endosc 2013;77(2):167–74.

113. Wu LM, Jiang XX, Gu HY, et al. Endoscopic ultrasound-guided fine-needle aspiration biopsy in the evaluation of bile duct strictures and gallbladder masses: a systematic review and meta-analysis. Eur J Gastroenterol Hepatol 2011;23: 113–20.

114. Kim MH, Moon SH, Kamisawa T. Major duodenal papilla in autoimmune pancreatitis. Dig Surg 2010;27:110–4.

115. Kalaitzakis E, Webster GJ. Review article: autoimmune pancreatitis–management of an emerging disease. Aliment Pharmacol Ther 2011;33:291–303.

116. DeWitt J, Misra VL, Leblanc JK, et al. EUS-guided FNA of proximal biliary strictures after negative ERCP brush cytology results. Gastrointest Endosc 2006;64: 325–33.

117. Eloubeidi MA, Varadarajulu S, Desai S, et al. Value of repeat endoscopic ultrasound-guided fine needle aspiration for suspected pancreatic cancer. J Gastroenterol Hepatol 2008;23:567–70.
118. Kamisawa T, Egawa N, Nakajima H, et al. Morphological changes after steroid therapy in autoimmune pancreatitis. Scand J Gastroenterol 2004;39:1154–8.
119. Hopkins RL, Leinung MC. Exogenous Cushing's syndrome and glucocorticoid withdrawal. Endocrinol Metab Clin North Am 2005;34:371–84.
120. Chari ST. Current concepts in the treatment of autoimmune pancreatitis. JOP 2007;8:1–3.
121. Maire F, Le Baleur Y, Rebours V, et al. Outcome of patients with type 1 or 2 autoimmune pancreatitis. Am J Gastroenterol 2011;106:151–6.
122. Kamisawa T, Shimosegawa T, Okazaki K, et al. Standard steroid treatment for autoimmune pancreatitis. Gut 2009;58:1504–7.
123. Choi EK, Kim MH, Kim JC, et al. The Japanese diagnostic criteria for autoimmune chronic pancreatitis: is it completely satisfactory? Pancreas 2006;33: 13–9.
124. Sandanayake NS, Church NI, Chapman MH, et al. Presentation and management of post-treatment relapse in autoimmune pancreatitis/immunoglobulin G4-associated cholangitis. Clin Gastroenterol Hepatol 2009;7:1089–96.
125. Alexander S, Bourke MJ, Williams SJ, et al. Diagnosis of autoimmune pancreatitis with intraductal biliary biopsy and treatment of stricture with serial placement of multiple biliary stents. Gastrointest Endosc 2008;68:396–9.
126. Hirano K, Tada M, Isayama H, et al. Long-term prognosis of autoimmune pancreatitis with and without corticosteroid treatment. Gut 2007;56:1719–24.

Palliation of Pancreatic Ductal Obstruction in Pancreatic Cancer

Reem Z. Sharaiha, MD, MSc, Jessica Widmer, DO,
Michel Kahaleh, MD*

KEYWORDS

- Pancreatic cancer • Pain • Duct obstruction • Palliation • Pancreatic stenting

KEY POINTS

- Pancreatic stenting for patients with obstructive pain secondary to a malignant pancreatic duct stricture is safe and effective, and should be considered a therapeutic option.
- Although pancreatic stenting does not seem to be effective for patients with chronic pain, it may be beneficial in those with obstructive type pains, pancreatic duct disruption, or smoldering pancreatitis.
- Fully covered metal stents may be an option, but data on their use are limited.
- Further studies, including prospective randomized studies comparing plastic and metal stents in these indications, are needed.

INTRODUCTION

Pancreatic cancer affects 25,000 new people per year in the United States.[1] It is the fifth most common cause of cancer-related death in the western world.[2] It is estimated that only approximately 30% of patients diagnosed with pancreatic cancer have operable disease, and half of those cancers are deemed inoperable at the time of surgery. As a result, a large percentage of patients have inoperable disease at the time of diagnosis. Estimates show that fewer than 20% of the patients will survive 1 year after diagnosis, with an overall 5-year survival rate of less than 3%.[3,4] Palliative management, therefore, is the primary concern. The most common symptoms that require treatment are obstructive jaundice, intestinal obstruction, and pain. Pain occurs in 85% of patients with advanced disease.[5] Pain in pancreatic cancer is distressing and often poorly controlled.[6,7] As a result, its management is an integral part of palliative care.[8]

Division of Gastroenterology & Hepatology, Department of Medicine, Weill Cornell Medical College, Street 1305 York Avenue, Fourth floor, New York, NY 10021, USA
* Corresponding author.
E-mail address: mik9071@med.cornelledu

Gastrointest Endoscopy Clin N Am 23 (2013) 917–923
http://dx.doi.org/10.1016/j.giec.2013.06.010
1052-5157/13/$ – see front matter © 2013 Elsevier Inc. All rights reserved.

PAIN IN PANCREATIC CANCER

The mechanism of pain in pancreatic cancer is multifactorial. It may be the result of neoplastic infiltration of the neural tissue and peripancreatic tissue,[6] or a result of obstruction of the main pancreatic duct, resulting in upstream dilation beyond a stricture with ductal hypertension, called *obstructive pain*.[9] Classically pain caused by obstruction is postprandial. It is mainly located in the epigastrium or left hypochondrium, and occasionally radiates to the back, lasting 1 to 2 hours.[10] This pain is similar to that which occurs in large duct chronic pancreatitis (CP).[11,12] CP with pain is characterized by poor vascularity with severe periductal and arterial fibrosis.[13] A main theory that has been tested in animal models and humans is that of increased pancreatic interstitial and ductal pressure causing a compartment syndrome, leading to a relative ischemia, as the source of pain.[14] Normal pressure has been estimated to be between 7 and 15 mm Hg. Intraoperative measurements of ductal pressures range between 20 and 80 mm Hg in patients with CP.[15] The thought is that continuous secretin excretion against a proximal obstruction from single or multiple strictures and/or calculi causes an increase in pressure, leading to decreased vascularity. The fibrosis that surrounds the chronically inflamed pancreas and its lobules plays a role in pancreatic tissue pressures. It does so by limiting the ability of pancreatic tissue to expand during periods of exocrine secretion, causing a situation similar to the compartment syndrome.[14] The increase in ductal and interstitial pressure is associated with diminished basal pancreatic blood flow, as shown in experimental studies.[16] This concept is further supported by the fact that decompression of a dilated pancreatic duct through stent insertion or, more often, surgical decompression (Puestow procedure) is frequently associated with pain relief.[17] This theory also explains the "burnt out" phenomenon that intraductal hypertension decreases as the disease advances, because acinar tissue atrophies and pancreatic secretion does not increase on eating.[13,15]

DUCTAL DISRUPTION

Another complication of pancreatic cancer is ductal disruption.[18,19] This leads to numerous complications such as pancreatic ascites, fistula, pseudocyst, abscess formation, and necrosis. Pancreatic duct disruptions and associated fluid collections can be treated by surgical interventions such as: roux loop cystoenterostomy and resection of the tail of the pancreas often combined with splenectomy, percutaneous, or endoscopic procedures, which include cystgastrostomies or pancreatic stenting as described subsequently.[18]

SMOULDERING PANCREATITIS

Pancreatic cancer produces obstructive pancreatitis upstream from a constricted portion of the pancreatic duct, acute pancreatitis is a less common manifestation of pancreatic cancer.[20] Histologically pancreatic cancer is usually identified around the stenosis or stricture of the main duct.[21]

PAIN MANAGEMENT

The management of pain remains a significant problem. Given that pain may be multifactorial, one single treatment is unlikely to result in complete resolution.

It is estimated that most patients have chronic, continuous, dull pain radiating to the back, and that this is the result of neoplastic infiltration. Celiac plexus block either endoscopically or percutaneously has been reported to have an 85% success rate.[22] In the minority of patients (≈15%), pain is postprandial, located in the epigastrium and left upper quadrants, and usually associated with ductal abnormalities. Postprandial pain is defined as obstructive.[5,6]

Endoscopic stenting of the main pancreatic duct may be considered to decompress obstructive-type pain that occurs after meal stimulation. Similar to the experience gained with large duct CP, inserting a stent will allow free pancreatic juice to flow into the duodenum with minimal obstruction.[17]

Stenting the pancreatic duct can be technically challenging. These challenges may be from the presence of strictures that make wire advancement difficult or from the presence of complete or partial pancreatic divisum, which occurs in 15% to 20% of cases.[10,23] If the patient is jaundiced, then simultaneous biliary sphincterotomy and stenting should be performed.

TECHNIQUE OF PANCREATIC STENTING

Other than the reasons cited earlier, pancreatic duct stenting does not differ from biliary stenting. However, access, when challenging, may be gained with a hydrophilic wire, angled tip, or a smaller wire, such as the PathFinder or Roadrunner, 0.018-in diameters. The stricture can then be dilated with a Soehendra bougie (Wilson Cook, Winston-Salem, NC, USA) or wire-guided balloon dilation. After this, large-caliber stents should be placed for drainage. Stents larger than 5F are preferred to prevent stent occlusion and provide adequate pancreatic decompression.[10] Plastic stents are thought to remain patent for up to 2 months, likely because of their small diameter. The Johlin-JPWS (Johlin Pancreatic Wedge Stent, Cook Endoscopy, Winston Salem, NC, USA) has also been used. It is a plastic multiperforated stent with a tapered distal tip. In a comparative retrospective study addressing feasibility and efficacy of this stent, the Johlin stent had a significantly reduced rate of painful relapse as well as a lower rate of ductal obstruction compared to conventional plastic stents.[24,25] Self-expanding metallic stents have been described in this indication, with the major advantage of longer patency, fewer repeat procedures, and better cost-effectiveness for patients expected to survive longer than 6 months (**Figs. 1–3**).[26] However, few reports have been published on their use in pancreatic strictures of malignant origin.[5,27]

EFFICACY AND OUTCOMES

A few studies have examined the efficacy and safety of pancreatic stent placement in patients with obstructive pain. In 1989, Harrison and Hamilton[28] reported pain relief in 1 patient after pancreatic stent placement. This report was followed by a case series by Costamagna[29] of 12 patients with obstructive pain. Technical success occurred in

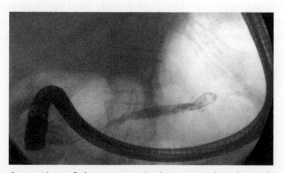

Fig. 1. Malignant obstruction of the pancreatic duct crossed with a sphincterotome.

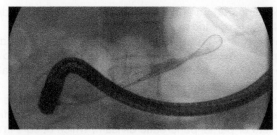

Fig. 2. Deployment of a fully covered 8 × 60-mm metal stent.

8 of 12 patients (66%), and pain resolution occurred in 7 of 8 patients (87%). In another retrospective study by Costamagna,[29] 55 patients (15%) had 1 or more indications for endoscopic stenting, including pain, brachyradiotherapy, and pancreatic iatrogenic infections. Technical success occurred in 81%. Only plastic stents were used in these studies, mainly for pain control and intraluminal brachytherapy, and one for pancreatic infection. Pain control was achieved in 61.7%.[29] In a study by Tham and colleagues[5] pancreatic stents were placed in 10 patients with malignant obstruction and pain. Of those patients, 70% had a reduction in pain after stent placement. In another series, 100% of patients experienced pain improvement after pancreatic stenting.[30] In a prospective study of 20 patients with unresectable pancreatic cancer and postprandial pain thought to be secondary to obstruction, pancreatic stenting was successful in 19 patients, with significant pain relief by 8 weeks. Quality of life improved, but it was not statistically significant.[9] Tham and colleagues[5] used 3 metallic stents with successful outcomes. Previously, metallic stents were used successfully by Keeley and Freeman[27] in patients with obstructive complications of pancreatitis cancer, including simultaneous biliary and pancreatic metallic stents for the indications of smoldering pancreatitis and 2 disrupted pancreatic ducts.

DISCUSSION: CURRENT CONTROVERSIES/FUTURE CONSIDERATIONS

For a selective group of patients, endoscopic pancreatic duct decompression has been shown to be effective in the few studies mentioned earlier. Both pain scores and opioid treatment were reduced after stent insertion. No postprocedure-related complications were seen.[5,9,30] Whether metal stent can provide better results than plastic and which kind of metal should be used remain to be determined. Most of the data are from patients with CP.[31–34] Although in benign settings uncovered metal stents are not an acceptable option based on the available data, because of the development of intimal hyperplasia and stent dysfunction, they may function adequately for pancreatic decompression in patients with malignant pancreatic obstruction, analogous to biliary metallic stents.[33] Fully covered metal stents (FCSEMS) have been

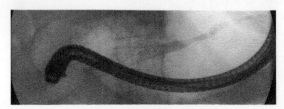

Fig. 3. Good decompression of the main pancreatic duct.

Table 1
Results of endoscopic pancreatic stenting in patients with pancreatic cancer

Author	Number of Patients	Type of Stents	Technical Success	Symptom Resolution
Harrison & Hamilton,[28] 1989	1	Plastic 7F	1	Yes
Costamagna et al,[30] 1993	12	Plastic 7F Plastic 10F	8	7 total 1 partial
Costamagna et al,[29] 1999	55	Plastic 7F–11.5F	45	28 total 12 partial
Tham et al,[5] 2000	10	Plastic 7F Plastic 10F Metal	10	7 total
Keeley & Freeman,[27] 2003	3	Metal	3	3

used; however, they have a high rate of migration (39%), although improvement and/ or resolution of stricture was seen in all patients (**Table 1**).[34] Covered metal stents with fins do not seem to provide long-term patency, with most patients experiencing a recurrence after removal.[31] Moon and colleagues[32] assessed the safety and efficacy of a modified FCSEMS, and although the rate of migration was decreased, they found focal stent-induced strictures in 16% of patients. The only currently available covered metal stents have a diameter of 8 or 10 mm. Although these stents may be appropriate for patients with very dilated pancreatic ducts, stents 6 mm in diameter might be more suited to patients with smaller ducts.

SUMMARY

In conclusion, pancreatic stenting for patients with obstructive pain secondary to a malignant pancreatic duct stricture is safe and effective, and should be considered a therapeutic option. Although it does not seem to be effective for patients with chronic pain, it may be beneficial in those with obstructive-type pain, pancreatic duct disruption, or smoldering pancreatitis. FCSEMS may be an option, but data are limited. Further studies, including prospective randomized studies comparing plastic and metal stents in these indications, are needed.

REFERENCES

1. Yeo C, Cameron L. The pancreas. In: Text book of surgery. The biological basis of modern surgical practice. Philadelphia: WB Saunders Company; 1991. p. 1093–7.
2. DiMagno EP, Reber HA, Tempero MA. AGA technical review on the epidemiology, diagnosis, and treatment of pancreatic ductal adenocarcinoma. American Gastroenterological Association. Gastroenterology 1999;117(6):1464–84.
3. HAR. Pancreas. In: Schwartz ST, Spencer F, editors. Principles of surgery. 6th edition. New York: McGraw Hil; 1994. p. 1401–32.
4. Weir HK, Thun MJ, Hankey BF, et al. Annual report to the nation on the status of cancer, 1975-2000, featuring the uses of surveillance data for cancer prevention and control. J Natl Cancer Inst 2003;95(17):1276–99.
5. Tham TC, Lichtenstein DR, Vandervoort J, et al. Pancreatic duct stents for "obstructive type" pain in pancreatic malignancy. Am J Gastroenterol 2000; 95(4):956–60.
6. Lebovits AH, Lefkowitz M. Pain management of pancreatic carcinoma: a review. Pain 1989;36(1):1–11.

7. Foley KM. Pain syndromes and pharmacologic management of pancreatic cancer pain. J Pain Symptom Manage 1988;3(4):176–87.
8. Gouma DJ, Busch OR, Van Gulik TM. Pancreatic carcinoma: palliative surgical and endoscopic treatment. HPB (Oxford) 2006;8(5):369–76.
9. Wehrmann T, Riphaus A, Frenz MB, et al. Endoscopic pancreatic duct stenting for relief of pancreatic cancer pain. Eur J Gastroenterol Hepatol 2005;17(12): 1395–400.
10. Costamagna G, Mutignani M. Pancreatic stenting for malignant ductal obstruction. Dig Liver Dis 2004;36(9):635–8.
11. DiMagno MJ, Dimagno EP. Chronic pancreatitis. Curr Opin Gastroenterol 2006; 22(5):487–97.
12. Sakorafas GH, Farnell MB, Nagorney DM, et al. Surgical management of chronic pancreatitis at the Mayo Clinic. Surg Clin North Am 2001;81(2):457–65.
13. Sakorafas GH, Tsiotou AG, Peros G. Mechanisms and natural history of pain in chronic pancreatitis: a surgical perspective. J Clin Gastroenterol 2007;41(7): 689–99.
14. Karanjia ND, Widdison AL, Leung F, et al. Compartment syndrome in experimental chronic obstructive pancreatitis: effect of decompressing the main pancreatic duct. Br J Surg 1994;81(2):259–64.
15. Bradley EL 3rd. Pancreatic duct pressure in chronic pancreatitis. Am J Surg 1982;144(3):313–6.
16. Reber HA, Karanjia ND, Alvarez C, et al. Pancreatic blood flow in cats with chronic pancreatitis. Gastroenterology 1992;103(2):652–9.
17. Cahen DL, Gouma DJ, Nio Y, et al. Endoscopic versus surgical drainage of the pancreatic duct in chronic pancreatitis. N Engl J Med 2007;356(7):676–84.
18. Shrode CW, Macdonough P, Gaidhane M, et al. Multimodality endoscopic treatment of pancreatic duct disruption with stenting and pseudocyst drainage: how efficacious is it? Dig Liver Dis 2013;45:129–33.
19. Varadarajulu S, Noone TC, Tutuian R, et al. Predictors of outcome in pancreatic duct disruption managed by endoscopic transpapillary stent placement. Gastrointest Endosc 2005;61:568–75.
20. Minato Y, Kamisawa T, Tabata T, et al. Pancreatic cancer causing acute pancreatitis: a comparative study with cancer patients without pancreatitis and pancreatitis patients without cancer. J Hepatobiliary Pancreat Sci 2013.
21. Mujica VR, Barkin JS, Go VL. Acute pancreatitis secondary to pancreatic carcinoma. Study Group Participants. Pancreas 2000;21:329–32.
22. Levy MJ, Chari ST, Wiersema MJ. Endoscopic ultrasound-guided celiac neurolysis. Gastrointest Endosc Clin N Am 2012;22(2):231–47, viii.
23. Dumonceau JM, Deviere J, Le Moine O, et al. Endoscopic pancreatic drainage in chronic pancreatitis associated with ductal stones: long-term results. Gastrointest Endosc 1996;43(6):547–55.
24. Boursier J, Quentin V, Le Tallec V, et al. Endoscopic treatment of painful chronic pancreatitis: evaluation of a new flexible multiperforated plastic stent. Gastroenterol Clin Biol 2008;32:801–5.
25. Quentin JB V, Le Tallec V, Person B, et al. Endoscopic treatment of Painful Chronic Pancreatitis Evaluation of a New Flexiable Multiperforated Plastic Stent. Volume 2013. Available at: http://www.cookmedical.com/esc/educationArticle.do?id=2591, 2008.
26. Yeoh KG, Zimmerman MJ, Cunningham JT, et al. Comparative costs of metal versus plastic biliary stent strategies for malignant obstructive jaundice by decision analysis. Gastrointest Endosc 1999;49(4 Pt 1):466–71.

27. Keeley SP, Freeman ML. Placement of self-expanding metallic stents in the pancreatic duct for treatment of obstructive complications of pancreatic cancer. Gastrointest Endosc 2003;57(6):756–9.

28. Harrison MA, Hamilton JW. Palliation of pancreatic cancer pain by endoscopic stent placement. Gastrointest Endosc 1989;35(5):443–5.

29. Costamagna G, Alevras P, Palladino F, et al. Endoscopic pancreatic stenting in pancreatic cancer. Can J Gastroenterol 1999;13(6):481–7.

30. Costamagna G, Gabbrielli A, Mutignani M, et al. Treatment of "obstructive" pain by endoscopic drainage in patients with pancreatic head carcinoma. Gastrointest Endosc 1993;39(6):774–7.

31. Sauer B, Talreja J, Ellen K, et al. Temporary placement of a fully covered self-expandable metal stent in the pancreatic duct for management of symptomatic refractory chronic pancreatitis: preliminary data (with videos). Gastrointest Endosc 2008;68(6):1173–8.

32. Moon SH, Kim MH, Park do H, et al. Modified fully covered self-expandable metal stents with antimigration features for benign pancreatic-duct strictures in advanced chronic pancreatitis, with a focus on the safety profile and reducing migration. Gastrointest Endosc 2010;72(1):86–91.

33. Gupta R, Reddy DN. Stent selection for both biliary and pancreatic strictures caused by chronic pancreatitis: multiple plastic stents or metallic stents? J Hepatobiliary Pancreat Sci 2011;18(5):636–9.

34. Park do H, Kim MH, Moon SH, et al. Feasibility and safety of placement of a newly designed, fully covered self-expandable metal stent for refractory benign pancreatic ductal strictures: a pilot study (with video). Gastrointest Endosc 2008;68(6):1182–9.

Index

Note: Page numbers of article titles are in **boldface** type.

Gastrointest Endoscopy Clin N Am 23 (2013) 925–934
http://dx.doi.org/10.1016/S1052-5157(13)00106-2
1052-5157/13/$ – see front matter © 2013 Elsevier Inc. All rights reserved.

Printed and bound by CPI Group (UK) Ltd, Croydon, CR0 4YY

19/10/2024

01776488-0001